GUIDE TO
Minimally Invasive
Aesthetic Procedures

GUIDE TO

Minimally Invasive
Aesthetic Procedures

M. Laurin Council, MD

Associate Professor of Dermatology
John T. Milliken Department of Internal Medicine
Division of Dermatology
Washington University School of Medicine in St. Louis
St. Louis, Missouri

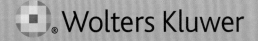 Wolters Kluwer

Philadelphia • Baltimore • New York • London
Buenos Aires • Hong Kong • Sydney • Tokyo

Acquisitions Editor: Colleen Dietzler
Development Editor: Eric McDermott
Editorial Coordinator: Cody Adams
Production Project Manager: Kim Cox
Design Coordinator: Steve Druding
Manufacturing Coordinator: Beth Welsh
Prepress Vendor: TNQ Technologies

9 8 7 6 5 4 3 2 1

Printed in China

Library of Congress Cataloging-in-Publication Data

ISBN-13: 978-1-975141-28-8

Cataloging in Publication data available on request from publisher.

shop.lww.com

To my mentors: Elizabeth McBurney, Murad Alam, and George Hruza.

Thank you for your unending support, guidance, and friendship.

Preface

Minimally invasive aesthetics is one of the fastest growing fields of medicine today. A 2017 survey by the American Society for Dermatologic Surgery (ASDS) revealed that over 8 million cosmetic procedures were performed by its members alone, a 19% increase from data the previous year. As the demand for and variety of these procedures continues to climb, it is paramount that one remains abreast of the advancements in the field of aesthetic medicine.

The purpose of this handbook of minimally invasive aesthetic procedures is to provide the fundamentals one needs to understand how botulinum toxin, soft-tissue fillers, deoxycholic acid, laser and light devices, sclerotherapy, and minimally invasive surgical procedures can be utilized in cosmetic medicine. We hope you enjoy reading it as much as we enjoyed putting it together.

M. Laurin Council

Contributors

Marc Avram, MD
Clinical Professor
Dermatology
Weill Cornell Medical College
New York, New York

John J. Chi, MD, MPHS
Associate Professor
Co-Director, AAFPRS Fellowship in Facial Plastic &
    Reconstructive Surgery
Division of Facial Plastic & Reconstructive
    Surgery
Department of Otolaryngology – Head & Neck
    Surgery
Washington University in St. Louis – School of
    Medicine
St. Louis, Missouri

Dillon Clarey, MD
Post-Doctoral Research Fellow
Department of Dermatology
University of Nebraska Medical Center
Omaha, Nebraska

M. Laurin Council, MD
Associate Professor of Medicine (Dermatology)
Department of Internal Medicine, Division of
    Dermatology
Washington University in St. Louis
St. Louis, Missouri

Charles E. Crutchfield III, MD
Adjunct Professor
University of Minnesota
Department of Dermatology
Minneapolis, Minnesota

Jessica B. Dietert, MD
Snyder Dermatology
Austin, Texas

Ronda S. Farah, MD
Assistant Professor
University of Minnesota
Department of Dermatology
Minneapolis, Minnesota

Dee Anna Glaser, MD
Professor
Departments of Dermatology
Internal Medicine, and Otolaryngology
Interim Chair
Department of Dermatology
Saint Louis University School of Medicine
St. Louis, Missouri

Katherine Glaser, MD
Micrographic Surgery and Dermatologic
    Oncology Fellow
Department of Dermatology
University of California
Irvine School of Medicine
Irvine, California

Rachit Gupta, BS
Medical Student
University of Minnesota
Department of Medicine
Minneapolis, Minnesota

Michelle Henry, MD
Clinical Instructor
Department of Dermatology
New York-Presbyterian Hospital/Weill Cornell
    Medical Center
New York, New York

Deirdre Hooper, MD
CoFounder
Audubon Dermatology
Clinical Associate Professor
Department of Dermatology
Tulane and Louisiana State University
New Orleans, Louisiana

Maria K. Hordinsky, MD
Professor, Chair
University of Minnesota
Department of Dermatology
Minneapolis, Minnesota

Eva A. Hurst, MD
Distinctive Dermatology
Fairview Heights, Illinois

Noora S. Hussain, BS
Medical Student
University of Minnesota
Department of Medicine
Minneapolis, Minnesota

Ethan C. Levin, MD
Golden State Dermatology
Mountain View, California

Christopher J. Rizzi, MD
Facial Plastic Surgeon
Premier ENT Associates
Dayton, Ohio

Frankie G. Rholdon, MD
Associate Clinical Professor
Department of Dermatology
Louisiana State University Health Sciences Center
New Orleans, Louisiana

Nazanin Saedi, MD
Associate Professor
Department of Dermatology and Cutaneous
  Surgery
Thomas Jefferson University
Philadelphia, Pennsylvania

Neil S. Sadick, MD
Adjunct Professor
University of Minnesota
Department of Dermatology
Minneapolis, Minnesota

Samantha L. Schneider, MD
Skin Cancer and Dermatology Institute
Reno, Nevada

Javed A. Shaik, PhD, MS
Assistant Professor
University of Minnesota
Department of Dermatology
Minneapolis, Minnesota

Nikhil Shyam, MD
Board-certified Dermatologist
Long Island, New York

Hema Sundaram, MA, MD
Board Certified Dermatologist
Medical Director
Sundaram Dermatology, Cosmetic & Laser
  Surgery
Rockville, Maryland and Fairfax, Virginia

Lindsey M. Voller, BA
Medical Student
University of Minnesota
Department of Medicine
Minneapolis, Minnesota

Jordan V. Wang, MD, MBE, MBA
Dermatologist
Department of Dermatology and Cutaneous
  Biology Thomas Jefferson University
Philadelphia, Pennsylvania

Ashley Wysong, MD, MS
Founding Chair and Associate Professor
William W. Bruce MD Distinguished Chair of
  Dermatology
Department of Dermatology
University of Nebraska Medical Center
Omaha, Nebraska

Contents

1

Approach to the Aesthetic Patient

Deirdre Hooper, MD

Chapter Highlights

- Train your staff extensively. Consider creating a cosmetic team to educate patients on the products and services you provide.
- Book appointments effectively with clear expectations.
- Make an impeccable first impression with a functional and engaging waiting room and consult room.
- Conduct a confident and friendly introduction.
- Listen and gain a more in-depth understanding of the patient's needs and wants.
- Assess your patients' personality as well as their anatomy.
- Educate and give clear recommendations.
- Be transparent as you work with budgets.
- Clearly outline next steps.
- Always follow up.

Skilled assessment and effective, safe technique are lifelong learning processes and crucial to your success as an aesthetic dermatologist. However, to successfully build an aesthetic practice, you need more than just skilled hands and eyes, you need to be able to reach and retain the type of patients you want to treat. Realize that the experience your aesthetic patients have with you encompasses many touchpoints, many of these occurring before the two of you ever meet. When you market effectively, set up your office attractively, and train your staff well, you make the entire experience of the patient one they will want to return to for a lifetime. It is also important to find patients who will have success with you and not treat those who will not be a success for varying reasons. This chapter should serve as a guide in creating successful consultations that lead to lifelong patients.

Begin by considering what services you will offer and what sort of patients you would like to treat. Ask yourself: what do I enjoy doing? What are my costs in offering these procedures? You may want to offer products, procedures, and devices to improve texture, pigment, and overall quality of skin. If you like to use your artistic eye and skilled hands to restore youthfulness or improve facial proportions, you will offer injectable neuromodulators and fillers. The cosmetic market is enormous. There are many potential patients out there and the market is growing. Based on 2019 data,[1] 65 million people in the United States are "considerers", meaning that they have thought about having a cosmetic procedure. In 2019, four million people were treated with injectables, a number that is predicted to double by 2025. The patient population is diversifying as well, with more men being treated every year as well as a widening of the age distribution we are treating—both younger and older patients are coming in. This means the patients are out there. Do not focus on competition, focus on being great and there will be patients for you.

How do you recruit patients? Chances are, many of your best aesthetic patients are already in your office seeing you as patients or bringing a family member in to see you. Healthy skin and beautiful skin are interchangeable terms, and no one understands skin health better than a dermatologist does. Doing aesthetic procedures is a natural evolution from the care you are giving your existing patients. Consider using a questionnaire (Table 1.1) to screen for patients' interest or lack thereof in your cosmetic services. This information can be very helpful in uncovering patient needs and wants and in previewing appropriate options for the patient. Marketing what you do internally (to patients in your office or your database) is very effective. You can put information on fliers or screens in your office, have a menu of services so people know what you offer, and of course have an attractive, informative website. You can host events at your office to tell people about what you offer. To reach new patients, word of mouth will help you, but you should consider

TABLE 1.1   Patient Questionnaire
What would you like to discuss today? (circle all that apply)   • Skin care   • Fillers   • Other injectable treatments   • Sunspots   • Broken blood vessels   • Scars   • Wrinkles   • Unwanted hair   • Other_____
What treatments have you had in the past? (circle all that apply)   • Fillers   • Microneedling   • Toxins/neuromodulators   • Laser hair removal   • Photofacial   • Other laser treatment   • Chemical peels   • Cosmetic surgery (explain_____)
What are your expectations for downtime after a procedure? (circle one)   • I can have minimal to no downtime   • I can have 1-2 d of downtime   • I can have 1 wk of downtime
How did you hear about us?   • My physician_____   • My friend or family member_____   • The Internet   • Advertisement

some sort of external marketing. Social media is effective and inexpensive when done with care and authenticity. In addition to social media, actually be social! Be active in your medical and local community, you are your own best advertisement. Be cautious before turning to paid advertising including paid ads online, paper media ads, billboards, and so on. Whatever marketing device you employ, be sure you have some way to track whether it is profitable for you. As you design any marketing material, keep your brand in mind. Credential yourself as an expert, use language and imagery that convey the experience people will have with you, and be consistent. A brand (in this case, you and your practice) is not a logo or a tagline. It is truly what people think of when they hear your name, and every touchpoint your aesthetic patient has with you and your practice should intentionally reflect your brand.

Train your staff well. Realize the aesthetic patients' experience with you begins well before you walk into the exam room. If you have marketed effectively, the patient has an idea of your aesthetic practice and your style. Your staff is a direct reflection of you as well. Effective staff training will help the right patient get to you and make the entire experience more successful for everyone. Start by making sure your staff gets to know you. I recommend you have all of your employees shadow you regularly. In my practice, I require each employee who is not regularly in the rooms to spend a half day each quarter just following me and observing. This helps my employees better understand my personality and how I interact with patients, and they learn about the products I recommend and the procedures I do just by listening. The questions your patients are asking you are often the same ones they ask your staff. Watching you inject or use devices demystifies the procedures and gives your staff an inside peek at what you do and how you do it. You should treat all of your employees and make sure they are on effective skin care regimens, as they are a reflection of your expertise and can also teach you about the day-to-day patient experience of your recommended regimens and procedure.

When considering training for specific roles, start with the person booking appointments. This employee is incredibly powerful. Often this is a patient's first contact with the practice and the experience should be friendly, warm, professional, and informative. The goal is to make patients feel welcome and confident in their choice to come see you. Train those booking appointments to credential you, to book patients for the proper amount of time they need, and to set expectations for the visit. To properly credential you, your staff should know your education, years of experience, and the number of procedures you have performed. They should know about your ongoing education including articles published, lectures given, and special talents you have. In teaching your staff to credential you, teach them that the goal is to differentiate you and your practice and to let patients know why your office is the place they want to be. They can give feedback on you, your technique, or on their personal experiences from the procedure. As the staff member and patient discuss what type of appointment to book, they can say, "Oh Dr X just came back from a conference on this topic, or they can say Dr X is amazing at injections! She just published an article on this technique." Ask your staff to try to work one credential of you or your practice into every conversation.

When it comes to putting the patient on your book, be sure your staff captures exactly why the patient is coming in and educates the patient on what to expect during the visit. You can separate consultations and services or offer same day services. Many patients want to be treated the day they come in. They have done their research, estimated a budget, and are ready to go. Others are completely in the dark about what they want, and many are somewhere in the middle. Train your staff to ask pertinent questions and to educate patients about what to expect from their appointment. We provide average costs and average time spent in the office, noting that these things are always variable. If patients do not have the budget for procedures, they can book a skin care consult only. If patients want to have procedures done that day, we provide a pretreatment planning document that includes contraindications to treatment and downtime expectations. When patients are fully informed, most of the time those that book same day consults and procedures end up being treated, but we always advise patients that it is completely up to the physician's discretion to treat that day. As I will discuss later in this chapter, you may determine it is in neither of your best interests when the time comes. Once the patient is booked, your staff should wrap up the booking with an overview of what to expect of the time they will spend in the office. For example, in my practice, I utilize a skin care expert and aestheticians who operate devices, so most cosmetic visits involve meeting with more people than just me. My staff will tell the patient, you will spend about 60 minutes in the office. You will start by speaking to a medical assistant about your medical history. You will be photographed. The doctor will come in, listen to you, and discuss your goals. She will assess you and make recommendations. Next, you will meet our skin care concierge and aestheticians who will review details and make sure you get every question answered. Finally, we review our policies and payment expectations. Patients who know what to expect are always happier, better patients, and you will have more fun doing what you love.

Finally, it is time for the appointment! At this point, your patient has probably looked at your website and social media. He or she has spoken to your staff. He or she has an expectation of what is going to happen and how he or she is going to feel. Be sure your office environment supports these expectations—this is your brand. As patients enter your office, it takes only a few seconds to form either a positive or a negative impression. You do not have to spend a fortune, but your reception area must be clean and attractive. Consider working with an interior designer to choose colors and make sure your furniture is scaled for the space. Fresh flowers, water, and tea can complete the mood. The office décor should be clean and in excellent condition, showing the patient (and your staff) that details are important to the practice.

Remind your front desk employees regularly that they are the CEO of first impressions and be sure you thank them for their attitude when you hear them being kind, or when patients give you good feedback. The front desk should know they are there to welcome patients and answer any questions. Hopefully you are not running behind, but if you are, your front desk can give your patients the Wi-Fi password, a cold or warm beverage, and of course you will have information on the services you provide available for them to read. Information should be available about the philosophy of the practice, the physicians and their backgrounds, and the services provided. Crisp-looking patient information forms are a must! This shows that the practice cares about details. Patients can interpret sloppy documents as a sign that the practice is careless about medical details also.

When the time comes, your assistant should check your patient in, welcome them, and get a sense of their expectations. Part of the check-in process should include quality photography. Good photos require good equipment and consistency.[2] Reproducing the settings of before photos after interventions allows more accurate evaluation of treatment outcomes. Standards for the studio, cameras, photographer, patients, and framing are all part of the process. Your background should be a solid color (I prefer black) with no equipment or furniture in the background. Only artificial light should be used. Natural light is subjected to weather conditions and seasonal changes. Ask the patient to remove earrings and makeup. Use a headband to pull the hair back from the face and have the patient sit or stand in front of your background. Align the patient's face; it should be straight. Take a series of pictures, employing protocols for photos depending on the patient's concerns and treatment you will be providing. Generally, for injection patients, take frontal and lateral pictures (45° and 90° to the left and right). For the lateral pictures (45°), the nose can be aligned with the malar eminence or zygomatic cheek (Figure 1.1) to facilitate the reproduction of the photos. When photographing the entire face, the photographer must focus at the area between the hairline and the lower edge of the chin (Figure 1.2). For photos of the upper third, the photographer must focus at the area between the nasal tip and

FIGURE 1.1 **Standard of lateral photographs (45°). The tip of the nose should be aligned with the cheek.**

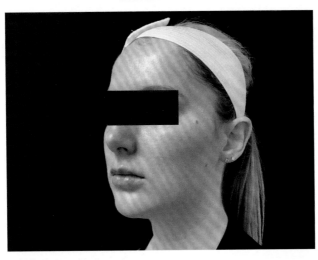

the hairline (Figure 1.3A); for midface, between the brows and mouth (Figure 1.3B); and for photos of the lower third, between the nasal tip to the lower edge of the chin (Figure 1.3C). Other pictures of specific areas can also be taken. Of note, when the goal of the photographs is to record the evolution of a treatment for dynamic wrinkles, two sequences of photographs with all the different positions have to be done: one with facial muscles relaxed and another with facial muscles of each area contracted at a time (Table 1.2). Set up a photography room with a dedicated employee if possible. Photography is essential when evaluating results with a patient and when publishing or presenting data. It is (usually) fun to show the patients their before and after images, and in the case of an unhappy patient, you will thank yourself over and over again when the patients come back saying they look exactly the same. If you are good at natural results, their face will be totally familiar—just from 5 years ago! Photography is also helpful in showing the patient where they have come from over years of visits.

FIGURE 1.2 **Standard of photographs of the entire face. The tag can be positioned elsewhere. The face should be aligned and centralized.**

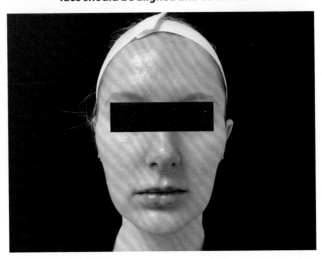

FIGURE 1.3 Standard set of photographs of each third of the face separately: (A) upper, (B) middle, and (C) lower face.

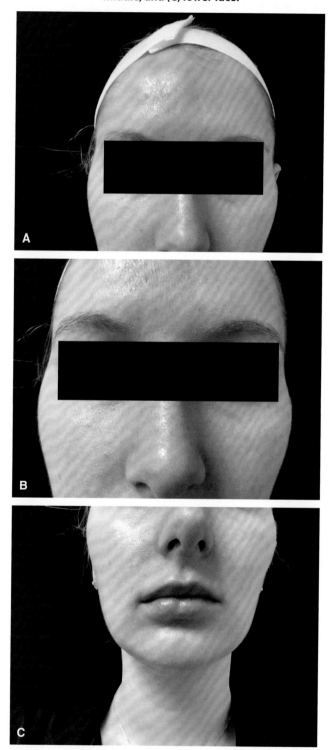

TABLE 1.2	Photography Checklist
Area	**Facial Expression**
Full face	Relaxed (no muscle movement)
Glabella	Frown
Forehead	Raise brow
Crow's feet	Squint
Bunny lines	Wrinkle nose
Perioral lines	Pucker lips
Neck	Clinch teeth

When you come in the room to meet your patient, remember that they are evaluating you as well. Take an interest in your own personal appearance. Always remember to be kind and gracious to your staff. Your interaction with office personnel will be noted by patients. Introduce yourself and welcome the patient to your practice. This is the time to establish rapport and trust. Be yourself and remember first impressions count. As you begin your meeting with the patient, realize that a crucial part of your consultation is listening to the patient. Taking a history from an aesthetic patient is really no different from other patient interviews you have performed. The medical interview is a pillar of medicine partly because it allows you to build a relationship with your patient. Eliciting and understanding the patient's agenda enhances and facilitates communication. When you understand what the patient is looking for, and your patient understands what you can offer, it is easier to make a plan that leads to focused, efficient, and patient-centered care. Unfortunately, basic communication skills are sometimes lost on physicians as we interrupt and make recommendations before really listening. In a landmark clinical communication study[3] published in 1984, Beckman et al. found that in 69% of the visits to a primary care practice, the physician interrupted the patient, with a mean time to interruption of 18 seconds. Twenty years later Dyche et al.[4] found that in general medicine visits, only 26% of the patients completed their initial statement uninterrupted, and that the mean time to interruption was 16.5 seconds. Failure to elicit the patients' agenda was associated with a 24% reduction in the physician's understanding of the main reasons for the consultation. These studies, performed decades apart, suggest that clinicians often fail to elicit the patient's agenda and even when they do, they often promptly interrupt patients, and this results in less successful consultations. In an aesthetic setting, not realizing what the patient wants can lead to unhappy patients. When surveyed[4] as to what they want from health care providers in general, patient goals included timeliness, kindness, hope, and certainty. They want to be taken seriously and first to be understood, then to understand. Listening is a critical step in this process, because it forms the basis of all communications. If done well, it will provide the information needed from the patient to enable you to address patient needs and discover patient values and motivations. Rarely will patients who feel that they have not been heard schedule a procedure. Keys to good listening include suspending judgment, avoiding interrupting, and providing eye contact to the patient. Use nonverbal behavior, such as smiling and nodding while the patient is talking. These cues let the patient know that you are engaged in listening and are encouraging the communication. Ask open-ended questions to gather information and engage the patient in the process. The most important part of asking open-ended questions is the listening required after the question is asked. Examples of open-ended questions include: "What are you trying to achieve?" "What bothers you the most?" "Can you help me understand that a little better?" "Would you mind telling me a little bit about your current skin care regimen?" Acknowledging the patient's concerns communicates to the patient that you understand his or her thoughts and serves to reduce patient anxiety. Acknowledging includes summarizing and verbally repeating the patient's statements, using phrases such as, "I heard you say...." or "Let me make sure I understand what you are saying...", and empathizing with the patient's concerns, using statements such as "I can understand how you might be concerned about that..." If the patient truly feels understood, he or she will be much more likely to be receptive to the information imparted to them.

It is important to elicit what is motivating your patient to help guide your recommendations. Aesthetic patients have a variety of goals. In a study surveying motivation for seeking cosmetic treatments,[5] the most common reasons given were reaching tipping point of frustration with a problem, unable to cover up a problem, or an upcoming event. Patients frequently give a psychosocial basis for coming and many of these reasons have a direct anatomical reference you can assess. When patients say, "I look angry", it is often their forehead/glabella that needs treatment, whereas those that say they look tired or sad often need their mid- or lower face treated, respectively. Listening to cues from the patient can help you effectively consider which treatment will make the biggest impact for them. As you create your plan, keep your patients' goals in mind. If you give them something they do not want, even if it is a good outcome, they will not be happy. If you disagree with your patients' goals, or prioritize them differently, make that part of the conversation. If you do not see eye to eye, remember you can always say no and refer the patient to someone else. When considering what to do first, there are some general commonalities among patients that may help guide you. In a survey[6] led by Narurkar of aesthetically oriented women, analysis revealed that features that were most bothersome to patients were also the ones most likely to be treated first, underscoring the idea that you should listen to and address the patients' primary concern. Crow's feet lines were most likely to be both most bothersome and treated first (82%), followed by oral commissures (74%), tear troughs (72%), forehead lines (66%), and glabellar lines (65%). In women younger than 45 years, features of the upper face were more likely to be treated first, whereas women aged 50 years or older had an increased preference for treating features of the lower face, with a reduction in preference for upper face treatment. Interestingly, in this study only 22% of patients complained about their cheeks, an area I frequently address early in treatment.

As you continue your consultation, be sure you are assessing the patients' personality as well as their anatomy. Remember, there are many potential patients out there, and you want to cultivate a group that will happily visit you for many years. Whom do you most enjoy working with? Who will happily pay what you are worth? Who will get great results from the services you offer? Cultivate these people and those who they refer, and you will minimize the patients you dread seeing. This is aesthetics and you have permission (as well as a responsibility in some cases) to weed out trouble. Some groups you may want to avoid include button pushers, negative/forever-unsatisfied patients, and deal makers/returners. When you are starting out a practice, it is tempting to take on every patient that walks in the door but remember that part of doing procedures is being able to handle the complications. If someone tells you they have seen every injector in town, and no one has been able to please them, you might not be able to please them either! If a patient is constantly returning products, asking for discounts, or trying to make deals with you, realize this will never change and decide if this is a patient you want to continue to treat. If someone pushes your buttons in any way, use the acronym PURR: pause, understand what is happening, reflect on whether this is a patient you want to form a relationship with, and then respond with a plan, which may be to refer the patient out.

You must be able to recognize body dysmorphic patients. Body dysmorphic disorder (BDD) is a psychological disorder in which the patient is obsessed with perceived or imaginary flaws in their appearance. We need to be aware of BDD to identify and refer these patients to mental health professionals. Those with BDD seem to primarily seek out treatment from someone other than a psychiatrist, most often a dermatologist.[7] BDD patients are frequently unsatisfied with the results of cosmetic treatment because in fact, they seek a cosmetic solution for a psychiatric issue. Although the prevalence of BDD in population-based samples is around 2%,[8] among dermatologic patients it ranges from 8.5% to 15.0%, and among patients who seek cosmetic treatments from 2.9% to 53.6%. Therefore, the first physician to have contact with these patients is very likely to be a dermatologist or a plastic surgeon. There is a growing need for awareness of this disorder among professionals who perform cosmetic medical procedures, as nonpsychiatric treatments are generally not considered beneficial for these patients. Treating these patients will likely not be beneficial for your business, either. In a recent review,[9] there was a high prevalence rate (14.2 %) of BDD in aesthetic procedure seekers, and it seemed that those patients suffering from BDD were more likely to be dissatisfied with the results of the aesthetic medical procedures. Treating patients with BDD can be frustrating. Patients with BDD have frequently seen a number of physicians for their perceived defect and are often dissatisfied with prior treatment. They may ask for inappropriate and, at times, overly aggressive treatment for their perceived defects. They are frequently seen as difficult or demanding, especially in light of their minimal or even nonexistent defect. How to detect BDD? The body dysmorphic disorder examination (BDDE)[10] is a specific measurement that deals solely with body image dysfunctions (Figure 1.4). The full questionnaire includes 34 items that assess the degree of dissatisfaction and assists physicians in the diagnosis of BDD. Consider utilizing this screening questionnaire to minimize dissatisfaction and complaints, and at a minimum, be aware of this disorder and be prepared to recommend psychiatric referral for these patients. When you screen out BDD and patients who are a poor fit for your practice, you can look forward to a fulfilling day! Cosmetic procedures can be so helpful to improve self-esteem in the right patient. In the same study,[9] when patients did not have BDD, they showed improvement not only in appearance, but also in self-esteem and quality of life. When asked about motivations for cosmetic procedures,[5] patients often report their motivation is not simply to look attractive, but to address psychological and emotional issues. Emotional considerations can be severe or milder, such as insufficient social confidence. The need to bolster confidence, the complete absence of which can be crippling, was noted by 69.5% of respondents in this survey.

If you decide this is a patient you want to treat, and you feel you have listened and understood your patients' goals, now is the time to complete your assessment and make treatment recommendations. Your physical assessment of the patient should begin when you walk in and continue as you converse with your patient. Notice how the face changes in animation and what features are prominent, in a good or bad way. Use a mirror to help illustrate what you notice. Some physicians keep props in the room, including examples of filler gel materials, anatomy illustrations, and before and after photos. When making your recommendations, always be kind and positive. Everyone has good qualities, be sure to point these out. Explain the why behind your recommendations. Often patients come in with a preconceived notion of what they need to achieve their goals, and your recommendation, while helping them achieve their goal, is a completely different product or procedure. For example, some patients want their lips treated, when really they need chin augmentation, or they request filler to their nasolabial folds when actually it is more lateral midface augmentation that is needed. As aesthetic procedures become more popular and

FIGURE 1.4   Body dysmorphic disorder questionnaire.

Are you very concerned about the appearance of some part of your body,which you consider especially unattractive?   Y   N

if no, thank you for your time and attention. You are finished with this questionnaire.

****

If yes, do these concerns preoccupy you? That is, you think about them a lot and they're hard to stop thinking about?   Y   N

What are these concerns? What specifically bothers you about the appearance of these body parts?_____
_____
_____
_____

What effect has your preoccupation with your appearance had on your life? _____
_____
_____

Has your defect often caused you a lot of distress, torment or pain? How much? (circle best answer)

1	2	3	4	5
No distress	Mild and not too disturbing	Moderate and disturbing but still manageable	Severe and very disturbing	Extreme and disabling

Has your defect caused you impairment in social, occupational or other important areas of functioning? How much? (circle best answer)

1	2	3	4	5
No limitation	Mild interference but overall per-formance not impaired	Moderate, definite interference, but still manageable	Severe, causes substantial impairment	Extreme, incapacitating

Has your defect often significantly interfered with your social life?   Y   N
If yes, how? _____
_____

Has your defect often significantly interfered with your school work, your job, or your ability to function in your role?   Y   N

Are there things you avoid because of your detect?   Y   N
_____
_____

(Reprinted with permission from Defresne RG, Phillips KS, Vittorio CC, et al. A screening questionnaire for body dysmorphic disorder in a cosmetic dermatologic surgery practice. *Dermatol Surg.* 2001;27(5):457-462.)

are increasingly referenced in the media and on the Internet, patients can develop mis-conceived ideas and unrealistic expectations about such procedures. It is imperative to set realistic expectations and educate patients regarding which cosmetic procedure might be best for their individual needs. Frequently, the cosmetic procedures that patients are ini-tially considering are in reality not the most efficient modalities to achieve the outcomes they seek. In the 2014 American Society for Dermatologic Surgery (ASDS) consumer sur-vey,[15] consumers gave the highest overall satisfaction ratings to injectable wrinkle treat-ments (93%) and injectable filler treatments (91%). In this survey, the procedures patients were actually most satisfied with (injectables) were not the procedures they were initially considering (energy-based devices). As you make recommendations, credential your aes-thetic vision and use words like natural, refreshed, and conservative. This will help you overcome a common barrier to patients receiving treatment: the fear of looking unnatural. Emphasize that you do not want your patients to look overdone. Be sure to talk about another common concern—pain. Discuss anesthesia options and what to expect during and after any procedures. Recognize that patients have some fears and be sure that you make them comfortable.

As you recommend treatment options, realize that different patients respond better to different styles of conversation. One way of looking at this is to think of four basic personality types[11] that you will encounter, each requiring a slightly different style of interaction. "Security" patients are skeptical, detail-oriented, and technical. They need data, availability, guarantees, and statistics. They want to know the practice and the physician's qualifications. Statements you will hear from security patients are: Are there any complications? Are there any side effects? How long is recovery? Where did the physician complete his/her training? Will the physician perform the procedure? How many of these procedures has the provider done? Affiliative patients, on the other hand, are very interested in their relationship with you. These people tend to be very friendly, family-oriented, and trusting. They often want to be on a first name basis with you. They like emotional nourishment and will avoid confrontation. Identify these patients when you hear: Your eyelashes look great, how do you do it? My friend came to you last month and she thinks you are great. Do you know my friend Leslie Crane? These patients need contact—they want that connection. They need to feel that you are genuinely interested in them. "Actualizers" are bottom-line oriented. Relationships are important to them (they want to know others that you treat) and they want to be up on trends. These patients need openness and sincerity, an acknowledgment of being first. You will hear statements from these patients like: How quickly will I see results? What is the latest technique being used? Finally, "power" patients. These people are aggressive, authoritative, and focus on themselves. They tend to dominate a conversation. Their needs include external approval, recognition, and high-profile service. Your consult with these patients needs to exude confidence. Power patients' statements include "I have a meeting/event to attend and must look my best. My job requires that I look my best. Will Dr Smith personally monitor my progress?". If you can tailor your conversations and style of recommendations to each patient type, you will have more success. This requires work on your "EQ", or emotional intelligence quotient, and is worth your research outside of this chapter.

Male patients require a different approach than your female patients. While men still comprise a small minority (approximately 10%-20%) of those pursuing nonsurgical cosmetic procedures, this sector is growing, in particular for injection of neurotoxins.[16] Of course, you must be familiar with gender-specific anatomical and physiological features of male aesthetics. Additionally, behavioral and psychological factors will affect your consults with men. Men are less tolerant of downtime, perhaps due to a combination of social stigmatization and career issues. Men also tend to be more conservative and tend to elect for only one procedure at a time, particularly with their first treatment sessions. Although it has not yet been studied, a higher percentage of male cosmetic patients may be naïve and may therefore have a less clear understanding of procedures from which they may benefit. They are less likely to have heard about specific procedures from same-gender peers. It is therefore possible that new male cosmetic patients may require more counseling than their female counterparts. The main barriers to trying aesthetic treatments, such as concerns regarding an unnatural outcome and side effects, stem from a lack of education. Thus, providing in-office education to men on the effectiveness and safety of cosmetic treatments is needed. This may be particularly important for dermal fillers, as men have the lowest level of awareness for this cosmetic treatment. In addition, another main barrier to undergoing treatment was "thinking they do not need it yet." Some explanations for this include that men may not focus on age-related changes as much as women, and/or they may be unaware of the benefits of beginning botulinum toxin type A treatment at earlier ages to aid in the prevention of wrinkles.

Men tend to focus on specific concerns, commonly body contouring, hair loss, or facial aging. Listen to the man's chief concern and always treat that first, and as you form a relationship you can introduce other issues and ask if he would like those treated as well. In making specific injectable recommendations, realize that the periorbital areas, in particular crow's feet and tear troughs, are of most concern and likely to be prioritized for treatment among aesthetically oriented men. In a survey of aesthetically oriented men,[17] crow's feet and tear troughs were rated as the most likely to be treated first (80% of first preferences) followed by forehead lines (74%), double chin (70%), and glabellar lines (60%). When I consult with a male patient, I find they are looking for specific language and numbers predicting efficacy. They require more guidance and less back and forth conversation than my female patients. When you establish a relationship in which you make a male patient comfortable, they can be some of the most rewarding and compliant patients to treat.

One other population that requires variations in approach is the millennial population, those born between 1982 and 2000. The largest generation in United States history, they are outspending Baby Boomers 2 to 1 on self-care, and the ASDS 2016 annual survey reported that, in the prior year, patients under 30 saw 20% growth in neuromodulators and 100% growth in injectable filler procedures. As such, they represent a significant segment of the dermatology patient base and understanding how best to communicate with this group is key to delivering the best quality and experience of care in your aesthetic practice.[18] Millennials tend to see the brands with which they choose to surround themselves as important identifiers in their life. They will want to understand your values and what value you in turn add to them. Millennials do a lot of online research and will question your expertise more than other patients. They like to feel a partnership with you. Self-care is an important part of daily life for millennials. At each appointment, you should discuss caring for their skin in general and themselves as a whole. Be confident and specific with your recommendations for products and procedures. Realize that this group seeks preventive treatment and are more likely to be dual users of neuromodulators and fillers than other populations. They represent a great opportunity for beautiful results when you form a solid relationship. If you want to build your millennial practice, loyalty programs, samples, and discounts are appreciated by this group.

I break my recommendations down into three main areas: skin care, injectables, and other procedures. As a dermatologist, I emphasize that a healthy complexion is truly the foundation of looking youthful and beautiful. I discuss the ways environmental stressors are impacting skin health and address any medical conditions that are impacting complexion. In recommending procedures, I present a concise plan with a short-term and a long-term component. There are a tremendous amount of techniques, products, and issues. It can feel overwhelming to the patient and to you. Beware the "everything" patient who wants all of it, right now. This is a marathon, not a sprint. Your short-term plan needs to be problem focused and create a wow. Examples include glabella or crow's feet neuromodulator, an intense pulsed light treatment, or cheekbone filler. The long-term plan needs to focus on prevention and maintenance. The long-term plan should reference the number of visits you expect each year, emphasizing your role as the guidance expert. I consider my long-term plan to be comprehensive over time. It allows predictable, natural results. I talk to patients about looking their best over time—not just for one event or a big birthday. An example of a long-term plan is: see me every 3 to 4 months for neuromodulators. At each visit, I will check in with you about your skin care regimen, at every other visit we will do one to two syringes of filler at various sites where you need it the most. Additionally, I want you to book three sessions of laser for existing lentigines and telangiectasia and a series of radiofrequency treatments to your jawline. The possibilities are endless, of course.

Editing the options for your patients be appreciated and will lead to success.[12] Your recommendations are based on your experience, your expertise, and what you hear from the patient. Discuss alternatives for the sake of completeness but recommend what you think will be best. You are the expert and patients want an expert opinion from you.

I recommend that you not discuss a specific budget before presenting your overall recommendations. Of course, not all patients have unlimited time and money, but I believe they are best served by hearing your expert opinion before discussing limitations. After you present your plan, get a sense of the patients' general limitations. Barriers to getting the treatments you offer are not just limited to cost, but also the amount of time spent in the office and the amount of downtime and discomfort the patient will tolerate. When I present my ideal short-term and long-term plan, I prioritize for the patient which aspects of the plan I recommend more highly. I always tell them I am respectful of their money and time and that I do not want my patients dissatisfied or disappointed. As mentioned previously, patients who know what to expect are always happier.

Sobanko et al.[13] showed that financial limitations were the greatest hindrance to patients' pursuing treatment. Most of the time you will be working with financial constraints and managing expectations within those constraints. Be clear if you cannot address the patients' concerns within their budget. Part of your aesthetic expertise is to prioritize your recommendations and to give clear, realistic expectations. Patient education becomes even more crucial when working within the constraints of a budget. When working with budgets, one tip is to always address your patients' primary concern.[14] You must balance creating an immediate effect and treating the underlying cause. Consider treating one area fully to avoid spreading resources too thin. It is always an option to defer treatment until budget allows. It is important to tell patients that if they do not spend enough, they may not be satisfied. If someone can only afford one syringe of filler and they need six, it is your job to say "well, let us look at doing something else."

Do not allow consultations to become an enormous waste of your time. Utilize your team for efficiency. I think of myself as the big picture guide/aesthetic expert and my support staff is there to provide details, supporting information, prices, and scheduling. If you appropriately credential your team, your patient will trust them to provide helpful information and you can spend your time doing what you are best at—assessing and treating. I present my short- and long-term plan briefly, covering what I would prioritize if time or money limits my options, then tell the patient that I am going to turn them over to my skin care concierge and an aesthetician who will answer every question they have on scheduling, costs, how, when, and why to use the products, and what to expect from your procedures. I make sure the patient knows that I am always available for additional questions, I try to be accessible and accommodating without being taken advantage of. I do give a rough estimate of prices, especially if the patient asks directly, but I allow my aesthetic team to sit with the patient, discuss prices, and finalize the plan. I believe this gives the patient time to feel less pressured and to ask questions of my team to help them make decisions. Of course, this requires training your team well.

Once the patient has a chance to discuss all the details with my team, we can implement the reality plan and actually (finally!) treat the patient or schedule the appointment. After any consultation or treatment, it is essential that the patient leaves the office knowing what the next steps are. I always tell the patient that they should call me at any time with any concern. First and foremost, I do not want to miss a complication, but also, I want my patients to be complaint and know that they should come to me or my staff (and not the Internet or their friends) with any questions. Before the patient leaves, have your assistants answer any questions and provide written instructions. If the patient is having a procedure, thoroughly explain what they will feel or see over the next few hours or days. If a product is purchased, provide specific instructions for use including how often and how much of the product to use and in what order. Print or email skin care regimens, pre- and postop recommendations, and prices. Providing both verbal and written communication is important, as information retention rates soar when both methods are employed. Additionally, educating your patient well will limit the number of postvisit questions and phone calls. Finally, I recommend that every patient book his or her next appointment before leaving the office. This increases compliance, allows the patient more flexibility in coming at the time or day they want, and provides a path to continuity.

Always follow up with patients. The time frame of the follow-up will depend on the treatment performed. Develop a follow-up protocol for each treatment offered. Follow up on new products as well, this helps increase compliance as well as patient satisfaction. Review before and after photographs and as you get to know the patient, you will understand better what motivates them to see you. Some patients want to chase perfection, some are happy as long as you keep their lentigines under control. Annually compare current photographs to those from the initial visit. This can be very beneficial, as patients are reminded of how they originally looked and realize the improvements have been achieved. The most successful consultations end up creating a patient for life.

In conclusion, your approach to aesthetic patients involves much more than a good, safe technique. Never underestimate the power of a well-trained staff and well-appointed office to enhance your patient experience. Patients who guided to make good choices and who know what to expect will look better, feel more confident, and send you great referrals. Enjoy your aesthetic practice!

REFERENCES

1. Allergan. *Allergan 360° Aesthetic Report*. 2019. Available at https://www.allergan.com/medical-aesthetics/allergan-360-aesthetics-report.
2. Hexsel CL, Dal'Forno T, Schilling de Souza J, Silva AF, Siega C. Standardized methods for photography in procedural dermatology using simple equipment. *Int J Dermatol*. 2017;56(4):444-451.
3. Beckman HB, Frankel RM. The effect of physician behavior on the collection of data. *Ann Intern Med*. 1984;101:692-696.
4. Dyche L, Swiderski D. The effect of physician solicitation approaches on ability to identify patient concerns. *J Gen Intern Med*. 2005;20:267-270.
5. Maisel A, Waldmen A, Furlan K, et al. Self-eported patient motivations for seeking cosmetic procedures. *JAMA Dermatol*. 2018;154(10):1167-1174.
6. Narurkar V, Shambam A, Sissins P, et al. Facial treatment preferences in aesthetically aware women. *Dermatol Surg*. 2015;41:S153-S160.
7. Wang Q, Cao C, Guo R, et al. Avoiding psychological Pitfalls in aesthetic medical procedures. *Aesth Plast Surg*. 2016;40:954-961.
8. Phillips KA, Dufresne RG Jr, Wilkel CS, Vittorio CC. Rate of body dysmorphic disorder in dermatology patients. *J Am Acad Dermatol*. 2000;42:436-441.
9. Conrado LA, Hounie AG, Diniz JB, et al. Body dysmorphic disorder among dermatologic patients: prevalence and clinical features. *J Am Acad Dermatol*. 2010;63:235-243.
10. Dufresne RG, Phillips KA, Vittorio CC, Wilkel CS. A screening questionnaire for body dysmorphic disorder in a cosmetic dermatologic surgery practice. *Dermatol Surg*. 2001;27:457-462.
11. VGuin. Personality types and the patient consultation. Allergan Presentation.
12. Swenson SL, Buell S, Zettler P, White M, Ruston DC, Lo B. Patient-centered communication: do patients really prefer it? *J Gen Intern Med*. 2004;19:1069-1079.
13. Sobanko JF, Tagleint AJ, Wilson AJ, et al. Motivations for seeking minimally invasive cosmetic procedures in an academic outpatient setting. *Aesthet Surg J*. 2015;35(8):1014-1020.
14. Black JM, Pavicic T, Jones DH. Tempering patient expectations and working with budgetary constraints when it comes to a single versus multimodal approach. *Dermatol Surg*. 2016;42(suppl 2):S161-S164.
15. American Society for Dermatologic Surgery Survey. *ASDS Survey: 52 Percent of Consumers Considering Cosmetic Procedures*. 2014. Available at http://www.asds.net/consumersurvey/.
16. Frucht CS, Ortiz AE. Nonsurgical cosmetic procedures for men: trends and technique considerations. *J Clin Aesthet Dermatol*. 2016;9(12):33-43.
17. Jagdeo J, Keaney T, Narurkar V, et al. Facial treatment preferences among aesthetically aware men. *Dermatol Surg*. 2016;42:1155-1163.
18. Sherber NS. The millennial Mindset. *J Drugs Dermatol*. 2018;17(12):1340-1342.

Botulinum Toxin

Katherine Glaser, MD, and Dee Anna Glaser, MD

Chapter Highlights

- Botulinum toxin inhibits acetylcholine release from the neuromuscular junction, resulting in flaccid paralysis of muscles, with numerous applications for medical and aesthetic use.
- There are four commercially available botulinum toxins available in the United States for aesthetic use: onabotulinumtoxinA (Botox®), prabotulinumtoxinA (Jeuveau®), abobotulinumtoxinA (Dysport®), and incobotulinumtoxinA (Xeomin®).
- Absolute and relative contraindications to therapy include known hypersensitivity to formulation and infection at injection site, as well as pregnancy, lactation, age younger than 18 years, neuromuscular disorders, and drug interactions.

▶ HISTORY

The advent of neurotoxins has revolutionized modern-day medicine with numerous clinical and cosmetic applications across many specialties. The discovery of neurotoxins dates back to the early 1800s when the often lethal outbreak of food poisoning known as "sausage poison" swept across Europe. In 1895, Emile Pierre Van Ermengem identified the gram-positive, anaerobic, spore-forming bacteria *Clostridium botulinum* as the culprit of botulism. Of the seven distinct botulinum toxin serotypes, the most potent serotype Botulinum toxin A (BoNT-A) was first isolated and purified in 1946 by Dr Edward Shantz.[1]

Historically, botulinum toxin ingestion led to flaccid paralysis and thus was proposed for use in small quantities in disorders of hyperfunctional muscles. Dr Alan Scott initially tested BoNT-A on humans with strabismus in 1980 with very promising results. The onabotulinumtoxinA product, then called Oculinum, was approved by the United States Food and Drug Administration (FDA) in 1989 for several muscular disorders including strabismus, blepharospasm, and hemifacial spasms. Soon after, the formulation was acquired by Allergan Inc. and renamed Botox®.[1-3]

While utilizing BoNT-A for blepharospasm, astute ophthalmologist Dr Jean Carruthers began to recognize its secondary effects of wrinkle reduction which she followed up with two landmark confirmatory clinical trials.[2,3] Numerous additional trials corroborated the safety and efficacy of Botox® for wrinkle reduction leading to the FDA approval for the treatment of moderate to severe glabellar lines in 2002.[4,5] Since then, the product has gained multiple additional indications and is utilized off-label for a variety of cosmetic uses.

▶ BASIC SCIENCE

Seven serotypes of botulinum toxin termed A through G have been isolated from various strains of *C. botulinum*.[1,3,6,7] While each serotype produces chemodenervation, there are some differences in their cellular structure and mechanisms of action.[6,7] The most potent types, A and B, are predominantly used in clinical practice.[7]

Structurally, botulinum toxins are all 150-kDa polypeptides composed of a 100-kDa heavy chain and a unique 50-kDa light chain which are linked by heat-labile disulfide bonds. The toxin is then complexed with nontoxic proteins, mainly hemagglutinins, by covalent bonds and dimerized to form the larger final compound.[3,6,7] In the United States, there are four commercially available BoNT-A: onabotulinumtoxinA (Botox®) weighing 900-kDa, prabotulinumtoxinA (Jeuveau®) weighing 900-kDa, abobotulinumtoxinA (Dysport®) weighing 500-kDa, and incobotulinumtoxinA (Xeomin®) weighing 150-kDa as it is a monomeric protein free of any complexing proteins.[4,5,8-10] Herein these products will be referred to as onabotA, prabotA, abobotA, and incobotA, respectively.

The mechanism by which botulinum toxin inhibits skeletal muscle contraction is due to the inhibition of acetylcholine release from the neuromuscular junction (NMJ).[1,3,6,7] After injection, the complex rapidly and irreversibly binds to synaptotagmin, a docking receptor on the presynaptic terminal of the NMJ. The toxin is then internalized via endocytosis, and the disulfide bonds are cleaved allowing the free light chain to translocate into the cytoplasm. Inhibition of acetylcholine release occurs when the free light chain fuses with proteins in the synaptic fusion complex and deactivates it by a proteolytic zinc-dependent endopeptidase. Several key proteins make up the synaptic fusion complex, known as SNARE (soluble *N*-ethylmaleimide-sensitive factor attachment protein receptors). Specifically, botulinum toxin types A, C, and E cleave the 25-kDa synaptosomal-associated protein (SNAP25), while toxin types B, D, F, and G cleave synaptobrevin, also known as vesicle-associated membrane protein.[6,7] Ultimately, the docking, fusion, and release of acetylcholine vesicles are permanently disrupted inhibiting downstream muscular contraction (Figure 2.1).

Clinically, muscle weakness is often apparent 2 to 3 days after injection with full response seen by 8 to 10 days, although timing can vary based on dose, treatment area, and the individual.[3] Despite the fact that chemical denervation is considered permanent, muscular activity typically returns 3 to 6 months after injection due to neurogenesis.[3,7] Peripheral axonal sprouts form, making new connections with the muscle, and to a lesser degree SNAP25 proteins regenerate in the original NMJ, allowing regained muscular function.[7] For this reason, injections of botulinum toxin are performed at 3 to 6 month intervals for facial rhytides.[3] Some data suggest that with repeated treatments, there is a tendency toward greater interval's of time between future treatments.[11]

Immunogenicity is a controversial topic in the literature, but generally speaking, although neutralizing antibody formation against BoNT-A has been reported, the phenomenon is rarely, if ever, witnessed with doses used for cosmetic purposes.[3,7] However, patients treated with 150 to 300 units for other neuromuscular diseases have developed resistance to the toxin's effects.[7] In these cases, switching to botulinum toxin type B (BoNT-B), available in the United States as rimabotulinumtoxinB (Myobloc®), may be helpful.[3,6,7] Using the lowest effective doses and longer intervals between injections may minimize the possibility of antibody formation.[3,7]

FIGURE 2.1   Mechanism of action of botulinum toxins. (A) The assembly of the SNARE mechanism that mediates fusion of acetylcholine-containing vesicles with the cell membrane and release of acetylcholine into the neuromuscular junction after normal excitatory stimuli. (B) The actions of botulinum toxins: proteolytic cleavage of either synaptobrevin, syntaxin, or SNAP-25 (the main components of the SNARE complex).

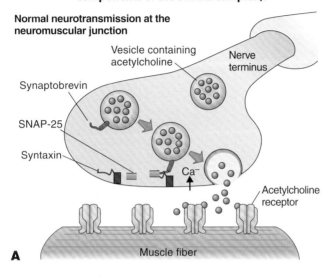

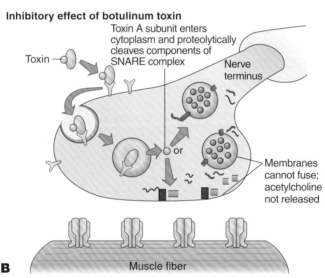

(With permission from Engleberg C, Dermody T, DiRita V. *Schaechter's Mechanisms of Microbial Disease.* 5th ed. Philadelphia, PA: Lippincott Williams and Wilkins; 2013.)

▶ COMMERCIALLY AVAILABLE TOXINS IN THE UNITED STATES

There are four BoNT-A products and one BoNT-B approved by the US FDA to date (Table 2.1).[4,5,8-10,12] Several similarities exist, but each formulation has unique chemical properties and therefore are not interchangeable. Dosing among products cannot be standardized or calculated with any exact conversion ratio as one unit of toxin corresponds

TABLE 2.1   Commercially Available Botulinum Toxins in the United States

	OnabotulinumtoxinA	AbobotulinumtoxinA	IncobotulinumtoxinA	PrabotulinumtoxinA	RimabotulinumtoxinB
Trade names®	Botox, Botox Cosmetic	Dysport	Xeomin	Jeuveau	Myobloc
Manufacturer	Allergan Inc.	Galderma, Ipsen Biopharmaceuticals	Merz Pharmaceuticals	Evolus	Solstice Neurosciences
Initial year of approval	1989	2009	2010	2019	2000
Units per single-dose vial	50, 100, 200[a]	300, 500	50, 100, 200	100	2500, 5000, 10,000
Ingredients	BoNT-A, human albumin, sodium chloride	BoNT-A, human albumin, lactose (may contain trace cow's milk protein)	BoNT-A, human albumin, sucrose	BoNT-A, human albumin, sodium chloride	BoNT-B, human albumin, sodium chloride, sodium succinate
FDA-approved indications	Glabellar lines, lateral canthal lines, forehead lines, overactive bladder, chronic migraines, cervical dystonia, spasticity, axillary hyperhidrosis, blepharospasm, strabismus	Glabellar lines, cervical dystonia, spasticity	Glabellar lines, cervical dystonia, spasticity, blepharospasm, chronic sialorrhea	Glabellar lines	Cervical dystonia, chronic sialorrhea

BoNT-A, botulinum toxin type A complex; BoNT-B, botulinum toxin type B complex; FDA, Food and Drug Administration.

[a]Only available as Botox, not available as Botox Cosmetic.

to the calculated median lethal intraperitoneal dose (LD50) in mice which varies across manufacturers.[7] It is critical that physicians understand these differences in order to achieve safe and clinically effective results.

OnabotA (Botox®), initially approved in 1989, is a sterile lyophilized botulinum A exotoxin distributed as a vacuum-dried single-use vial without preservative. Each vial contains 0.5 mg of human albumin and 0.9 mg of sodium chloride. OnabotA has the most FDA indications including the treatment of glabellar lines, lateral canthal lines, forehead lines, and axillary hyperhidrosis.[4,5]

AbobotA (Dysport®), initially approved in 2009, is also a sterile lyophilized botulinum A exotoxin but manufactured with different purification techniques. Each vial contains 0.125 mg of human albumin and 2.5 mg of lactose.[8] Most studies suggest similar efficacy using a conversion ratio of 2-3:1 (abobotA:onabotA).[13] The only aesthetic FDA indication is the treatment of glabellar lines.[8]

IncobotA (Xeomin®), approved in 2011, is a sterile lyophilized botulinum A exotoxin that is free of any complexing proteins making it theoretically less immunogenic. Each vial contains 1 mg of human albumin and 4.7 mg of sucrose.[9] Clinical and preclinical data suggest similar potencies between incobotA and onabotA using a conversion ratio of 1:1 or 1.2:1.[13] Like abobotA, the only cosmetic FDA indication is the treatment of glabellar lines.[9]

PrabotA (Jeuveau®), approved in 2019, is another sterile lyophilized botulinum A exotoxin distributed as a vacuum-dried single-use vial without preservative. Similar to onabotA, each vial contains 0.5 mg of human albumin and 0.9 mg of sodium chloride.[10] Limited data exist comparing its potency to onabotA, but noninferiority has been established using a 1:1 conversion ratio in phase 3 clinical trials for glabellar and lateral canthal lines.[14,15] The only FDA indication is for the treatment of glabellar lines.[10]

RimabotulinumtoxinB (Myobloc®), approved in 2000, is the sole BoNT-B available and the only nonlyophilized stable liquid formulation. Depending on the vial size, each vial contains concentrations of human albumin, sodium chloride, and sodium succinate.[12] Dosing is variable with conversion ratios as high as 1:100 (onabotA:rimabotB) being reported for muscular diseases. RimabotB injections are typically more painful, offer a shorter duration of action, and have more autonomic side effects.[16] There are no cosmetic indications.[12,16]

Diffusion

Neurotoxin diffusion refers to the slow dispersion of toxin beyond the original site of injection.[17] In some cases, higher diffusion is desirable such as with the treatment of hyperhidrosis. In comparison, minimal diffusion may be preferred for injections of facial muscles to minimize unwanted adverse effects. Several factors contribute to the rate of diffusion including dose, type of skin, anatomical location, and the density of botulinum toxin receptors.[17] Definitive data are lacking, although some studies using forehead anhidrosis as the end point have suggested innately higher diffusion with abobotA compared to onabotA with equivalent injection volumes.[18,19]

Reconstitution

All products available in the United States, except rimabotB, require reconstitution prior to injection.[4,5,8-10,12] Reconstitution with preservative-free saline is recommended by the FDA; however, most injectors prefer bacteriostatic saline due to the preservative benzyl alcohol and its anesthetic properties.[20] The amount of diluent added varies greatly among injectors. The most common reconstitution volumes for onabotA, prabotA, and incobotA

TABLE 2.2   Common Reconstitution Volumes for Botulinum Toxins

(A) OnabotulinumtoxinA, IncobotulinumtoxinA, and PrabotulinumtoxinA	
Diluent[a] Added per 100 Unit Vial (mL)	Concentration (units per 0.1 mL)
1	10
2	5
2.5[b]	4
4	2.5
5	2
(B) AbobotulinumtoxinA	
Diluent[a] Added per 300 Unit Vial (mL)	Concentration (units per 0.1 mL)
0.6	50
1.5[b]	20
2.5[b]	12
3	10
6	5

FDA, Food and Drug Administration.
[a]Preservative-free 0.9% sodium chloride is the only FDA-approved diluent.
[b]On-label dilution per FDA guidelines.

ranges from 1 to 5 mL per 100 unit vial compared to abobotA wherein volumes range from 1.5 to 6 mL per 300 unit vial (Table 2.2). Several studies have evaluated the association between reconstitution volume and diffusion, but the results are rarely clinically significant or reproducible in patients.[17] Since clinical efficacy and result duration do not seem to be correlated with dilution, it may be easiest to pick one dilution initially.

To add the diluent to the botulinum toxin, first remove the plastic cap covering and wipe the top of the vial with alcohol, allowing it time to thoroughly dry. Then, use an 18 to 23 gauge needle to pierce through the bottle top. As the bottle is vacuum sealed, the diluent should be easily pulled into the vial.[4,5,8-10] After the diluent is added, gently swirl the vial in a circular motion until all particulate matter is well mixed. Avoid vigorous shaking or foaming of the product.[3,17] Record the date and time of reconstitution as well as the final concentration on the label. All of these data in addition to the lot number and vial expiration date should be included in the patient's record during treatment.

Safe Handling

Unopened vials of neurotoxin should be kept frozen or refrigerated in temperatures ranging from 2°C to 8°C and used prior to the label's expiration date.[4,5,8,10,12] IncobotA is the exception which can be stored at room temperatures (20°C-25°C) for up to 36 months or until the expiration date.[9] After reconstitution, the package insert for all neurotoxins suggests storage in a refrigerator (2°C-8°C) and administration within 24 hours.[4,5,8-10,12] These narrow shelf life guidelines have been viewed as impractical and are rarely followed. Recent clinical studies have proven maintained safety and product efficacy for up to 6 weeks post reconstitution with appropriate storage techniques.[71] Although this reduces product waste and consequently costs, it is still necessary to utilize safe handling and storage techniques to prevent contamination.

Contraindications

Only two absolute contraindications are listed in the FDA-approved package inserts: (1) known hypersensitivity to any botulinum toxin preparation or any of the components in the formulation and (2) infection at the injection site.[4,5,8-10,12] However, there are multiple relative contraindications which should be considered especially when weighing the risks and benefits of cosmetic use. Limited safety data are available in humans for use during pregnancy, lactation, or in children younger than 18 years, so it is generally recommended to avoid in these patient populations. Based on animal data, neurotoxins are labeled pregnancy category C.[4,5,8-10,12]

Caution is advised in patients with known neuromuscular disorders, swallowing or breathing difficulties due to the predisposition for severe muscle weakness, dysphagia, and respiratory compromise.[4,5,8-10,12] These potentially life-threatening events have been reported hours to weeks after treatment and in nearly all cases were seen in the setting of noncosmetic indications.[22] Regardless, a black box warning has been issued by the FDA outlining the risks of inadvertent neurotoxin spread and should be discussed with all patients. Medication reconciliation is also important as there are several drug interactions that may potentiate the toxins effects. Common culprits include aminoglycosides, anticholinergics, systemic anesthetics, and muscle relaxants.[4,5,7-10,12]

▶ INJECTION TECHNIQUES

Pretreatment preparation is overall minimal both for the patient and for the physician. Traditionally, patients are advised to avoid nonessential use of aspirin, nonsteroidal anti-inflammatory drugs, vitamin E, and other supplements for one week prior to treatment to minimize the risks of bruising.[23] Regardless, botulinum toxin can still be utilized in patients who are taking these medications. If neuromodulator injections are the only procedure planned for the visit then anesthetics are ordinarily not required. Ice packs or topical anesthetics may be applied prior to injections to minimize discomfort in more sensitive individuals.

After appropriate consultation with the patient, all treatment sites should be identified with intended doses outlined per treatment area. Use of a marking pen or a white eyebrow pencil to pinpoint each injection site may be considered, especially for novice injectors. The reconstituted botulinum toxin is then drawn up using an 18 to 23 gauge needle on a 1-mL Luer-Lok syringe. The product may either be kept in this syringe for injection or transferred to an ultrafine BD insulin syringe, both of which have clear markings to allow for easy observation of smaller injection volumes. Syringes are available that have a plunger designed to reduce wasting and are used by the authors (Figure 2.2). Withdrawing all product from the needle bevel will help minimize product waste before transitioning to a 30 to 32 gauge half-inch needle for the actual injection. An additional pearl to minimize product waste is to remove the vial's cap and stopper and tilt the vial 45° to draw up any remaining droplets (Figure 2.3). Separating syringes by treatment site can allow for more efficient and accurate injections and decreases the possibility of needle dulling which ultimately leads to improved patient satisfaction.

The areas to be treated should be cleaned with an alcohol wipe or other antiseptic and allowed to dry completely before proceeding with injections. Patients are typically seated upright with their head rested against the procedure chair.[3] It is essential for both the patient and the injector to be in an ergonomically comfortable position throughout the treatment. Typically, syringes are held perpendicular to the skin surface, although technique certainly varies based on the treatment area and injector preference (Figure 2.4). Injections are delivered slowly into the intramuscular plane or in some areas intradermally or subcutaneously.[3,22] Gauze or cotton tip applicators should be easily accessible in the advent of bleeding at which time gentle pressure can be applied to minimize bruising.

FIGURE 2.2   Syringes used by the authors for botulinum toxin injections. From left to right: 1-mL Luer-Lok, 1-mL Luer-Slip with zero dead space plunger, and 1-mL BD Insulin.

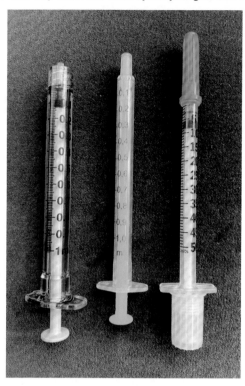

FIGURE 2.3   Removal of the botulinum toxin stopper minimizes product waste when drawing up reconstituted product.

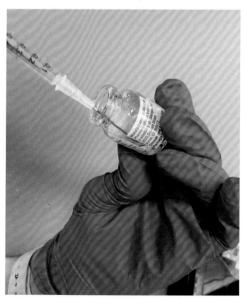

FIGURE 2.4   **Botulinum toxin injection technique in the glabellar complex. The nondominant hand is used to support the patient and syringe for optimal injection placement.**

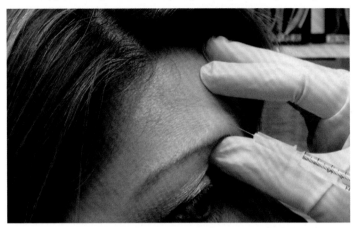

A routine follow-up 2 to 4 weeks after the procedure may be considered as a standard practice in cosmetic indications to allow for any small touch-ups. Patients should also be provided the office contact information and office protocols if they develop questions or complications.

▶ TREATMENT OF DYNAMIC RHYTIDES

Rhytides form due to repeated contraction of hyperdynamic facial muscles. Generally, wrinkles develop perpendicular to the vector of the muscle's force.[3,7] Weakening the muscles with botulinum toxin can help smooth dynamic rhytides and even prevent future formation. However, it is important to remember that static rhytides, wrinkles visible at rest, are typically unaffected and may require additional treatment modalities to address the aging skin's loss of elasticity.[24]

Understanding facial anatomy is critical for safe and appropriate injection placement (Figure 2.5). Nevertheless, anatomic variations exist among individuals of different ages, sex, and ethnicities, so clinicians should carefully observe each patient's muscle movement before designing their treatment strategy.[25] The muscle groups targeted in the most commonly encountered cosmetic treatment areas for rhytides are outlined in Table 2.3. Each treatment area will be discussed separately, although many patients desire and warrant the treatment of multiple sites simultaneously. Again, many of the treatments are considered off-label uses of botulinum toxin. OnabotA has gained FDA approval for the treatment of glabellar, forehead, and lateral canthal lines, whereas abobotA, incobotA, and prabotA are approved only for the glabella.[4,5,8-10] In this section, the dosing recommendations are outlined in onabotA units unless otherwise specified, but in clinical practice, other neurotoxins are used just as effectively with appropriate conversion ratios.

Glabellar Complex

The muscles of the glabellar complex serve as the primary brow depressors which contribute to the horizontal and vertical wrinkles between the eyebrows. The complex is composed of the procerus, bilateral corrugator supercilii, depressor supercilii, and some contribution of the orbital portion of the orbicularis oculi.[26]

FIGURE 2.5   **Anatomy of facial muscles commonly treated with botulinum toxin.**

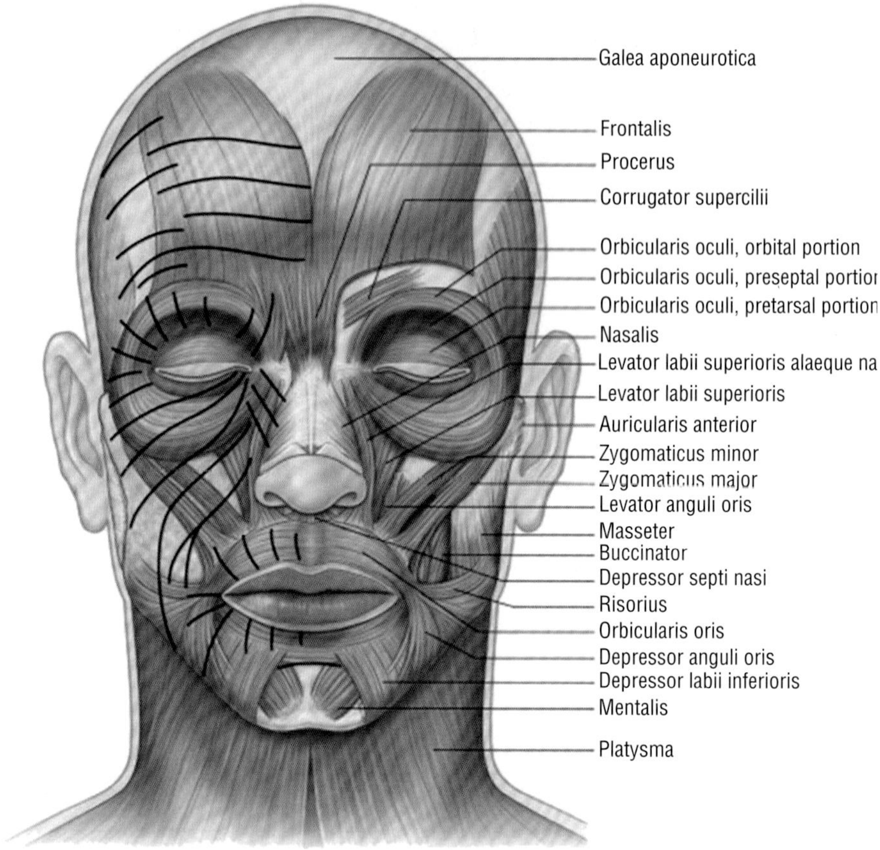

Galea aponeurotica

Frontalis

Procerus

Corrugator supercilii

Orbicularis oculi, orbital portion
Orbicularis oculi, preseptal portion
Orbicularis oculi, pretarsal portion
Nasalis
Levator labii superioris alaeque na
Levator labii superioris
Auricularis anterior
Zygomaticus minor
Zygomaticus major
Levator anguli oris
Masseter
Buccinator
Depressor septi nasi
Risorius
Orbicularis oris
Depressor anguli oris
Depressor labii inferioris
Mentalis

Platysma

(Used with Permission from Giordano CN, Matarasso SL, Ozog DM. Injectable and topical neurotoxins in dermatology: basic science, anatomy, and therapeutic agents. *J Am Acad Dermatol.* 2017;76(6):1013-1024.)

TABLE 2.3	Muscle Groups Targeted in Botulinum Toxin Cosmetic Treatments	
Upper face injections	Glabellar complex	Corrugator supercilii, depressor supercilii, procerus, and orbital portion of the orbicularis oculi
	Forehead lines	Frontalis
	Lateral canthal lines, "crow's feet"	Lateral portion of the orbicularis oculi
Midface injections	Nasal "bunny lines"	Nasalis
	Nasal tip droop	Depressor septi nasi
Lower face injections	Perioral lines	Orbicularis oris
	Gummy smile	Levator labii superioris alaeque nasi
	Frown lines "Marionette lines"	Depressor anguli oris
	Masseter hypertrophy	Masseter
	Mental crease	Mentalis
	Dimpled chin	Mentalis
Neck injections	Platysmal bands	Platysma

Located midline is the pyramidal-shaped procerus which originates on the nasal bone, inserts superiorly to the dermis, and interdigitates with fibers of the other aforementioned glabellar muscles. Lateral to the procerus are the deeper corrugator supercilii muscles which originate on the frontal bone just above the orbital rim, insert superiorly to the deeper dermis, and interdigitate with other glabellar complex muscles as well as the frontalis muscle. The corrugator muscles are long, narrow, and oriented at an oblique angle.[26] Although the thin depressor supercilii is reportedly located just superficial and medial to the corrugator muscles with a vertical orientation, it can be cumbersome to locate even on cadaver dissections.[27] Palpation of the orbital rim and observation of muscle movement during scowling is necessary to identify the glabellar complex muscles. The eyebrows should not serve as a substitute landmark as they often droop with age and can be manipulated with grooming.[28]

Treatment of the glabellar complex muscles consists of three to seven injection sites, each performed intramuscularly with the syringe held horizontal to the skin surface.[3] The first injection point is central to inactivate the procerus, typically determined by marking the intersection point between two drawn lines extending from the medial brow to the contralateral medial canthus.[25] One to three injection points per side is then performed to inactivate the corrugators and depressor supercilii muscles.[25] The more medial injection is typically 1 cm above the orbital rim in line with the medial canthus, placed just above the periosteum. The most lateral injection, if performed, is positioned slightly more than 1 cm above the orbital rim in the midpupillary line (Figure 2.6).[26] An individualized approach allows for variability in the number of injection sites which is determined by the shape, length, and strength of the corrugators, as well as the needs of the patient.

Dosing varies significantly, but generally speaking, men are thought to require higher doses than women.[3,25] Although the package insert of onabotA recommends a total of 20 units into the glabellar complex with 4 units in each of the five sites, physicians may use higher doses.[4] Several well-known authors published a consensus paper suggesting starting doses of 10 to 30 units for females and 20 to 60 units for males.[25] Similar practices were outlined for the other FDA-approved toxins.

FIGURE 2.6   Injections for glabellar frown rhytides. A man during movement (A) and at rest (B) with five planned injection points. Patients with this degree of muscular activity would require higher starting doses such as 25 units onabotA or 60 units abobotA.

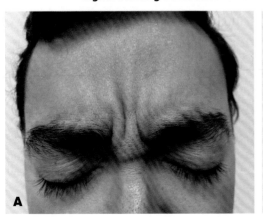
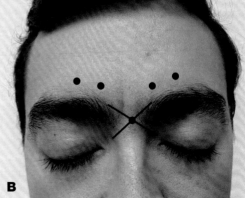

Forehead Lines

Horizontal forehead lines develop from the vertical tension vectors of the broad bifid frontalis muscle which functions as the main eyebrow elevator. Superiorly it originates on the galea aponeurotica, inserts inferiorly on the frontal bone, and interdigitates with muscles of the glabellar complex.[26] Variability exists in the diameter of muscle activity; some individuals have predominantly central forces, while others have contractions and resultant rhytides extending beyond the lateral eyebrows.[29]

Treatment of this region can be challenging as slight overtreatment can lead to eyebrow drooping and improper toxin placement can lead to rather obvious asymmetries. Based on the breadth of muscle activity, 4 to 10 injection points are scattered across the forehead with superficial intramuscular or subcutaneous injections aimed horizontally to the skin surface.[25] Injections should generally be placed at least 2 cm above the orbital rim to prevent eyebrow depression.[25,26] Classic teaching is to inject above the lowest forehead wrinkle. Extra caution should be taken over the lateral eyebrows as both extremes can have consequences. High doses or low placement can lead to significant brow drooping, but undertreatment can result in an unnatural expression which many have termed "spock eyebrows."[30] For this reason, it is best to start with small doses, higher injection sites, and close follow-up arranged for any potential touch-ups.

Dosing again varies based on muscle activity and patient desires. The onabotA package insert recommends 20 units total injected into five sites with 4 units per injection.[4] Many authors suggest lower starting doses around 5 to 15 units divided among 4 to 10 injection sites.[25] These injections should be implemented simultaneously or shortly after glabellar treatments to help maintain neutral eyebrow position and minimize unopposed elevation or depression.[26]

Lateral Canthal Lines

"Crow's feet," a term used to describe lateral canthal lines, are a result of tension from the lateral fibers of the orbicularis oculi. The muscle is a large, superficial circular band which encircles the orbit to assist in closing the eyes and eyebrow depression. Some variability in muscle size and distribution around the eye is noted among patients.[26]

Treatment of this area is often intradermal with two to five small blebs per side spaced approximately 1 cm apart in an arcuate orientation placed at least 1 cm lateral from the lateral orbital rim (Figure 2.7).[25] Superficial injections allow for adequate muscle paralysis while minimizing the risk of bruising which is innately high given the abundance of nearby vessels.[31] Caution should be taken at the inferior aspect to avoid unintentional injection of the zygomaticus complex which can inadvertently lead to upper lip ptosis.[31] An additional superficial injection can be placed in the midpupillary line approximately 0.3 cm below the lower lash line which may help decrease the infraorbital fold and offer a wider appearance of the eye.[32] If this technique is utilized, patients should be counseled on the risk of dry eyes, inability to completely close the eye, and potential for infraorbital puffiness.

The onabotA package insert recommends a total of 24 units divided among three injection sites per side with 4 units injected at each site.[4] Authors of the aforementioned consensus paper agree that 10 to 30 total units divided among 2 to 5 injection sites per side is likely sufficient.[25] Injections at the midpupillary line are entirely off-label and should not exceed 2 to 3 units per side.[32]

FIGURE 2.7   **Injections for lateral canthal rhytides or "crow's feet." It is important to observe natural variations in muscle activity, not only between patients but also in the same patient. As seen in this man, the pattern of movement differs between the left (A) and right (B) sides. Numerals indicate the number of onabotA units used at each injection point.**

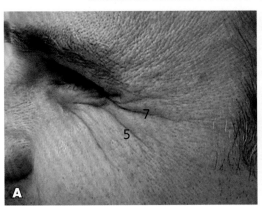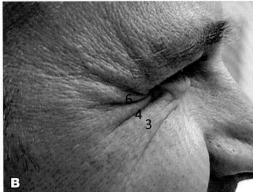

Brow Lift

An interplay of the frontalis, glabellar complex, and orbicularis oculi muscles helps establish natural eyebrow position.[26] Elevation of the eyebrows especially in the mid and lateral aspects can offer a more youthful aesthetically pleasing appearance. Botulinum toxin can be utilized as a temporary chemical brow lift.[31] Botulinum toxin injections into the eyebrow depressor muscles will shift the balance of forces toward unopposed eyebrow elevation. Beyond treatment of the glabellar complex, an extra injection into the lateral superior fibers of the orbicularis oculi muscle can provide additional benefit.[30] In one study, an average measured gain of 1-mm elevation at the midpupillary line and 4.8-mm elevation at the lateral canthus was achieved with this technique.[33] A superficial injection of 2 to 4 units into the lateral tail of the eyebrow bilaterally is typically sufficient.[25]

Nasal Lines

"Bunny lines" over the lateral aspects of the nasal root are a result of underlying nasalis muscle contraction. The muscle is divided into two regions including the proximal transverse portion and alar portion which are responsible for bunny lines and nasal flaring, respectively.[26] Bunny lines may be softened by injecting 2 to 4 units of botulinum toxin superficially into the proximal portion of the nasalis typically with only one injection point needed per side (Figure 2.8).[22,34] Injections should be placed above the nasofacial sulcus to minimize inadvertent treatment of the levator labii superioris resulting in lip ptosis.[30] Treatments for bunny lines are often combined with glabellar complex injections to prevent additional nasal muscle recruitment.[26]

Nasal Tip Droop

Descent of the nasal tip is common with advancing age and can lead to a more pronounced columellar show. Overuse or repeated contraction of the depressor septi nasi muscle may further accentuate the drooping nasal tip. The muscle originates from the

FIGURE 2.8   Injections for nasal rhytides or "bunny lines." A woman with movement (A) and at rest (B). Numerals indicate the number of onabotA units injected which is placed medial to the nasofacial sulcus in order to minimize diffusion into the levator labii superioris and unwanted lip ptosis.

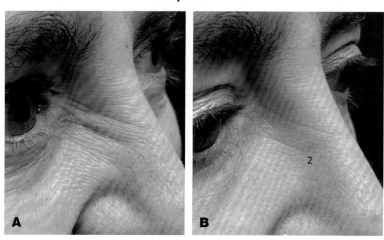

maxilla, courses along the columella, and inserts into the alar portion of the nasalis.[22,26] Proposed treatments for nasal tip droop include hyaluronic acid injections, surgical cutting of the depressor septi nasi muscle, or botulinum toxin into the depressor septi nasi.[35] Injection of 2 to 3 units of botulinum toxin placed at the base of the columella is typically sufficient to achieve subtle, temporary, but appreciable nasal tip elevation.[22,35] Injections in this sensitive area can be painful and so may warrant ice packs or anesthetics.

Perioral Lines

Vertical perioral rhytides, nicknamed "smoker's lines" or "barcode lines," are often more pronounced on the upper cutaneous lip. Although there are some genetic and environmental factors contributing to perioral line development, the primary culprit is a hyperfunctional orbicularis oris. The elliptically shaped orbicularis oris muscle encircles the oral aperture with lateral insertions at the modiolus and anterior insertions at the wet-dry lip border. The muscle is critical for speech and helps with numerous actions that require pursed lips.[22,26] For this reason, overtreatment with botulinum toxin should be avoided.

Dosing and injection techniques vary, although typically small 1 unit aliquots are injected superficially along the vermillion border using 2 to 4 injection points per lip (Figure 2.9).[22] Avoidance of the midline upper lip can help prevent cupids bow flattening, an aesthetically displeasing look for most patients. Caution should also be taken around the corners of the mouth to minimize lateral lip drooping or in severe cases drooling.[22,26] Patients should be notified that injections around the lip may be more painful and may require increased treatment intervals compared to those of the upper face. Additionally, those with a combination of deep and superficial rhytides may not achieve substantial correction with neurotoxins alone and may warrant additional treatment modalities such as soft-tissue fillers or resurfacing procedures.[22]

FIGURE 2.9   Injections for perioral rhytides. A female pursing her lips (A) and at rest (B). The authors injected 5 units total of onabotA into the upper lip just above the vermilion border. Note that the pattern and dosing are based on the individual's muscle activity.

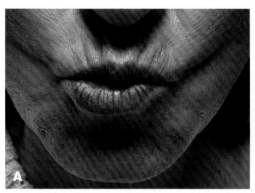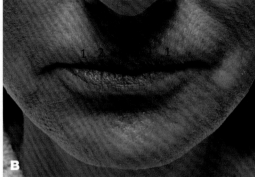

Gummy Smile

Gummy smiles are defined as excessive (>3 mm) gingival show while smiling.[36] Several muscles contribute to lip elevation including the levator labii superioris alaeque nasi (LLSAN), levator labii superioris, and zygomaticus major.[26] Hyperactivity of these muscles leads to a gummy smile which can be cosmetically bothersome for patients. Treatments are commonly focused on inactivating the LLSAN which can be achieved with 1 to 2 unit injections placed deeper on each side of the nasolabial fold approximately 1 cm lateral and inferior to the nasal ala.[22]

Mazzuco et al classified gummy smiles into four different subtypes, each pattern ultimately dictating which muscles require botulinum toxin injections. Patients were found to have either anterior, posterior, mixed, or asymmetric gummy smiles. Those with anterior gummy smiles received 2.5 to 5 units of abobotA on each side of the nasolabial fold using the previously mentioned injection point into the LLSAN. Posterior gummy smiles were treated with two injection points per side into the zygomaticus muscles: 2.5 units of abobotA per site were placed into the lateral nasolabial fold and approximately 2 cm laterally and superiorly in the malar cheek at the level of the tragus. Mixed gummy smiles were treated with the same four injection points as the posterior patients but with a 50% dose reduction. Asymmetric smiles were also treated similarly with 2.5 units of abobotA into two injection points on the stronger side but only one injection point in the lateral nasolabial fold on the contralateral side.[36] Regardless of technique or neurotoxin preference, lower doses should be implemented in the perioral areas.[22]

Frown Lines

"Marionette lines" or frown lines refer to the accentuated melomental fold which develops from an overactive depressor anguli oris (DAO) muscle. The DAO is a deeper fan-shaped muscle which originates on the mandible just lateral to the oral commissure and inserts superiorly onto the modiolus. The muscle functions to depress the corners of the mouth, and thus, treatment with botulinum toxin leads to unopposed elevation via the zygomaticus.[22,26] Injections of 2 to 7 units per side are placed into the DAO just above the angle of the mandible, approximately 1 cm lateral to the oral commissure (Figure 2.10).[22] Asking the patient to show their lower teeth or frown will allow easy visualization of the

FIGURE 2.10   Injections for frown lines or "marionette lines." A female frowning (A) and at rest (B). The authors injected 4 units of onabotA into each depressor anguli oris (DAO) muscle. A more lateral injection helps avoid effect on the more medial depressor labii inferioris.

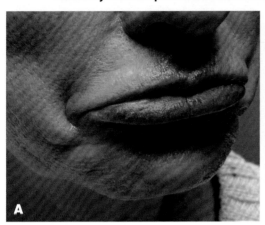 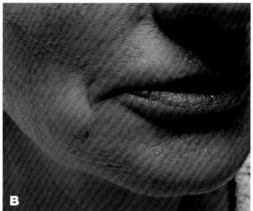

DAO and minimize unwanted injections into the more medial depressor labii inferioris (DLI).[25,26] Over time, patients are frequently noted to have a softer resting expression; however, similar to perioral rhytides, results are best achieved using a combination of treatment modalities.[22]

Masseter Hypertrophy

The width of the lower face is determined by the size of the mandibular bone, the thickness of the masseter muscle, and the volume of overlying subcutaneous tissue.[37] Widening of the lower face is often correlated with a more masculine and less youthful appearance. Women, especially of Asian descent, are often cosmetically bothered by a rounded facial contour and are more likely to seek treatment.[30] Botulinum toxin injections into the hypertrophic masseter muscle are considered a safe, noninvasive, and readily available treatment option with extremely high patient satisfaction scores.[37]

The masseters are larger diamond-shaped masticatory muscles which originate deep from the mandibular angle and insert superiorly on the zygomatic bone.[26] Identification of the muscle can be made more accurately when patients are asked to clench their teeth. Injections should be placed lateral to the DAO and inferior to the risorius which can be arbitrarily identified with a line extending from the earlobe to the oral commissure.[30] Typical starting doses of 20 to 30 units per side are injected into 3 to 6 points within the masseter depending on muscle volume. Both the deep and superficial components need to be treated.[38] Repeated treatment with neurotoxin can lead to muscle atrophy even after muscle tone returns, evident by ultrasonogram measurements.[37] Uncommon side effects to monitor include hematoma formation, headaches, weakness with chewing, paradoxical muscle bulging, asymmetric smiling, dry mouth, and sunken lateral cheeks.[38]

Mental Crease

Horizontal creasing at the junction between the cutaneous lower lip and chin is termed the mental crease. Deeper mental grooves may result from a hyperactive mentalis muscle which assists in lower lip elevation and eversion. The two mentalis muscles originate at the midline mandible and form a V-shaped triangle interdigitating with the orbicularis oris and DLI muscles.[26] Softening of this crease can be achieved with botulinum toxin injections and is often combined with soft-tissue filler augmentation.[22] Typically 3 to 5 units of botulinum toxin are placed into the inferior portion of the mentalis over the bony prominence of the chin.[22] Caution should be taken near the mental crease itself as a weakened orbicularis oris or DLI can result in an incompetent mouth.[22,25]

Dimpled Chin

Similar to the mental crease formation, overactivity of the mentalis muscle can also lead to a dimpled or "peau d'orange" appearance of the chin which may be accentuated while talking.[22,26] Botulinum toxin injections can be very effective at softening the dimpled skin texture and may be used in combination with soft-tissue fillers.[22] Like the mental crease treatments, botulinum toxin should be injected inferiorly and medially over the bony prominence of the chin to minimize diffusion into the surrounding orbicularis oris or DLI.[22,25] Total doses of 5 to 10 units are injected into one or two points within the mentalis and massaged into place.[22]

Platysmal Bands

Treatments of the aging neck are constantly evolving. Several less invasive treatment modalities have been identified to hopefully postpone the need for more costly surgical techniques like a face lift. However, the most appropriate treatment option varies based on the predominant aging feature which ranges from cutaneous photoaging to skin laxity to muscle banding.[28] Botulinum toxin injections can be helpful to combat platysmal muscle banding, sharpen the jawline, and soften horizontal neck rhytides.[22] These features typically arise in the setting of platysma overactivity making it amenable to treatment with neurotoxins.

The platysma is a thin muscle draped in a fan like distribution over the neck and décolleté regions. Inferiorly, it originates from the superficial fascia of the upper chest, inserts superiorly onto the mandible, and interdigitates with many muscles of the lower face including the superficial musculoaponeurotic system (SMAS).[26] Beneath the platysma are several important anatomic structures including the deglutition muscles, larynx, and neck flexors.[22,26] Treatment in this area is considered generally safe, but it is important to be aware of the risks of botulinum toxin diffusion which can result in neck weakness and dysphagia.[4,5,22] Most authors recommend dosing not exceed 75 to 100 units of onabotA into the neck; however, case reports do exist with adverse events seen even at lower doses.[22,39] Individuals in occupations that require strong neck musculature such as musicians or athletes and patients already prone to breathing or swallowing difficulties would not be good candidates for the procedure.[22]

If platysmal bands are the main focus of treatment, then typical starting doses of 30 to 60 units divided among multiple injection points are required.[25] Platysmal banding is best appreciated when the patient is asked to grimace. Many patients will have two larger distinct bands near the midline neck, while others have multiple smaller bands laterally. Larger bands are more easily treated by grasping the band between the thumb and pointer finger. While lifting the band away from deeper structures, injections of 2 to 5 units are placed superficially into the band. Commonly three injection sites are used per band separated by 1 to 2 cm intervals, but individual patient assessment is important.[22]

For the treatment of horizontal superficial neck rhytides, a slightly different approach is recommended. Small 1 to 2 unit aliquots are injected intradermally at approximately 1-cm intervals along each horizontal neck line and then gently massaged.[22] Injections should stay superficial to minimize diffusion to the deeper anatomic structures. A total dose of 15 to 20 units is routinely used per treatment session.[22] Platysmal bands may be treated in the same session; however, extreme caution is recommended when using higher doses. Overall, horizontal lines do not improve as much as the bands do with botulinum injections.

Lastly, a newer botulinum toxin injection technique has been described to further sharpen the jawline. The Nefertiti lift is named after the Egyptian queen, Nefertiti, who is portrayed to have the perfect mandibular contour.[40] Treatments are focused on the platysmal insertions along and underneath the mandible. By weakening the upper posterior platysma fibers, the elevator muscles of the lower face are left unopposed to tighten and lift.[30,40] To implement the Nefertiti lift, injections of 2 to 3 units are placed along the mandible and into the superior aspect of the posterior platysmal bands. In one study, seven injection sites were chosen per side with two placed into a band and five sites along the mandible starting just posterior to the melomental fold and finishing at the mandibular angle. Total doses of 15 to 20 units were utilized per side with only minor adverse events.[40]

▶ TREATMENT OF HYPERHIDROSIS

Hyperhidrosis (HH) affects approximately 5% of the population.[41] Primary focal hyperhidrosis can affect several different body locations including the axilla, palms, soles, inframammary, groin, scalp, and face.[41,42] Sweat reduction and improved quality of life can be achieved with botulinum toxin injection.[41] OnabotA is FDA-approved to treat axillary HH, but all BoNT-A products along with BoNT-B can reduce sweating.[4,5] As previously discussed, the presynaptic release of acetylcholine is blocked by BoNT-A and BoNT-B. This occurs not only at the neuromuscular junction but also at the neuro-eccrine junction.[43]

The key to treating any hyperhidrotic body site is to identify the area involved and to inject the botulinum toxin at the level of the eccrine gland, which is generally found at the dermal-subcutaneous junction.[42] Injections are spaced roughly 1 to 1.5 cm apart, allowing for diffusion of the drug.[42,43] A Luer-lock syringe and a 30 to 31 gauge needle are commonly used. The starch iodine test is a simple colorimetric method to identify the area of sweating (Figure 2.11).[41,42] The intensity of the color does not correlate with severity. It is helpful to document photographically for future reference.

For axillary HH, 100 units onabotA is the FDA-approved dose wherein 50 units are injected into each axilla (Table 2.4).[4,5] Reconstitution with 4 mL of saline per 100 units is recommended, and the authors use preserved saline.[4,5] Injections should be roughly 1.5 cm apart: the number of injections will vary based on the size of the axilla and the area identified by the starch iodine test.[41,42] If the starch iodine test is negative, or is not performed, the hair-bearing area is usually treated. Results typically last around 6 months with some increase in duration of efficacy with repeated injections.[44] If the duration is significantly less, the authors will increase the dose to 100 units per axilla for a total of 200 units.

Nonaxillary HH can be treated off-label with any of the BoNT-A products, although the authors have the most experience using onabotA. Palms and soles will sweat from the entire volar surface; thus, a preinjection starch iodine test is not relevant. However, it can be useful if the patient does not have adequate improvement with injections to identify which areas are still sweating and would benefit from focal retreatment. Pain control is key.[41-43] Nerve blocks can be performed prior to injection, but authors use ice and pressure most commonly (Figure 2.12).[45] Doses range from 100 to 200 units per palm or sole based on the size (Table 2.4).[41,43] Injections are placed every 1 cm for best results.[41,43] The thenar eminence needs to be injected very superficially to help reduce muscle affect and potential thumb weakness.[43] Complications include pain, bruising, and muscle weakness, especially of the finger-thumb which can last for a few weeks to months.[41,43]

FIGURE 2.11   Step-by-step instructions to perform the starch iodine test. This same process can be used in any treatment area.

Starch Iodine Test Overview

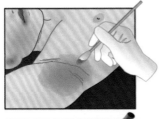

1. Clean and dry the axilla thoroughly and completely.
2. Paint the entire underarm area with an iodine solution or povidone-iodine, or with premoistened Betadine® swabs or swabsticks.

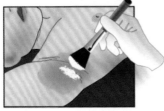

3. Evenly dust site with fine starch powder using sifter, guaze pad, or makeup brush. Wipe off any excess.

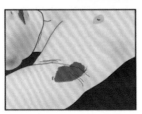

4. Wait several minutes (10-15 minutes). Presence of sweat will cause mixture to turn dark blue-purple color, making location of sweat discernible.

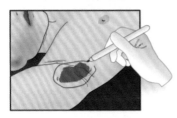

5. With marker, mark/identify regions of the sweating area with center points that are 1.5 cm apart. Do this in a zigzag or staggered pattern. You will have a grid.

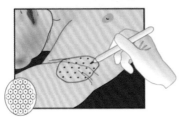

6. With marker, outline areas of excessive sweating. May be a circle, oval, or "islands". Wipe off excess starch and iodine solution.

© 2020 Albert Ganss for the International Hyperhidrosis Society

Illustration by Albert Ganss for the International Hyperhidrosis Society (www.SweatHelp.org). Used with permission.

Craniofacial sweating is another area commonly treated with botulinum toxin.[42] It is helpful to get the patient to identify where the sweating starts since the sweat will eventually spread throughout the scalp and face. The most common patterns seen by the authors are forehead (usually includes frontal scalp and temples), ophiasis pattern (usually includes the forehead), or a more global sweating. Dosing varies by location (Table 2.4). When treating the forehead, superficial injections will help to reduce muscular affect. Regardless, decreased and or asymmetric frontalis movement is possible with resulting brow ptosis.[42] Gustatory sweating or Frey syndrome responds very well to botulinum

TABLE 2.4   Areas of Hyperhidrosis Treated With Botulinum Toxins

Area of Treatment	OnabotulinumtoxinA Dose per Side (Units)	AbobotulinumtoxinA Dose per Side (Units)	Pain Control	Unique Considerations
Axilla	50[a]	150	Not usually necessary	Shaving not needed
Palms	100-150	300-450	Ice Vibration Nerve block	Inject every 1 cm Thumb pincer weakness
Soles	150-200	450-600	Ice Vibration Nerve block	Inject every 1 cm Depth varies with stratum corneum thickness
Forehead/ temples	100 total	300 total	None	Brow ptosis Asymmetric forehead movement
Forehead/ temples + ophiasis pattern	200 total	600 total	None	Inject 4-6 cm width in ophiasis pattern
Global scalp	300 total	900 total	None	Inject every 2 cm
Face such as nose, upper lip, cheeks	Variable 1-2 per cm	Variable 2-6 per cm	Topical anesthetic if needed	Underlying facial musculature and potential weakness
Inframammary	100-150	250-400	None	Inject superior and inferior to crease
Inguinal	100	250-300	Topical	Inject 4-6 cm lateral to crease and 2-3 cm medial to crease
Buttocks	Variable	Variable	Topical	Avoid perirectal

FDA, Food and Drug Administration; HH, hyperhidrosis; onabotA, onabotulinumtoxinA.
[a]Only FDA-approved HH indication is for onabotA into the axillae with 50 units injected per side.

toxin therapy.[42,46] A starch iodine test is performed to help determine the area affected and to calculate the necessary number of units. The entire cheek should be painted with iodine and dusted with starch prior to having the patient eat a food most likely to induce sweating.[42] The area of sweating can range from a few centimeters to >50 cm^2. The authors use approximately 2.5 units of onabotA or an equivalent, injected every 1 to 2 cm superficially to avoid underlying facial muscle affect. The duration of benefit can vary from 6 months up to 3 years.[42]

For other body areas such as the groin, inframammary, lower back, and buttocks, the starch iodine test is very helpful to outline where to inject and how many units will likely be needed (Table 2.4).[42] The authors use an average of 2.5 units every 1.5 cm. If the starch iodine test is negative, we will use around 200 units of onabotA or an equivalent for the

FIGURE 2.12   Use of ice to control pain during botulinum toxin injections for palmar hyperhidrosis. The ice is applied with pressure and is advanced ahead of each injection.

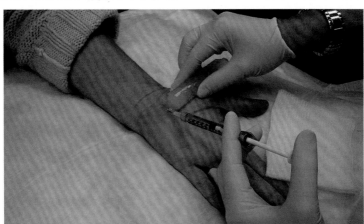

bilateral groin. Injections are performed 4 to 6 cm lateral to the inguinal crease and 2 to 3 cm medial.[42] Similarly, the skin superior and inferior to the mammary crease is treated, and doses vary based on the starch iodine test findings, but typically 200 to 300 units onabot or an equivalent are divided between the right and left sides.[42] Buttock sweating may be the most variable in our practice and usually involves the intergluteal cleft. A starch iodine test is particularly helpful and will require an assistant to hold the buttocks apart during the application and drying of the iodine. Rectal incompetence and fecal leakage can occur if the injections are too close to the rectal muscle.[42]

▶ COMPLEXION ENHANCEMENT

The cosmetic toolbox is ever expanding with countless products, devices, and treatment modalities to choose from. Although neuromodulators are an extremely popular treatment tool, they do not address all aspects of facial aging.[28] Soft-tissue fillers and many laser or light-based therapies have been used in combination with neuromodulators to better address volume loss and skin texture abnormalities.[30] The combination of treatment modalities can offer synergistic and longer-lasting improvements that may not be achieved with monotherapy.[22] This is especially true for static rhytides, increased skin laxity, and poor skin complexion.

Optimization of skin complexion aims to decrease sweat and sebaceous gland activity, decrease pore size, and improve skin texture. Several studies have demonstrated the use of diluted neurotoxin with an intradermal microdroplet delivery technique to achieve an enhanced skin complexion.[47-49] Injections into the intradermal plane, where the muscle fibers attach to the undersurface of the dermis, allow for superficial muscle fiber weakening without complete paralysis producing subtle skin tightening. Atrophy of the sebaceous and sweat glands is also seen with intradermal injections resulting in smoother, cleaner skin texture.[47]

Microtox is a term coined for the microdroplet neurotoxin technique. In one study, the toxin was prepared using 20 units of onabotA (0.5 with 2.5 mL per 100 unit vial) and an equivalent volume of lidocaine with epinephrine (0.5 mL). Each 1-mL syringe was estimated to deliver 100 to 120 separate injections with 2 to 3 syringes used per treatment session. Injections were placed extremely superficially in the intradermal plane and staggered at approximately 1-cm intervals. The patients were pretreated with a topical anesthetic to reduce pain.[47] Treatments have been implemented in the upper face, midface, lower face, and neck, all with promising results and high rates of patient satisfaction. Neurotoxins can be used alone for the microdroplet technique or in combination with hyaluronic acid.[49]

❱ COMPLICATIONS

Neurotoxins have consistently proven to be safe in-office procedures with extremely low complication rates.[22,25,30] Fortunately, most complications can be avoided with appropriate patient selection, proper injection technique, and a sound understanding of anatomy. Generally speaking, most adverse events are considered mild and transient with a continually declining incidence.[30] Many patient concerns pertain to treatment efficacy such as persistent muscle action, sweating, or rhytides and thus are not true complications.[25] Consultation prior to the procedure can help set expectations and provides an opportunity to review intended and unintended outcomes. Pretreatment photographs at rest and in motion are critical so that any subjective adverse events can be compared to baseline (Figure 2.13).[22,25] For example, many facial asymmetries are present at baseline but only noticed by the patient after neurotoxin injections.

Common side effects of neurotoxins include injection site discomfort, erythema, bruising, and temporary headaches.[22,25,30,31] As previously discussed, several techniques can be utilized before and during the procedure to minimize pain and bruising. If bruising does occur, use of a pulsed dye laser can accelerate recovery.[50]

Each treatment area is also associated with its own unique risks, many of which have been reviewed within the preceding sections. Briefly, uncommon side effects of neurotoxins into the upper face include eyelid ptosis, diplopia, brow ptosis, and unnatural or "spock eyebrows.[30,31] Injections into the midface and lower face can rarely lead to lip ptosis, asymmetric smiling, dry mouth, or an incompetent mouth (ie, difficulty chewing,

FIGURE 2.13 Consultation photographs of a woman requesting treatment of her horizontal forehead lines. Photographs obtained at rest (A) and with movement (B). Appreciable asymmetries in eyebrow height and resting eyebrow ptosis are noted along with upper eyelid dermatochalasis. Botulinum toxin injections were not performed in the forehead to minimize further brow ptosis. Instead, injections were placed in the glabella and lateral eyebrows to optimize eyebrow height.

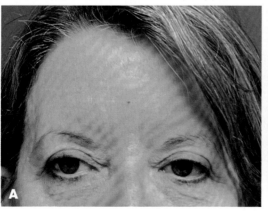
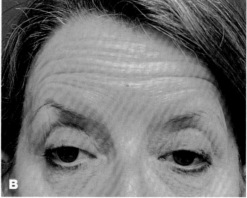

speech difficulty, drooling, etc).[22,30] Treatments in the neck region can infrequently cause neck weakness, dysphagia, or difficulty breathing.[22,30] Again, appropriate dosing and precise injection placement can drastically reduce the risks of these sometimes serious events.

Eyelid ptosis, a rare complication, is most frequently due to levator palpebrae superioris muscle paralysis which occurs from toxin diffusion through the orbital septum. Injection placement at least 1 cm above the orbital rim and medial to the midpupillary line can minimize this risk.[25,30] If eyelid ptosis occurs, watchful waiting is a reasonable option. Some patients prefer treatment which can be implemented with alpha adrenergic eye drops to temporarily stimulate contraction of the Müller muscles of the eyelid.[30] Prescription strength drops are the most effective including apraclonidine or phenylephrine drops. Over-the-counter options such as Naphcon-A® or Lumify® are available, but the authors find them to be slightly less effective.

Finally, although exceedingly rare, serious allergic hypersensitivity reactions have been reported to botulinum toxin and its inactive ingredients.[4,5,8-10,12] If a reaction develops, patients should be treated accordingly and closely monitored under direct medical supervision. Avoidance of any future injections with botulinum toxin products is strongly recommended. Nevertheless, true allergic reactions are extremely rare and most complications are a result of the injector.

▶ ON THE HORIZON

The future of neuromodulators is exciting and rapidly evolving. Current research demonstrates many interesting biological behaviors of botulinum toxins on various cellular processes.[6,7] The expansive mechanisms of action indicates many future applications including roles in scarring, sebum production, and ultraviolet-induced skin pigmentation.[51-53] Additionally, several unique injectable products are coming down the pipeline. DaxibotulinumtoxinA, NivobotulinumtoxinA, LetibotulinumtoxinA, and a new BotulinumtoxinE are among the most promising.[54] As the global expansion of botulinum toxins becomes more pronounced, pharmaceutical companies will be incentivized to develop products with deliberate advantages in order to stay competitive which ultimately leads to alternative options and happier patients.

DaxibotulinumtoxinA (Revance Therapeutics) is a novel BoNT-A in clinical development with the promising potential for more extended durations of action up to 6 months. Two published multicenter, randomized, double-blind, placebo-controlled, phase 3 studies (SAKURA1 and SAKURA2) and one long-term safety study (SAKURA 3) support its efficacy and longer duration of action in the treatment of glabellar lines. The 150-kDa purified protein is devoid of any accessory proteins and formulated with a proprietary stabilizing peptide which allows the lyophilized powder to remain free of human albumin and safely stored at room temperatures prior to reconstitution.[55] A topical gel preparation of daxibotulinumtoxinA was also introduced with initially encouraging results in the treatment of lateral canthal lines; however, the phase 3 trial showed disappointing outcomes, and thus development was discontinued.[56,57]

NivobotulinumtoxinA, brand name Innotox®, is currently available in South Korea and marketed as the world's first liquid injectable BoNT-A. Previously owned by Medytox, the product license has more recently been purchased by Allergan.[58] The 900-kDa protein complex is free of albumin or other animal-derived materials and conveniently packaged in a sterile prefilled syringe. Trials within the United States have not yet been published but a double-blind, randomized, phase 3 study in Korea comparing nivobotulinumtoxinA to onabotA showed similar outcomes in the treatment of glabellar lines.[59] At the time of this writing, Galderma is also undergoing clinical trials for the treatment of glabellar and lateral canthal lines with a proprietary liquid toxin formulation that is free of albumin and other animal-based proteins.[60] Liquid formulations offer convenience, increased storage shelf life, and minimize any inconsistencies or contaminants during the reconstitution process. However, the obvious drawback is the inability to change dilutions based on the treatment area or injector preference.

LetibotulinumtoxinA (Hugel), brand name Botulax®, is another BoNT-A currently available in South Korea. The product is developed from a new bacterial strain, CBFC26, and is suggested to have a higher quality level due to additional enzyme-free purification processing steps which remove nucleic acids. Studies in the United States are lacking, but phase 3, double-blind, randomized, clinical trials in Korea have demonstrated noninferiority to onabotA in the treatment of glabellar lines.[61]

Botulinum toxin E shares many similarities to BoNT-A; however, subtle pharmacodynamic differences do exist. Literature suggests a faster onset of action, quicker time to peak activity, and a shorter duration of action compared to BoNT-A.[6] Ipsen manufactured the first and only recombinant botulinum toxin serotype E to make it to clinical trials. A small phase 1, randomized, placebo-controlled study conducted in Europe verified the safety and tolerability of the project when injected into the extensor digitorum brevis of healthy male subjects.[62] Trials for cosmetic indications are not yet underway.

▶ CONCLUSION

Botulinum toxins have revolutionized medicine since their approval in 1989. Injections of these toxins are now effectively utilized as a treatment for a plethora of medical and cosmetic indications. Importantly, these agents are safe, easy to use, minimally invasive, and well tolerated. However, a strong understanding of facial anatomy and an individualized approach is essential to achieve aesthetically pleasing outcomes. As the desire for a more youthful appearance continues to increase, the use of neuromodulators will remain a staple in everyday practice among many specialties. New neurotoxins are continuing to develop with many exciting future applications.

REFERENCES

1. Schantz EJ, Johnson EA. Botulinum toxin: the story of its development for the treatment of human disease. *Perspect Biol Med.* 1997;40(3):317-327.
2. Carruthers JD, Carruthers JA. Treatment of glabellar frown lines with *C. botulinum*-A exotoxin. *J Dermatol Surg Oncol.* 1992;18:17-21.
3. Carruthers A, Kiene K, Carruthers J. Botulinum A exotoxin use in clinical dermatology. *J Am Acad Dermatol.* 1996;34:788-797.
4. Allergan Inc. Botox Cosmetic (OnabotulinumtoxinA) [package insert]. US Food and Drug Administration; 2017. Available at https://www.accessdata.fda.gov/drugsatfda_docs/label/2017/103000s5303lbl.pdf. Accessed December 5, 2019.
5. Allergan Inc. Botox (OnabotulinumtoxinA) [package insert]. US Food and Drug Administration; 2017. Available at https://www.accessdata.fda.gov/drugsatfda_docs/label/2017/103000s5302lbl.pdf. Accessed December 5, 2019.
6. Peck MW, Smith TJ, Anniballi F, et al. Historical perspectives and guidelines for botulinum neurotoxin subtype nomenclature. *Toxins (Basel).* 2017;9(1):38.
7. Huang W, Foster JA, Rogachefsky AS. Pharmacology of botulinum toxin. *J Am Acad Dermatol.* 2000;43:249-259.
8. Ipsen Biopharmaceuticals and Galderma Laboratories. Dysport (AbobotulinumtoxinA) [package insert]. US Food and Drug Administration; 2016. Available at https://www.accessdata.fda.gov/drugsatfda_docs/label/2016/125274s107lbl.pdf. Accessed December 5, 2019.
9. Merz Pharmaceuticals. Xeomin (IncobotulinumtoxinA) [package insert]. US Food and Drug Administration; 2018. Available at https://www.accessdata.fda.gov/drugsatfda_docs/label/2018/125360s073lbl.pdf. Accessed December 5, 2019.
10. Evolus Inc. Jeuveau (PrabotulinumtoxinA-xvfs) [package insert]. US Food and Drug Administration; 2019. Available at https://www.accessdata.fda.gov/drugsatfda_docs/label/2019/761085s000lbl.pdf. Accessed December 5, 2019.
11. Carruthers A, Sadick N, Brandt F, et al. Evolution of facial aesthetic treatment over five or more years: a retrospective cross-sectional analysis of continuous onabotulinumtoxinA treatment. *Dermatol Surg.* 2015;41(6):693-701.

12. Solstice Neurosciences. Myobloc (RimabotulinumtoxinB) [package insert]. US Food and Drug Administration; 2019. Available at https://www.accessdata.fda.gov/drugsatfda_docs/label/2019/103846s5190lbl.pdf. Accessed December 5, 2019.
13. Scaglione F. Conversion ratio between Botox®, Dysport®, and Xeomin® in clinical practice. *Toxins (Basel)*. 2016;8(3):65.
14. Cheon HI, Jung N, Won CH, Kim BJ, Lee YW. Efficacy and safety of prabotulinumtoxin A and onabotulinumtoxin A for crow's feet: a phase 3, multicenter, randomized, double-blind, split-face study. *Dermatol Surg*. 2019;45(12):1610-1619.
15. Rzany BJ, Ascher B, Avelar RL, et al. A multicenter, randomized, double-blind, placebo-controlled, single-dose, phase III, non-inferiority study comparing prabotulinumtoxinA and onabotulinumtoxinA for the treatment of moderate to severe glabellar lines in adult subjects. *Aesthet Surg J*. 2020;40(4):413-429.
16. Bentivoglio AR, Del Grande A, Petracca M, et al. Clinical differences between botulinum neurotoxin type A and B. *Toxicon*. 2015;107(pt A):77-84.
17. Dover JS, Monheit G, Greener M, Pickett A. Botulinum toxin in aesthetic medicine: myths and realities. *Dermatol Surg*. 2018;44(2):249-260.
18. Trindade de Almeida AR, Marques E, de Almeida J, Cunha T, Boraso R. Pilot study comparing the diffusion of two formulations of botulinum toxin type A in patients with forehead hyperhidrosis. *Dermatol Surg*. 2007;33(1 spec no):S37-S43.
19. Hexsel D, Brum C, do Prado DZ, Soirefmann M, et al. Field effect of two commercial preparations of botulinum toxin type A: a prospective,double-blind, randomized clinical trial. *J Am Acad Dermatol*. 2012;67:226-232.
20. Alam M, Dover JS, Arndt KA. Pain associated with injection of botulinum A exotoxin reconstituted using isotonic sodium chloride with and without preservative: a double-blind, randomized controlled trial. *Arch Dermatol*. 2002;138:510-514.
21. Hexsel DM, De Almeida AT, Rutowitsch M, et al. Multicenter, double-blind study of the efficacy of injections with botulinum toxin type A reconstituted up to six consecutive weeks before application. *Dermatol Surg*. 2003;29(5):523-529; discussion 529.
22. Carruthers J, Carruthers A. Aesthetic botulinum A toxin in the mid and lower face and neck. *Dermatol Surg*. 2003;29(5):468-476.
23. Cox SE, Adigun CG. Complications of injectable fillers and neurotoxins. *Dermatol Ther*. 2011;24(6):524-536.
24. Glogau R, Kane M, Beddingfield F, et al. OnabotulinumtoxinA: a meta-analysis of duration of effect in the treatment of glabellar lines. *Dermatol Surg*. 2012;38(11):1794-1803.
25. Carruthers J, Fournier N, Kerscher M, et al. The convergence of medicine and neurotoxins: a focus on botulinum toxin type A and its application in aesthetic medicine – a global, evidence-based botulinum toxin consensus education initiative. Part II: incorporating botulinum toxin into aesthetic clinical practice. *Dermatol Surg*. 2013;39(3 pt 2):510-525.
26. Giordano CN, Matarasso SL, Ozog DM. Injectable and topical neurotoxins in dermatology: basic science, anatomy, and therapeutic agents. *J Am Acad Dermatol*. 2017;76(6):1013-1024.
27. Cook BE Jr, Lucarelli MJ, Lemke BN. Depressor supercilii muscle: anatomy, histology, and cosmetic implications. *Ophthalmic Plast Reconstr Surg*. 2001;17(6):404-411.
28. Cotofana S, Fratila AA, Schenck TL, et al. The anatomy of the aging face: a review. *Facial Plast Surg*. 2016;32(3):253-260.
29. Costin BR, Wyszynski PJ, Rubinstein TJ, et al. Frontalis muscle asymmetry and lateral landmarks. *Ophthalmic Plast Reconstr Surg*. 2016;32(1):65-68.
30. Giordano CN, Matarasso SL, Ozog DM. Injectable and topical neurotoxins in dermatology: indications, adverse events, and controversies. *J Am Acad Dermatol*. 2017;76(6):1027-1042.
31. Monheit G. Neurotoxins: current concepts in cosmetic use on the face and neck–upper face (glabella, forehead, and crow's feet). *Plast Reconstr Surg*. 2015;136(suppl 5):72S-75S.
32. Flynn TC, Carruthers JA, Carruthers JA. Botulinum-A toxin treatment of the lower eyelid improves infraorbital rhytides and widens the eye. *Dermatol Surg*. 2001;27(8):703-708.
33. Ahn MS, Catten M, Maas CS. Temporal brow lift using botulinum toxin A. *Plast Reconstr Surg*. 2000;105(3):1129-1135; discussion 1136-1139.
34. Tamura BM, Odo MY, Chang B, Cucé LC, Flynn TC. Treatment of nasal wrinkles with botulinum toxin. *Dermatol Surg*. 2005;31(3):271-275.
35. Redaelli A. Medical rhinoplasty with hyaluronic acid and botulinum toxin A: a very simple and quite effective technique. *J Cosmet Dermatol*. 2008;7(3):210-220.
36. Mazzuco R, Hexsel D. Gummy smile and botulinum toxin: a new approach based on the gingival exposure area. *J Am Acad Dermatol*. 2010;63(6):1042-1051.
37. Kim NH, Chung JH, Park RH, Park JB. The use of botulinum toxin type A in aesthetic mandibular contouring. *Plast Reconstr Surg*. 2005;115(3):919-930.
38. Peng HP, Peng JH. Complications of botulinum toxin injection for masseter hypertrophy: incidence rate from 2036 treatments and summary of causes and preventions. *J Cosmet Dermatol*. 2018;17(1):33-38.
39. Obagi S, Golubets K. Mild to moderate dysphagia following very low-dose abobotulinumtoxin A for platysmal bands. *J Drugs Dermatol*. 2017;16(9):929-930.
40. Levy PM. The 'Nefertiti lift': a new technique for specific re-contouring of the jawline. *J Cosmet Laser Ther*. 2007;9(4):249-252.
41. Nawrocki S, Cha J. Botulinum toxin: pharmacology and injectable administration for the treatment of primary hyperhidrosis. *J Am Acad Dermatol*. 2020;82(4):969-979.
42. Glaser DA, Galperin TA. Botulinum toxin for hyperhidrosis of areas other than the axillae and palms/soles. *Dermatol Clin*. 2014;32:517-525.

43. Solomon BA, Hayman R. Botulinum toxin type A therapy for palmar and digital hyperhidrosis. *J Am Acad Dermatol.* 2000;42:1026-1029.

44. Lecouflet M, Leux C, Fenot M, Celerier P, Maillard H. Duration of efficacy increases with the repetition of botulinum toxin A injections in primary axillary hyperhidrosis: a study in 83 patients. *J Am Acad Dermatol.* 2013;69:960-964.

45. Kang A, Burns E, Glaser DA. Botulinum toxin A for palmar hyperhidrosis: associated pain, duration, and reasons for discontinuation of therapy. *Dermatol Surg.* 2015;41:297-298.

46. Tugnoli V, Marchese Ragona R, Eleopra R, et al. The role of gustatory flushing in Frey's syndrome and its treatment with botulinum toxin type A. *Clin Autonom Res.* 2002;12:174-178.

47. Wu WT. Microbotox of the lower face and neck: evolution of a personal technique and its clinical effects. *Plast Reconstr Surg.* 2015;136(suppl 5):92S-100S.

48. Cao Y, Yang JP, Zhu XG, et al. A comparative in vivo study on three treatment approaches to applying topical botulinum toxin A for crow's feet. *Biomed Res Int.* 2018;2018:6235742.

49. Kim J. Clinical effects on skin texture and hydration of the face using microbotox and microhyaluronicacid. *Plast Reconstr Surg Glob Open.* 2018;6(11):e1935.

50. Mayo TT, Khan F, Hunt C, Fleming K, Markus R. Comparative study on bruise reduction treatments after bruise induction using the pulsed dye laser. *Dermatol Surg.* 2013;39(10):1459-1464.

51. Jung JA, Kim BJ, Kim MS, et al. Protective effect of botulinum toxin against ultraviolet-induced skin pigmentation. *Plast Reconstr Surg.* 2019;144(2):347-356.

52. Sayed KS, Hegazy R, Gawdat HI, et al. The efficacy of intradermal injections of botulinum toxin in the management of enlarged facial pores and seborrhea: a split face-controlled study. *J Dermatolog Treat.* 2020:1-7. [Epub ahead of print]

53. Xiao Z, Qu G. Effects of botulinum toxin type A on collagen deposition in hypertrophic scars. *Molecules.* 2012;17(2):2169-2177.

54. Hanna E, Pon K. Updates on botulinum neurotoxins in dermatology. *Am J Clin Dermatol.* 2020;21(2):157-162. doi:10.1007/s40257-019-00482-2.

55. Bertucci V, Solish N, Kaufman-Janette J, et al. Daxibotulinumtoxin A for injection has a prolonged duration of response in the treatment of glabellar lines: pooled data from two multicenter, randomized, double-blind, placebo-controlled, phase 3 studies (SAKURA 1 and SAKURA 2). *J Am Acad Dermatol.* 2020;82(4):838-845.

56. Glogau R, Blitzer A, Brandt F, et al. Results of a randomized, double-blind, placebo-controlled study to evaluate the efficacy and safety of a botulinum toxin type A topical gel for the treatment of moderate-to-severe lateral canthal lines. *J Drugs Dermatol.* 2012;11(1):38-45.

57. TCampbell,. Why Revance Therapeutics is Crashing 23% Today. Available at https://www.fol.com/investing/2017/04/12/investors-in-veeva-systems-cant-miss-this.aspx. Accessed December 10, 2019.

58. Allergan. *Allergan Highlights Key Growth Drivers for Medical Aesthetics.* PR Newswire: Press Release Distribution, Targeting, Monitoring and Marketing; 2018. Available at https://www.prnewswire.com/news-releases/allergan-highlights-key-growth-drivers-for-medical-aesthetics-300713038.html. Accessed December 10, 2019.

59. Kim JE, Song EJ, Choi GS, et al. The efficacy and safety of liquid-type botulinum toxin type A for the management of moderate to severe glabellar frown lines. *Plast Reconstr Surg.* 2015;135(3):732-41.

60. Galderma. Long-Term Treatment of Moderate to Severe Glabellar Lines and Lateral Canthal Lines (READY-4); 2020. Available at https://clinicaltrials.gov/ct2/show/NCT04225260?term=QM1114&draw=2&rank=1. Accessed February 23, 2020.

61. Kim BJ, Kwon HH, Park SY, et al. Double-blind, randomized non-inferiority trial of a novel botulinum toxin A processed from the strain CBFC26, compared with onabotulinumtoxin A in the treatment of glabellar lines. *J Eur Acad Dermatol Venereol.* 2014;28(12):1761-1767.

62. Pons L, Vilain C, Volteau M, et al. Safety and pharmacodynamics of a novel recombinant botulinum toxin E (rBoNT-E): results of a phase 1 study in healthy male subjects compared with abobotulinumtoxinA (Dysport®). *J Neurol Sci.* 2019;407:116516.

Soft Tissue Augmentation

Samantha L. Schneider, MD, Hema Sundaram, MD, and M. Laurin Council, MD

Chapter Highlights

- Soft tissue augmentation is currently the second most common minimally invasive aesthetic procedure in the United States.
- Numerous soft tissue fillers are commercially available, but the most commonly used products are made of hyaluronic acid.
- Soft tissue augmentation is most commonly performed on the face; other anatomic locations include the dorsal hands and genitalia.
- Common adverse events include edema and ecchymosis. Serious adverse events include vascular occlusion, resulting in tissue necrosis, blindness, and central nervous system sequelae.
- Strong understanding of anatomy and appropriate training of the injector are paramount to prevent complications and maximize aesthetic results.

Aesthetic medicine has continued to grow in the United States and worldwide. Patients are increasingly interested in minimally invasive procedures such as soft tissue augmentation with fillers, which has been shown to improve patients' psychosocial states.[1] In 2011, Americans spent $10.4 billion on elective surgical and nonsurgical procedures,[1] with soft tissue fillers representing the second most common minimally invasive procedure after botulinum toxin.[2] Physician administrations of soft tissue fillers have more than doubled from 1.3 million in 2007 to 2.7 million in 2017,[3] and the number of treatments performed annually has grown by over 300% from 2000 to 2017.[4] All of these statistics demonstrate the importance of fillers in the practice of dermatology.

❱ HISTORY

For almost a century, patients have been interested in soft tissue augmentation. As early as the early 20th century, clinicians were offering fat transplantation for augmentation; however, it was limited in its longevity and was a more invasive procedure compared to the soft tissue fillers that we have today. These limitations encouraged research into other options for tissue augmentation, which led to the utilization of liquid injectable silicone products in the 1950s.[5] With the early liquid injectable silicone products, there were issues with purity and the formation of granulomas, foreign body reactions, and extrusion of the product through the skin.[6] Due to these adverse events, the Food and Drug Administration (FDA) banned the sale of injectable liquid silicone for aesthetic purposes in the 1960s.[5] These issues prompted the search for other injectable products and ultimately the creation of collagen products in the 1970s.[6] The first collagen injectable was bovine collagen; however, it only had short-lived results. Additionally, skin testing was required prior to use of bovine collagen fillers to identify those at risk for allergic reactions. These concerns led to the development of additional soft tissue fillers, including some hyaluronic fillers, in the 1990s and early 2000s.[6]

▶ RHEOLOGY AND BIOPHYSICAL PROPERTIES

In order to choose the appropriate soft tissue filler products to address a particular patient's needs, it is important to understand the products' physical properties. Rheology is the study of how materials react and deform under mechanical stress, which ultimately helps physicians understand the rationale for the behavior of certain soft tissue fillers.[7] These include many of the fillers available for aesthetic use today, particularly hyaluronic acid (HA) and calcium hydroxylapatite (CaHA). There are four main parameters to consider—G′, Viscosity, G*, and tanδ, as well as a product's cohesivity.

G′ (elastic modulus) is a measurement of the product's elastic properties, which quantifies the ability of the filler to recover its initial shape when faced with applied force.[7] Another way to explain G′ is that it represents the fillers' ability to resist deformation once placed within the skin.[8] G′ is typically related to the amount of hyaluronic acid cross-linking present in a product, with more cross-linking leading to a higher G′ value.[9] Higher G′ products aid in lifting and volumizing and are particularly useful for subcutaneous implantation in areas with higher levels of muscular activity as they are more effective at resisting deformation.[10,11] Higher G′ products can be of value in areas such as the nasolabial folds, upper cheeks, nasal dorsum, and chin where these products provide outward projection.[12] Soft fillers, with lower G′, are less resistant to deformation and may provide a softer feel in thinner-skinned, mobile areas such as tear troughs and lips.[12] G″ (viscous modulus) is a measurement of a filler's viscosity.[10] Viscosity, which can also be measured as complex viscosity, determines how spreadable the product will be in the tissue, as well as its resistance to flow (extrusion force) during the injection. Higher viscosity products stay localized to the site of injection, whereas lower viscosity products are more likely to spread.[9,10] G* (complex modulus) measures viscoelasticity of the filler product. It is a measure of how much applied energy is stored versus how much is dissipated.[13] Fillers with higher G* represent harder fillers, which should be injected more deeply.[13] Tanδ is the ratio of a product's viscosity to its elasticity, which describes the filler's balance between fluidity (related to viscosity) and elasticity.[13] Finally, cohesivity describes the ability of the solid and fluid phases of the filler gel to remain together.[14,15] For hyaluronic acid fillers, the affinity between the solid and fluid phases may contribute to three-dimensional tissue expansion rather than outward tissue projection alone.[12] Keeping these concepts in mind can allow the physician to select the most appropriate product for a given injection location and patient goal.

▶ FILLERS

There are many options available on the market today for soft tissue augmentation including hyaluronic acid, poly-L-lactic acid (PLLA), CaHA, and permanent fillers including poly-methymethacrylate (PMMA). Table 3.1 provides a comprehensive overview of products available on the US market and their FDA indications.[16-19]

TABLE 3.1 Commercially Available Fillers in the United States

Trade Name	Company	Year of FDA Approval	Composition	Anesthetic	Cross-Linking	US FDA Aesthetic Indications
Bellafill® (previously known as Artefill)	Suneva Medical, Inc.	2015 (2006)	20% PMMA microspheres, 3.5% bovine collagen	0.3% Lidocaine	N/A	[a]Correction of nasolabial folds and moderate to severe, atrophic, distensible facial acne scars on the cheek
Belotero Balance®	Merz Pharmaceuticals	2011	22.5 mg/mL HA	None	BDDE-crosslinked cohesive polydensified HA	[a]Injection into facial tissue to smooth wrinkles and folds, especially around nose and mouth (e.g., nasolabial folds)
Juvéderm® Ultra™	Allergan	2006	24 mg/mL HA	None	BDDE-crosslinked Hylacross HA	[a]Moderate to severe facial wrinkles and folds
Juvéderm® Ultra Plus™	Allergan	2006	24 mg/mL HA	None	BDDE-crosslinked Hylacross HA	[a]Moderate to severe facial wrinkles and folds
Juvéderm® Ultra Plus XC™	Allergan	2010	24 mg/mL HA	0.3% Lidocaine	BDDE-crosslinked Hylacross HA	[a]Moderate to severe facial wrinkles and folds
Juvéderm® Ultra XC™	Allergan	2010	24 mg/mL HA	0.3% Lidocaine	BDDE-crosslinked Hylacross HA	[a]Moderate to severe facial wrinkles and folds
Juvéderm® Volbella XC™	Allergan	2016	15 mg/mL HA	0.3% Lidocaine	BDDE-crosslinked Vycross HA	[a]Lip augmentation [a]Perioral rhytids
Juvéderm® Vollure XC™	Allergan	2017	17.5 mg/mL HA	0.3% Lidocaine	BDDE-crosslinked Vycross HA	[a]Injection into mid to deep dermis for moderate to severe facial wrinkles and folds (i.e., NLF)
Juvéderm® Voluma™ XC	Allergan	2013	20 mg/mL HA	0.3% Lidocaine	BDDE-crosslinked Vycross HA	[a]Deep (subcutaneous and/or supraperiosteal) injection for cheek augmentation for age-related volume deficit in the midface
Radiesse®	Merz Pharmaceuticals	2006 (Approval in 2015 for hands)	Calcium hydroxylapatite	None	N/A	[a]Subdermal injection for moderate to severe facial wrinkles and folds (e.g., NLF) [a]Lipoatrophy in HIV-positive patients
Radiesse® (+)	Merz Pharmaceuticals	2015	Calcium hydroxylapatite	0.3% lidocaine	N/A	[a]Dorsal hands

Continued

TABLE 3.1   Commercially Available Fillers in the United States   (Continued)

Trade Name	Company	Year of FDA Approval	Composition	Anesthetic	Cross-Linking	US FDA Aesthetic Indications
Restylane®	Galderma Laboratories, L.P.	2011 (2003)	20 mg/mL HA	None	BDDE-crosslinked NASHA	[a]Lip augmentation
Restylane-L®	Galderma Laboratories, L.P.	2012	20 mg/mL HA	0.3% Lidocaine	BDDE-crcsslinked NASHA	[a]Injection into mid to deep dermis for moderate to severe facial wrinkles/folds (i.e., NLF) [a]Lip augmentation
Resty ane® Defyne	Galderma Laboratories, L.P.	2016	20 mg/mL HA	3mg/mL lidocaine	BDDE-crosslinked XpresHAn HA	[a]Injection into mid to deep dermis for moderate to severe deep facial wrinkles and folds (e.g., NLF)
Restylane® Lyft with l docaine (previously known as Perlane)	Galderma Laboratories, L.P.	2018	20 mg/mL HA	0.3% Lidocaine	BDDE-crosslinked NASHA	[a]Injection into deep dermis to superficial subcutis for moderate to severe facial folds and wrinkles (i.e., NLF), subcutaneous to supraperiosteal implantation for cheek augmentation and correction of age-related midface contour deficiencies in patients [a]Injection into subcutaneous plane of dorsal hand to correct volume deficit
Restylane® Refyne	Galderma Laboratories, L.P.	2016	20 mg/mL HA	3mg/mL lidocaine	BDDE-crosslinked XpresHAn HA	[a]Injection into mid to deep dermis for moderate to severe facial wrinkles and folds (e.g., NLF)
Restylane® Silk	Galderma Laboratories, L.P.	2014	20 mg/mL HA	0.3% Lidocaine	BDDE-crosslinked NASHA	[a]Lip augmentation [a]Dermal implantation for perioral rhytids
Restylane® Kysse	Galderma Laboratories, L.P.	2020	20 mg/mL HA	3mg/mL lidocaine	BDDE-crosslinked XpresHAn HA	[a]Lips and perioral rhytids in adults over 21 years of age

Product	Manufacturer	Year	Concentration	Lidocaine	Crosslinker	Indications
RHA2®	Teoxane SA/Revance Therapeutics	2017	23 mg/g	0.3% Lidocaine	BDDE-crosslinked Resilient HA	[a]Mid to deep dermis or correction of moderate to severe dynamic facial wrinkles and folds, such as nasolabial folds
RHA3®	Teoxane SA/Revance Therapeutics	2017	23 mg/g	0.3% Lidocaine	BDDE-crosslinked Resilient HA	[a]Mid to deep dermis for correction of moderate to severe dynamic facial wrinkles and folds, such as nasolabial folds
RHA4®	Teoxane SA/Revance Therapeutics	2017	23 mg/g	0.3% Lidocaine	BDDE-crosslinked Resilient HA	[a]Deep dermis to superficial tissue for correction of moderate to severe dynamic facial wrinkles and folds, such as nasolabial folds
Revanesse Versa	Prollenium Medical Techologies	2017	22-28 mg/mL	None	BDDE-crosslinked	[a]Injection into the mid to deep dermis for correction of moderate to severe facial wrinkles and folds, such as nasolabial folds
Revanesse Versa (+)	Prollenium Medical Techologies	2018	22-28 mg/mL	0.3% Lidocaine	BDDE-crosslinked	
Sculptra® Aesthetic	Galderma Laboratories, L.P.	2009 (2004 approval as Sculptra for HIV lipoatrophy)	367.5 mg PLLA (per vial)	None	N/A	[a]Shallow to deep contour modification for facial wrinkles [a]Lipoatrophy in HIV-positive patients

BDDE, 1,4-butanediol diglycidyl ether; HA, hyaluronic acid; NASHA, Nonanimal stabilized hyaluronic acid; NLF, nasolabial fold; PLLA, poly-L-lactic acid.
[a]All are US FDA-approved for patients > 21 years of age.

Hyaluronic Acid

Hyaluronic acid (HA) products were first approved for use in the United States in 2003.[6] Glycosaminoglycans occur naturally in the body to provide scaffolding and volume. With age and increasing exposure to ultraviolet radiation, a patient's natural HA decreases. There is also loss of all hard and soft tissues, including fat, prompting clinicians to supplement with soft tissue facial fillers.[20] A patient's decreasing facial volume due to loss of bone, fat, and other subcutaneous and cutaneous components results in the accentuation of facial lines and hollows.

HA fillers restore volume themselves and can potentially upregulate synthesis of new collagen and elastin. Volumizing with HA fillers predominantly relies upon their intrinsic ability for hygroscopic uptake of up to 1000 times their molecular weight in water, allowing hydration to augment tissue volume.[20] They are polysaccharides composed of alternating residues of monosaccharides D-glucuronic acid and N-acetyl-D-glucosamine.[6,7] *Streptococcal* bacteria fermentation processes are used to develop most HA fillers.[6] Because HA fillers do not have any protein components, typically there is little or no immunologic reaction when they are injected into patients.[20,21]

Non–crosslinked HA has a short half-life of in the skin approximately 1 to 2 days.[20] HA fillers have varying levels of crosslinking to slow their degradation.[20] Several commercially available products use a 1,4-butanediol diglycidyl ether (BDDE) cross-linking agent.[20]

Understanding of the properties of various HA fillers allows the provider to select the most appropriate product for each patient. In order to create the scaffolding network that leads to volume, many products have a combination of low molecular weight and high molecular weight HA. Products with a higher concentration of HA have a stiffer consistency and have been associated with increased duration in the tissue. Higher molecular weight HA allows for greater lift. Less cross-linked products are easier to inject into the patient but may be more quickly degraded, although newer methods of HA manufacture allow a decrease in cross-linking while preserving durability. As previously discussed, HA fillers rely upon hygroscopic water update to create maximal volume. Patient can therefore develop increased volume over the days and weeks following filler injection.[20] This is important to consider during the in-office procedure so as not to overvolumize patients.

HA products are highly versatile and can be used in most anatomic locations. They are highly malleable, and clinicians sometimes mold filler immediately after injection to optimize the appearance and minimize nodules.[20] Softer, less viscous HA products are useful in the lips, tear troughs, and superficial wrinkles, whereas harder, more viscous HA products are injected into areas of deep volume loss such as the cheeks and temples.[7,13] Most HA products are FDA-approved for correction of nasolabial folds. Because of the large variety of products, many providers develop a multifaceted, patient-centric approach where various products are used in layers to provide the best cosmetic outcomes. Using this technique, higher G′, more viscous products are placed deeper for maximal volume achievement, whereas fine lines are addressed with lower G′, less viscous products more superficially.[12] HA lasts anywhere from 6 to 18 months, or longer, depending on the product and the location of implantation.[6,7,22] HA products also have the advantage of being reversible with varying doses of hyaluronidase.[23-26]

Poly-L-Lactic Acid

PLLA was first developed by French chemists in the 1950s[5] and ultimately approved by the FDA in 2004.[6,27] It is a synthetic polymer that comes in powder form and is reconstituted using sterile water 48 to 72 hours before injection. Once injected, the particles settle into the subcutaneous tissue and the water is absorbed by the body.[7,28] The particles in the subcutis are treated as small foreign bodies similar to PMMA, which induces fibrosis and collagenesis.[5-7,28] It is important to keep this in mind as the injections are being performed because the patient will lose some volume initially as the water is resorbed and then will gain more volume over the following several months with collagenesis.[7,28] Techniques to avoid clogging the needle while injecting the PLLA suspension include using a 25-gauge needle or a wider cannula for injection, reconstituting the particles with larger volumes than recommended by the package insert, storage of the reconstituted product for 48 to 72 hours before injection, and thorough remixing of the product suspension just prior to injection.[7,28]

PLLA is injected into the subcutaneous tissue.[7] It was first approved by the FDA for HIV lipoatrophy where it has shown improvement in skin thickness, confidence, self-perception and quality of life, and decreased anxiety and depression.[5,6,29] For the cosmetic patient, PLLA is most frequently used in the cheeks but can be used in other facial areas.[6] After FDA approval for HIV lipoatrophy, the FDA indications of PLLA were expanded to include shallow to deep nasolabial fold rhytids and other facial wrinkles that are amenable to a deep dermal grid pattern of injection.[27] Patients typically require three injections spaced 4 to 8 weeks apart.[5,7,28] The durability of results from PLLA is, on average, 18 to 24 months,[5,6,28,29] though some report durability up to 3 years.[29]

PLLA has the potential side effect of delayed-onset nodules, which is why many clinicians consider this product to be contraindicated in the lips and tear troughs.[5,6] The incidence of nodules has decreased significantly with the use of larger reconstitution volumes, reconstitution 48 to 72 hours ahead of injection, and mixing well prior to injection.[29] In addition, some clinicians recommend that patients massage the injected areas five times daily for 5 days to prevent nodule formation.[5,7,28,30] Other clinicians recommend massage only on the day of injection.[28] No objective evidence exists to support massage as an effective method of preventing nodules.[30]

Calcium Hydroxylapatite

CaHA, a natural component of bone, is now also used as a commercial filler.[5,7] Similar to PMMA and PLLA, CaHA is a 30% concentration of small spherules (approximately 25-45 μm diameter) of synthetic CaHA in a neutral gel matrix composed of sodium carboxymethylcellulose which is resorbed after injection.[6,7] After the gel is resorbed, the microspherules remain in the tissue and stimulate collagen formation.[5,6] Over time, the body breaks down the microspherules into calcium and phosphate, which are excreted by the body.[5,6]

CaHA is injected into the deep subcutaneous tissue,[7] typically with a 27-gauge needle or blunt cannula.[6,31] CaHA is now FDA-approved with and without 0.3% lidocaine for use in patients with HIV lipoatrophy[6,32-34] as well as for moderate to several facial wrinkles and folds (such as the nasolabial folds) that would permit subdermal injection.[33] In 2015, CaHA became the first FDA-approved filler for the dorsal hands.[5,6,33,35] For the cosmetic patient, it can be used for the chin, mandibular line, nasolabial folds, marionette lines and midface as well as for atrophic scars. Mixing CaHA with lidocaine suspension and/or saline, to reduce its G' and viscosity and make it softer and more spreadable, is preferred by some when injecting the hands, face or other areas. CaHA can form subcutaneous nodules and is thus avoided in the lips and tear troughs. Since there has been no reversal agent, nodules have been addressed by saline or lidocaine dispersion or by excision.[5-7,10] Robinson reported in a proof-of-concept study that intralesional sodium thiosulfate, topical sodium metabisulfite under occlusion, or a combination of the two could potentially dissolve CaHA filler in cadaveric porcine skin samples.[36] Rullan et al. applied these concepts to two patient cases and illustrated the utility of intralesional sodium thiosulfate to dissolve CaHA nodules in vivo.[37] The durability of results from CaHA is typically 1 to 2 years depending on the site injected.[5-7,32] CaHA has a radio-opaque appearance on x-ray and CT images because it is composed of a constituent of the bone.[7]

Fat Grafting/Autologous Fillers

Autologous fat grafting has been a choice for soft tissue augmentation since the early 20th century. Fat grafting works on the principle that some of the fat cells harvested from the patient survive the transplantation and become revascularized in the recipient site. It is hypothesized that some of these fat cells are transplanted with pluripotent stem cells that can differentiate into additional fat cells once in place. This technique is most successful when smaller aliquots are injected to improve the chances of the individual cells obtaining a sufficient blood supply. Autologous fat grafting has the advantages of being cost-effective, efficacious for filling larger volume areas, and achieving significant improvement in tissue quality when performed appropriately. However, it requires that patients have fat deposits from which to harvest, as well as their consent to undergo this additional procedure.[6] Fat grafting is appropriate for areas including the nasolabial folds, cheeks, marionette lines, hands, jawline, and chin. It can last up to a year or more depending on the patient, the location treated, and the techniques of harvesting and performing injection.[38]

Permanent Fillers

PMMA is a permanent filler that was FDA-approved in 2006 for soft tissue augmentation.[7] The commercially available preparation is composed of a mixture of 20% PMMA microspheres suspended in 3.5% bovine collagen and 0.3% lidocaine. The microspheres are 30 to 50 μm in diameter.[5-7,39] Because the product is suspended in bovine collagen, skin testing is required at least 4 weeks prior to injection to rule out allergies.[5,6] The test is performed on the forearm and test syringes are provided along with the product. A positive reaction is considered as any degree of erythema, induration, tenderness, or swelling with or without associated pruritus that appears immediately following implantation and persists for more than 24 hours, or appears more than 24 hours following implantation following injection of the allergen. A positive test is a contraindication to using this product. An equivocal response (i.e., no localized skin reaction but possible systemic symptoms such as arthralgias or myalgias) at any point during the 4-week observation period requires an additional test on the opposite arm. Two equivocal tests are also contraindications for using this product.[5] PMMA products have been FDA-approved for use in the nasolabial folds as well as for moderate to severe atrophic facial acne scars. All other indications would be considered off FDA labeling.[5,6,39-41] PMMA is contraindicated for soft tissue augmentation in the lips.[6]

After injection of the product, the bovine collagen is resorbed within a month. The longevity of the product in the tissue results from fibrosis that occurs around the polymer beads. The microspheres of PMMA are too large for macrophage phagocytosis, so they remain in the tissue where they provide a nidus for collagenesis. This process leads to long-lasting or permanent volume augmentation.[5,6] For the best results, patients require two to three treatments spaced 8 to 16 weeks apart.[6]

Non–FDA-approved products for "permanent" or long-lasting soft tissue augmentation include liquid injectable silicone, a heterogeneous group of polymers of the element silicone.[5] Two liquid silicone products on the market are FDA-approved for use in retinal detachment, but not for soft tissue augmentation.[5] Initially, injectable silicone was not a pure product, which was thought to be the reason for granulomas, foreign body reactions, and product expulsion. If silicone is injected, it is recommended to utilize a microinjection technique as opposed to boluses, to minimize these side effects.[6] Additionally, the microdroplet injections are thought to contribute to the permanence of the filler as fibrosis is induced around the droplets of product.[6]

▶ TECHNIQUES FOR INJECTION

Clinicians employ a variety of techniques to place the filler product precisely where it is needed. All injections should be carefully performed with slow even pressure on the plunger to avoid high extrusion forces and bolus deposition. In addition the clinician must consider whether to inject the product in an anterograde or retrograde fashion. These techniques are often combined in the same patient and in the same area to achieve the desired effects.

Anterograde Injection

When a clinician injects the product while advancing the needle in the tissue, this is an anterograde injection. The aim is for the filler product to flow ahead of the needle and dissect through the tissue.[6,16] Advantages of an anterograde injection include a theoretical decrease in the amount of tissue trauma when a needle is used for injection since it is the filler product dissecting through the tissue as opposed to the needle creating a track.[16]

Retrograde Injection

In contrast to anterograde injection, a retrograde injection is when the clinician injects the filler product as the needle or cannula is being withdrawn from the tract that it had created in the tissue. The advantage to this technique is that it allows for more precision in the filler placement. Furthermore, because the filler is injected into a preformed tract, the injection requires less pressure.[16]

Linear Threading

Linear threading describes a method whereby the clinician injector inserts the needle into the skin at an acute angle (i.e., <90°) and advances the needle or cannula laterally underneath the skin. Once the needle or cannula is in place, the clinician can choose to inject the product in an anterograde or retrograde manner. Advantages of linear threading include fewer injection points and more uniform filler delivery. Additionally, because there are fewer insertions into the skin, there can be a lower risk of inadvertent dermal injection.[6,16]

Serial Puncture

As the name implies, serial puncture requires the clinician to perform multiple injection points that each receive a small microbolus of filler. This technique does not rely on any lateral movement of the needle once it is in the tissue. It has the advantages of less trauma as the needle is not traversing the tissue longitudinally. There is also substantial precision in product placement and this is particularly useful for smaller defects.[6,16]

Cross-Hatching

The cross-hatching technique describes the placement of rows of parallel threads of filler followed by a second perpendicular row of parallel threads of filler. This technique is most useful in larger areas and/or areas with deep soft tissue defects such as the cheeks. Often, injections will minimize the trauma to the tissue by fanning the needle as opposed to multiple insertions.[6,16]

Depot Injections

With depot injections, clinicians inject an aliquot of filler deep into the center of a defect. After withdrawal of the needle, the product is molded with the hands into the appropriate shape to achieve the desired outcome. This technique has been used in larger areas with deeper soft tissue defects such as the cheeks. Although the needle insertions are minimized, which limits bruising and pain, the molding of the product can be uncomfortable for patients and can lead to bruising.[6,16] Current thinking emphasizes the avoidance of large bolus injections as this can increase the risk of both nodular and vascular complications.

▶ ANATOMIC CONSIDERATIONS

The cosmetic consultation is paramount when treating a patient with fillers. It is critical to ascertain patients' concerns and the areas that they want to see improved. Preinjection and postinjection photos are also very helpful in demonstrating improvement and outcomes. Additionally, during the consultation, the clinician should keep in mind that multiple products may be necessary to achieve a patient's desired outcome. Injectors may need a higher G′, more viscous product to help with volume loss as well as a lower G′, less viscous product to use on more superficial rhytids. This is important to explain to the patient to manage expectations in terms of outcomes as well as cost.[16]

Upper Face

Soft tissue augmentation of the upper face includes the brow, forehead, and temples. The glabella is considered a higher risk area for vascular complications due to the underlying anatomy; however, understanding facial anatomy and utilizing good injection techniques can allow for meaningful results. At the glabella and in the forehead, the tissue planes from superficial to deep are as follows: epidermis, dermis, subcutaneous tissue, superficial fascia, muscle, subgaleal areolar tissue, periosteum, and bone.[42] The supraorbital neurovascular bundle emerges from the cranium through the supraorbital foramen, which is typically located 2.7 cm from midline, which correlates with the boundary between the medial third and the lateral two-thirds of the superior margin of the orbital bone (Figure 3.1).[42] Additionally, the supratrochlear nerve, a branch of the frontal nerve, is present medial to the supraorbital nerve, typically at 1.7 cm from midline[42] (Figure 3.2). The supraorbital and supratrochlear arteries, which are branches of

FIGURE 3.1   **Vasculature of the face.**

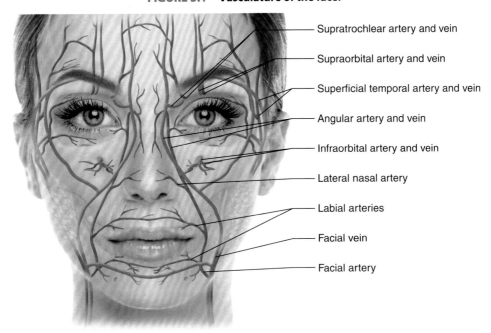

Supratrochlear artery and vein

Supraorbital artery and vein

Superficial temporal artery and vein

Angular artery and vein

Infraorbital artery and vein

Lateral nasal artery

Labial arteries

Facial vein

Facial artery

the ophthalmic artery, both emerge with their paired nerves. Because these vessels are branches of the ophthalmic artery, there is a concern for retrograde flow of a filler embolus if inadvertent intravascular injection were to occur, which could ultimately lead to blindness. Importantly, there is a relatively safe zone located in this region between the periosteum and the galea, which should be the targeted plane when injecting deeply in this area.[20]

Carruthers et al. recommend utilizing three injection points at the glabella and the lateral brows bilaterally. This area is most amenable to soft tissue augmentation using a cannula. The skin is lifted away from the periosteum during the injection to avoid the underlying supratrochlear and supraorbital arteries. The cannula or needle is inserted into the subgaleal glide plane and advanced for retrograde or anterograde injections, with postinjection molding to adjust the product.[43]

When filling the forehead, the suprabrow concavity is one area of interest. This is delineated by the superciliary ridge of the frontal bone inferiorly and the frontal eminence superiorly. Laterally, it can extend to the temple. Because of the underlying anatomy, it is important not to inject too medially so as to avoid the supraorbital nerve. This risk can potentially be decreased by the use of a cannula. It is recommended to stay at least 1 cm lateral to the anticipated location of the supraorbital notch and foramen, which are typically located 2.7 cm from midline.[42,44] This injection is placed deep to the galeal fat pad in all locations except those approaching the supraorbital foramen where the injection should be more superficial in the subcutaneous tissue plane (Figure 3.3).[44] Injections are recommended as retrograde with postinjection massage to mold the product (Figure 3.4).[42,44]

As with the brow, when filling the temple area, tenting the skin can help delineate the correct plane for filler insertion.[44] When considering injections in the temple area, there are three ideal planes to target: on the bone, over the deep temporal fascia, and subcutaneously. These planes avoid the important superficial temporal artery and vein and the

FIGURE 3.2   Facial innervation.

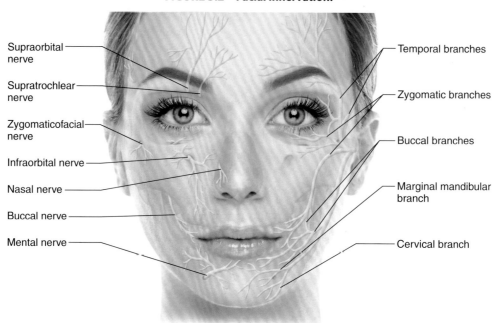

frontal branch of the facial nerve, which run within the temporoparietal fascia. If injecting in the subcutaneous plane or over the deep temporal fascia, a cannula should be used.[20] All injections in the temple should be within a certain boundary. The temporal fusion line, which is located at the lateral tail of the eyebrow, represents the superomedial border. 1.5 cm superior to the zygomatic arch represents the inferior boundary. Injections should remain outside of the orbital rim.[20]

FIGURE 3.3   A 62-year-old woman before (left) and after (right) injection of glabellar and forehead rhytids with 0.9 mL of cohesive polydensified matrix hyaluronic acid filler. Retrograde superficial blanch injection technique into the dermis and hypodermis was used. The pretreatment image shows an elevated resting position of the eyebrows caused by bilateral, partial compensation for age-related upper eyelid ptosis. After treatment, the forehead rhytids are improved, the eyebrows have a more natural resting position, and the eyelid ptosis is not worsened.

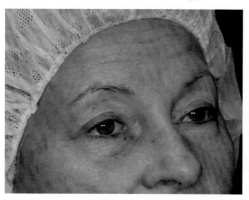
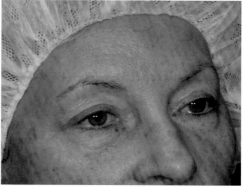

(Courtesy of Hema Sundaram, MD.)

FIGURE 3.4   A 56-year-old woman before (left) and after (right) injection of nasojugal folds and eyebrows with 2 mL of small particle nonanimal stabilized hyaluronic acid (NASHA) filler and midface with 1 mL of high G′, high viscosity large particle hyaluronic acid filler. Retrograde supraperiosteal and subcutaneous injection technique was used. Botulinum toxin type A was also injected to target the lateral and medial brow depressors for brow lifting and the pretarsal orbicularis oculi for eye opening, the lateral canthal region, and the glabella.

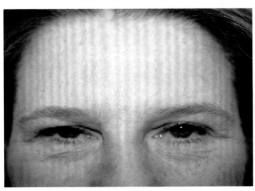 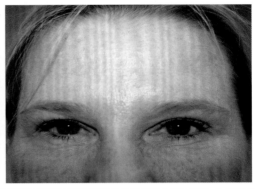

(Courtesy of Hema Sundaram, MD.)

Midface

The midface includes the tear troughs, cheeks, nasolabial folds, and nose. The tear trough deformity can be addressed in thicker, physiologically younger skin with a higher G′ and more viscous product than in thinner, physiologically older skin where there is greater risk of nodules and Tyndall effect (Rayleigh scattering). There are several techniques for addressing volume loss in this area, including linear threading using a cannula. This technique is thought to minimize bruising due to fewer injection points.[16] Serial puncture is another effective technique in this area, with microdroplets of filler deposited in the suborbicularis oculi fat pad.[45] In addition to technique, it is important to consider the patient's morphotype and characteristics. It has been proposed that the best outcomes arise in younger patients with thick skin and an apparent hollow.[45]

The cheeks are a common location for facial fillers. It is important to consider the goals of soft tissue augmentation in this area (Figure 3.5). If the treatment goal is to address volume loss, using a more viscous filler will provide greater contour stability and contribute to volumizing effects of the filler; however, if there are fine lines, the clinician may need to layer a less viscous product on top to address those concerns. Useful techniques in the upper cheeks include cross-hatching, fanning, and/or deep depot injections[16] (Figure 3.6). In addition to volume loss, the cheeks are a common location of acne scarring, which can be amenable to facial fillers. The types of scarring that can be effectively treated with facial fillers include atrophic or rolling acne scars.[6] Serial puncture with small aliquots injected into the reticular dermis and subcutis is a useful technique for treating acne scarring.[16]

The nasolabial folds are a popular area for soft tissue augmentation. Because of the decreased mobility compared with other areas of the face, patients often feel that they have increased product longevity in this location.[6] Useful techniques include linear threading, cross-hatching, or serial puncture[16] (Figures 3.7 and 3.8). Due to the variable subcutaneous course of the angular artery toward the medial canthus, there is a risk of vascular occlusion when injecting in the nasolabial folds.[20] This can result in cutaneous necrosis or blindness and other cerebrovascular sequelae if a filler embolus reaches the central retinal artery.

FIGURE 3.5   Before (A) and after (B) injection of midface and jawline with 4 mL of Vycross hyaluronic acid filler. Retrograde subcutaneous and supraperiosteal injection was performed with a 22G 50 mm cannula (C-E). Filler treatment is often staged to allow sequential tissue integration and to accommodate patients' financial constraints. This patient would benefit from subsequent filler injection to the temples, chin, perioral, and periocular regions.

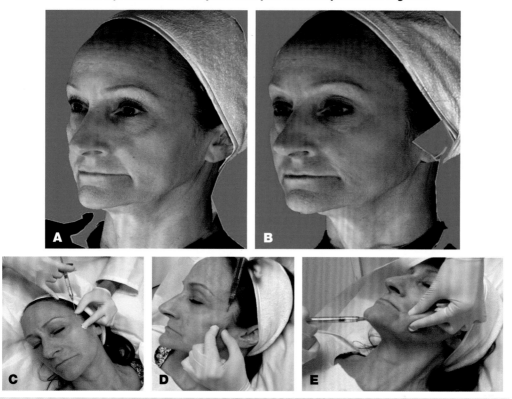

(Courtesy of Hema Sundaram, MD.)

The nose, including the radix, is a high-risk area for filler injection and clinicians should use caution. The thinner skin, numerous vascular anastomoses, and tight tissue compartments may lead to increased risk of complications such as occlusion and cutaneous necrosis in this area. Blindness and/or other cerebrovascular sequelae can also occur. Additionally, patients may report more unsatisfactory results due to visualizing the product under the thinner skin. On the nose, filler has been used to alter the profile and contour and to fill scars.[6]

Lower Face

The lower face includes the lips, chin, marionette lines, and mandibular line. Multiple techniques can be useful to achieve the desired cosmetic outcomes in this area, such as cross-hatching, fanning, and/or deep depot injections[16] (Figure 3.9). To address volume loss around the lips, clinicians should consider treatment of perioral rhytids, overall volume loss, and restoring the white roll at the vermilion border[6] (Figure 3.10). Filling of the marionette lines typically achieves high patient satisfaction[6] and can have long-lasting effects if the appropriate products are selected. For chin projection, fillers of high G′ can be effective in the right patient.[6] As patients age, bone resorption changes the mandibular angle. The profile can be restored using soft tissue filler.[6]

FIGURE 3.6   (A) Before (left) and after (right) injection of midface and chin with 3.6 mL of Vycross hyaluronic acid filler. Retrograde subcutaneous and supraperiosteal injection was performed with a 22G 50 mm cannula to create the effect of narrowing the midface and to increase chin projection. This patient would benefit from subsequent filler injection to the temples, radix, labiomental crease, and nasolabial folds. (B) Same patient in oblique view before (left) and after (right) injection of midface and chin with 3.6 mL of Vycross HA filler. Secondary improvement can be seen in the mandibular line and submental contour due to restoration of tissue support.

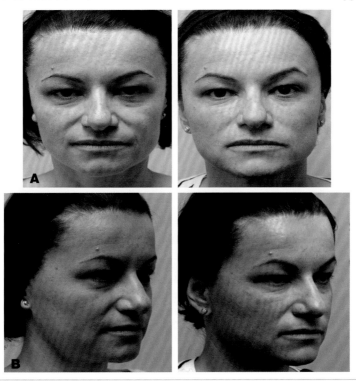

(Courtesy of Hema Sundaram, MD.)

FIGURE 3.7   Before (left) and after (right) injection of midface, nasolabial folds, and oral commissures with 2 mL of two cohesive polydensified matrix hyaluronic acid products indicated for subcutaneous and supraperiosteal injection. Retrograde injection was performed with a 22G 50 mm cannula. There is improved support and secondary improvement of the lips, although they were not injected with filler during this first treatment session. This patient would benefit from subsequent filler injection to the temples, tear troughs, vermilion borders of the lips, and the philtrum.

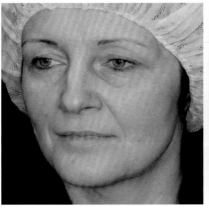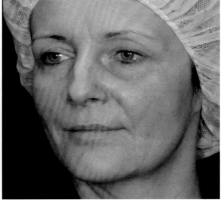

(Courtesy of Hema Sundaram, MD.)

FIGURE 3.8   After subcutaneous injection of the right nasolabial fold, midface, and oral commissure with 1 mL of large particle NASHA and before injection of the left side. Anterograde injection technique was used. This patient would benefit from subsequent filler injection to the chin, labiomental crease, and preauricular region.

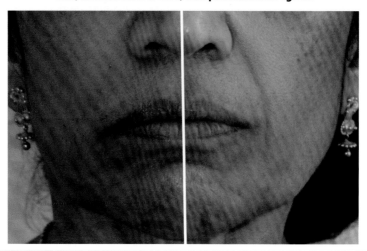

(Courtesy of Hema Sundaram, MD.)

FIGURE 3.9   (A) After subcutaneous injection of the right midface, nasolabial fold, preauricular region, and lower face with 1.5 mL of calcium hydroxylapatite injected subcutaneously and supraperiosteally, and 1 mL of cohesive polydensified matrix hyaluronic acid injected intradermally. Before treatment of the left side. Retrograde injection technique was used. Before (left) and after (right) bilateral injection with the same fillers. (B) Same patient in oblique view in facial repose before (left) and after (right) bilateral injection of the midface, nasolabial folds, preauricular region, and lower face with 3 mL of calcium hydroxylapatite subcutaneously and supraperiosteally and 2 mL of cohesive polydensified matrix HA injected intradermally. Retrograde injection technique was used. (C) Same patient in oblique view in facial animation before (left) and after (right) bilateral subcutaneous and supraperiosteal injection of the midface, nasolabial folds, preauricular region, and lower face with 3 mL of calcium hydroxylapatite and intradermal injection of 2 mL of cohesive polydensified matrix HA. Retrograde injection technique was used. Layering of fillers addresses multilevel volume loss and creates a natural effect both in repose and in animation.

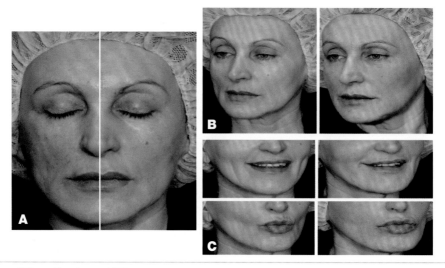

(Courtesy of Hema Sundaram, MD.)

FIGURE 3.10 Before (left) and after (right) intradermal injection of perioral rhytids and philtrum with 1 mL of resilient hyaluronic acid and subcutaneous injection of chin, jawline, and oral commissures with 2 mL of resilient hyaluronic acid.

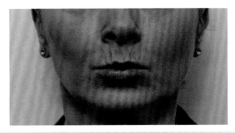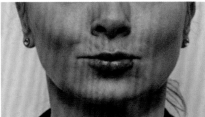

(Courtesy of Hema Sundaram, MD.)

Extrafacial

As the cosmetic interests and needs of patients continue to expand, soft tissue augmentation is evolving beyond the soft tissues of the face to include body areas such as the hands, neck, décolletage, and the genitalia. The dorsal hands appear more skeletal with obvious volume loss as patients age. CaHA was FDA-approved to treat the dorsal hands in 2015, and large particle NASHA followed in 2018.[5] To treat the dorsal hands, clinicians should tent the skin away from the underlying tendons and vasculature and advance the needle between the subcutaneous and superficial fascial layers. Clinicians should remain vigilant about their plane of injection to avoid placing the filler too deeply, which increases the risk of inflammation and swelling. Dispersal of small filler aliquots or threads with a cannula carries a decreased risk of filler displacement to the deeper tissue plane than the previously favored depot injections with massage (Figure 3.11).

Soft tissue augmentation of the male and female genitalia is off FDA labeling. Controlled studies are needed to fully evaluate safety, tolerability, and efficacy. Males tend to seek consultation to increase penile girth, which has been reportedly achieved with injection of soft tissue filler. The product is placed in the fascial layer of the penile body using a cannula and then is molded into place with a roller postinjection.[46] Hyaluronic acid filler is the more common filler choice; however, PMMA has been used in this area and nodules have been reported which are more readily apparent because of the lack of subcutaneous fat on the

FIGURE 3.11 Before (left) and after (right) superficial subcutaneous injection of the dorsal hand with 0.75 mL of calcium hydroxyapatite diluted 1:1 with 0.75 mL 1% lidocaine suspension. Retrograde fanning injection was performed with a 22G 50 mm cannula.

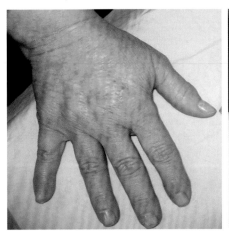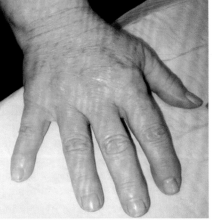

(Courtesy of Hema Sundaram, MD.)

penis to provide camouflage.[47] Patients typically receive 2 to 3 treatment sessions with injections every 6 weeks.[47] Females may have concerns regarding age-related volume loss from the mons pubis and the labia majora, which were previously addressed with fat grafting and now can be treated with HA filler.[48] As when treating the penis, some authors recommended using a cannula to minimize tissue trauma and vascular complications, with retrograde injections into the subcutaneous tissue. One injection point centrally in the mons pubis can treat this area as well as the superior aspect of the bilateral labia majora.[48] To address the posterior labia majora, one injection site per side can be performed at the location of a mediolateral episiotomy and the cannula advanced.[48] Given the potentially devastating risks of inadvertent intravascular injection, one should have a great understanding of anatomy and technique prior to attempting any off-label use of filler products.

▶ SPECIAL CONSIDERATIONS FOR MALES

Facial augmentation in men is gaining in popularity. Aesthetic procedures for the male patient increased 273% from 1997 to 2014, with botulinum toxins and fillers being the most commonly requested procedures.[49] When considering the male aesthetic patient, it is important to keep in mind the sexual dimorphism of male faces in comparison to females. Male faces are squarer in appearance with a broader forehead and flatter brow contour along the orbital rim.[11,49] The male nose ideally should be wide and straight.[49] Male cheeks are fuller anteromedially with wider frontal and zygomatic processes, which gives an overall flatter appearance to the cheeks.[49] Males have an upper lip that projects about 2 mm beyond the lower lip and a squarer lower jaw.[49] Additionally, the vasculature in the male face is more robust making male patients at higher risk for bruising postinjection.[49-52] Male patients have thicker epidermis and dermis compared with female patients, which makes fine rhytids and other manifestations of facial aging less readily apparent.[11,49] The thicker epidermis and dermis are also important to consider when selecting the appropriate product. In order to support the heaver tissue, male patients may require products with higher G'.[11]

The midface is the most common area for soft tissue augmentation in men.[49] Because men have a more even medial to lateral cheek projection,[11] placement of filler is important to optimize cosmetic outcomes. To find the malar eminence in the male patient, the Hinderer method or the Wilkinson method has been recommended. The Hinderer method draws a line from the intersection of the lateral commissure toward the ipsilateral lateral iris and a second line from the ala to the ipsilateral infratragal notch. The malar eminence is at the intersection of these two lines. The Wilkinson method draws a vertical line from the lateral canthus to the edge of the mandible with the malar eminence lying one-third of the way down this line.[11] If utilizing these techniques, care must be taken to avoid lateral overvolumization. Ideally, bony landmarks should be used for volumization techniques, as soft tissues shift with age.

When addressing the temples, the technique is the same as for females. Filling this area augments the brow to give it a more masculine appearance. Safe injection technique includes performing a slow injection in the temple area.[11]

Nasal filler can help create the ideal nose contour in the male patient. Because this is a high-risk injection site, clinicians should inject slowly with small volumes into the periosteal or perichondrial planes. Filler in this area can even out bumps on the nose via injections superiorly and inferiorly to the affected area. Additionally, wider noses can have the appearance of being narrower when filler is placed along the nasal dorsum.[11]

The lower face is a common area of cosmetic concern for the male patient. Chin projection can be corrected with facial fillers. The ideal outcome for chin projection has been described as the Riedel plane, which places the anterior chin projection in proportion with the lip and nasal tip projection.[11] Lateral projection of the jaw has been recommended to be in line with the lateral zygoma, which gives the male patient a squarer face.[11] For both males and females, it is important to note ethnic variations in ideals of facial morphotype and proportions.

▶ COMPLICATIONS OF FILLER INJECTION

The informed consent process for soft tissue augmentation is critical. Although all procedures have perceived risks and benefits, comprehension of the risk-benefit balance is essential for an elective procedure. It is important to disclose all risks to the patient, including rare but potentially serious adverse events. Risks to discuss include facial bruising, redness, swelling, pruritus, and pain as well as nodule formation, filler displacement, infection, and allergic reaction. Patients should be warned about scarring, intravascular injection, cutaneous necrosis, blindness, and stroke.[3,4,6] It is also recommended to disclose to the patient if the product will be used off FDA labeling.[6] Importantly, 10 out of 11 cases of malpractice associated with soft tissue augmentation were found to be associated with inadequate or no informed consent.[3]

When examining adverse events in cosmetic dermatologic procedures as a whole, certain trends emerged. The most common location reported was on the cheeks, followed by the lips, nasolabial folds, and eyelids.[3,53] The most common adverse events reported with filler use were lumps, nodules, and beading.[53] Hyaluronidase was used in 39.1% of reported complications.[3] Several informative publications exist regarding the avoidance and management of filler complications, of which a few are noted in the reference list for this chapter.[54-56]

Transient Sequelae

Transient sequelae of filler injection include injection site reactions, edema, ecchymoses, and pain. Swelling is the most commonly reported complication, encompassing 60.1% of complications. Swelling was significantly associated with HA products, but this is likely due to their greater utilization, in over 95% of filler procedures worldwide.[3] The extent of swelling depends on factors such as the volume of product, the technique used, the location of injection, and sometimes the rheologic properties of the product. To minimize swelling and other adverse events, it is recommended to inject smaller volumes with the plan to touch up any areas as needed in a few weeks.[7]

Ecchymoses occur more commonly in the perioral and periorbital areas due to the higher prevalence of smaller blood vessels.[7] To minimize bruising, cannulas have been recommended as they avoid sharp trauma.[7] Furthermore, vitamin K, arnica, and bromelain may help prevent and treat postinjection ecchymoses, although the data are largely anecdotal.[7,57-61] Using the pulsed dye laser (595 nm) at nonpurpuric settings for any immediate bruising may help expedite its resolution[61,62] treatment is recommended at postprocedure day 2 to 3[61] and even up to 10 days postprocedure.[63] The data on pulsed dye laser for ecchymosis resolution are somewhat mixed.[58,61,63] Narurkar has reported the use of intense pulsed light devices in the amelioration of postprocedure ecchymoses noted at 24 to 48 hours.[64,65] Patients can apply ice or cool packs after filler injections with the aim of minimizing bruising.[6]

Pain is a commonly reported outcome. It was reported as 22.6% of complications in a study examining over 2800 cases.[3] Most filler products, including those containing hyaluronic acid, CaHA, and PMMA, are available premixed with lidocaine to help mitigate the pain of subsequent injections.[7] As mentioned previously, PLLA can be reconstituted with lidocaine without alteration of its basic properties to mitigate discomfort.[31] Clinicians could consider using additional lidocaine to aid in anesthesia, though some recommend against adjacent lidocaine injections to minimize tissue distortion.[7] Other methods of minimizing pain during injection include using ice or cool packs, topical anesthetics (applied 30-60 minutes prior to procedure), vibration devices, regional nerve blocks, small gauge needles, possibly larger cannulas, and auditory distraction.[6,7,66-68] Wider cannulas may actually be less painful than thinner ones because they achieve a more precise tissue dissection and are less likely to bend within the tissue.

Asymmetry

Facial asymmetry is a common complaint of aesthetic patients. Most patients might not realize that they have asymmetry at pretreatment baseline, highlighting the importance of preprocedure photographs and counseling. A full set of standardized photographs is recommended prior to treatment, with photographic views head-on, oblique, and in profile.[6,7] Photography both in facial repose and in animation is recommended. Perfect symmetry can be challenging. It is important to set appropriate expectations with the patient prior to the procedure. If patients are concerned about asymmetry, it has been recommended to wait up to 2 weeks for any edema to resolve before attempting corrections.[7] These authors would recommend waiting up to 4 weeks.

Infections

Although signs of overt infections, such as frank abscesses, have been reported to be uncommon following filler injections, microbial contamination is a major and underdiagnosed cause of inflammatory complications. In a study examining over 2800 cosmetic procedures, infections were reported in 301 cases (representing 10.7% of complications).[3] Patients were prescribed antibiotics in 48.3% of reported complications.[3] The most common anatomic location for an infection is in the cheeks.[3]

Biofilms are presumed to be a cause of inflammatory complications after filler injection.[16] Biofilms are defined as an amalgamation of cells containing microorganisms located within a self-secreted extracellular substance.[69] Interestingly, biofilms, in general, do not elicit an immune response.[69] Within the confines of the polymeric extracellular substance, bacteria of a biofilm are able to avoid antibiotics and the immune system and lie dormant. During this dormancy, the cells within the biofilm in essence shut down and the biofilm enters a "persister" state.[69] This persister state is protective because it tends to cause negative bacterial cultures and it minimizes the effects of antibiotics, which target metabolically active cells.[69] Changes to the environment surrounding the biofilm are thought to contribute to its reactivation, which leads to granulomatous inflammation, abscesses, nodules, and infections.[55,69]

Microbial contamination should be considered as the first cause of any inflammatory nodule following filler injection, as the skin can never be sterilized and hence even filler injections performed with aseptic technique can introduce microbes below the epidermis.

Displacement

In order to minimize the risk of filler displacement, it is important to consider a product's rheologic characteristics in the context of the area to be treated. Patient should be advised against massaging or manipulating the injected areas as this may displace the product. Some practitioners anecdotally advise patients to avoid exercise immediately after treatment to minimize the risk of filler displacement.

Nodules

Soft tissue augmentation with facial fillers requires that clinicians consider the anatomic area to be treated as well as the rheological characteristics of the product to be used. More viscous filler should be placed deeper into the subcutaneous tissue. When injected too superficially (i.e., in the dermis), patients run the risk of developing nodules.[7,16] An additional risk factor for the development of nodules is injection of a larger bolus of product.[7]

Out of 2800 cases studied, nodules represented 33.7% of complications.[3] Fortunately, nodules often improve with massaging the area. They can also be treated with hyaluronidase, excision, radiofrequency devices, or laser, and oral antibiotics.[7,22,30,70] Treatment with steroids is advocated by some, while many recommend that it should be avoided until infection or contamination has been conclusively ruled out. This is because, when treating delayed-onset filler nodules from any product, subclinical infection, contamination, or presumptive biofilm should always be considered as possible etiologies. Oral antibiotics such as macrolides that have anti-inflammatory and multimodal immunomodulatory activities may be of value, as may hyaluronidase—even for non-HA fillers where it may facilitate nodule dispersal within the tissue.[69]

Delayed-onset nodules may be more resistant to treatment with hyaluronidase, requiring multiple treatments of several hundred units each.[7] In over 4700 treatments performed with hyaluronic filler utilizing Vycross technology, 23 patients reported delayed-onset nodules (0.5%).[71] The median time from injection to nodule formation was 4 months and most resolved at about 6 weeks.[71] Interestingly, 9/23 (39%) patients had an identifiable immunologic trigger such as flu-like symptoms or dental procedures.[71] When anecdotally attributing filler complications to any specific product, it should be taken into consideration that the most frequently used products will logically give rise to more reports of complications. Evidence-based comparisons between products with respect to risks of complications require prospective, controlled studies.

True granulomas, which require a histopathological diagnosis, can be treated with intralesional corticosteroids or excision.[6]

In summary, the risk of nodule formation can be decreased by selecting appropriate filler products for the desired tissue plane and performing small volume injections with product dispersal throughout the tissue.

Tyndall Effect

Superficial injection of HA or other translucent fillers can lead to the Tyndall effect, which is a bluish discoloration of the skin due to light scattering by the superficially placed filler product.[6,16,72] This is more likely to occur in areas of thinner skin such as the tear troughs and the perioral lines.[72] The Tyndall effect is more apparent when larger filler aliquots or boluses are deposited in the tissue. To minimize the risk of the Tyndall effect, it is recommended to avoid inappropriately superficial injections, to deposit small amounts of filler, and to select products with lower G' and higher cohesivity.[12,72] Treatment options include hyaluronidase, skin incision and extrusion of the product using a small gauge needle, and tissue massage.[6,72]

Serious Adverse Events

Serious adverse events that have been reported as related to facial fillers include vascular compromise or occlusion resulting in cutaneous necrosis, blindness, and central nervous system (CNS) events. Several anatomic sites put the patient at higher risk of these serious adverse outcomes, including the glabella, forehead, temples, nasolabial folds, and nose.[3,73,74] However, vascular occlusion, necrosis, and ocular sequelae can occur following injection into almost any area on the face.

Inadvertent intravascular injection has been well reported in the literature.[22,53,74-79] In 2015, the FDA issued a safety communication regarding unintentional intravascular injection.[73,80] Inadvertent canalization of an artery can permit filler injection into the vascular system leading to an ischemic or embolic response. It has been shown that intravascular injection can occur with needles and cannulas,[4] although appropriate use of a

22-gauge cannula is considered by many to decrease the risk. Tissue ischemia presents with a violaceous to bluish-gray discoloration with pain out of proportion to examination, followed by skin discoloration and/or erosions.[6,78] In an attempt to prevent intravascular injection, clinicians have recommended drawing back on the plunger to look for a flash of blood; however, due to the viscous nature of filler products and the small-gauge needles used for injection, this can give a false-negative result.[7,75,76] Other suggested methods to prevent intravascular injection include using digital pressure over higher risk areas,[73] minimizing injection pressure, injecting small volumes, using 22G cannulas wherever possible or otherwise small-diameter needles, concomitant epinephrine injection, and use of smaller syringes to lower injection pressure.[4,73,74,76] Injections should stop immediately at any complaint of severe pain.[76]

Recently, high-frequency ultrasonographic imaging has been advocated for use during filler procedures to aid in the avoidance of inadvertent intravascular injection.

Necrosis can result from intravascular injection as well as from tissue compression or injury related to the filler product.[81]

Visual symptoms are a feared adverse event with filler injections. The first case of blindness due to an injection in the scalp was reported in 1963.[76,82] The mechanism of visual compromise has been proposed as inadvertent intravascular injection[73] resulting in retrograde flow of the product into the ophthalmic and/or central retinal arteries, ultimately resulting in microemboli disseminating to the retina.[7,83] There have been a number of cases reported in the literature of partial or complete vision loss, some with concomitant CNS symptoms.[3,4,76] Beleznay et al. identified 48 new cases in the literature from January 2015 through September 2018. High-risk areas for visual compromise include the nasal region (56.3%), glabella (27.1%), forehead (18.8%), and nasolabial folds (14.6%) with hyaluronic acid filler being the most common product employed (81.3%)—a reflection of the fact that the great majority of filler injections worldwide are of hyaluronic acid. Previous studies identified autologous fat as the most common product to result in visual compromise,[4,74,76] which may be related to more traumatic techniques and larger boluses used in the early days of fat grafting. The most common symptoms of visual compromise included vision loss, pain, ophthalmoplegia, and ptosis. About 43.8% of patients had concomitant skin changes and 18.8% of patients also had CNS changes such as stroke-like features or brain infarction on imaging.[4] Ten patients had complete recovery and eight had partial recovery of their vision.[4] It is important to differentiate between vascular visual spastic events and vaso-occlusive/embolic events. Visual spastic events are similar to a migraine or migraine with aura and they resolve spontaneously, whereas vaso-occlusive/embolic events are more severe and often have long-lasting and devastating outcomes.[84]

The retina has been considered as able to survive for only about 90 minutes without adequate blood supply, though some argue as few as 15 minutes can lead to permanent damage.[4,85] As such, clinicians should have an action plan readily available to address any serious adverse outcomes. Retrobulbar hyaluronidase has been proposed as a method of treating blindness due to retinal artery occlusion; however, to date, there are no verifiable reports of high evidence level of blindness that was reversed with this technique.[56,86] Protocols that have been developed include breathing into a paper bag to promote vasodilatation, ocular massage, heparin injections, systemic steroids, and antibiotics.[4,87] Topical timolol has also been advocated. Additional options that ophthalmologists or other specialists could consider include anterior chamber paracentesis, sublingual glyceryl trinitrate, hyperbaric oxygen, direct intravascular or intravenous injection of hyaluronidase with urokinase, intravenous acetazolamide, mannitol, or prostaglandins.[4] The use of nitroglycerin paste is controversial with some recommendations for its application to the area two to three times daily as long as the patient does not develop headaches or light headedness[6,81,88] and other concerns that it may divert blood away from the ischemic area. Patients who suffer severe adverse events such as visual compromise should receive full ophthalmological and neurological evaluations, as there is recent concern that cerebral infarction and other CNS pathology may be more common than previously realized.[89-96] Where appropriate, patients who are not responding well to treatments should be transferred promptly to the emergency room.

Determination of which treatments are effective and which are not is hampered by the fact that the analysis of procedural complications is by nature retrospective and anecdotal.[97]

Protocol to Address Vascular Occlusion via Filler

Every clinician should have protocols in place to address intravascular injection of filler, cutaneous necrosis, and/or visual symptoms. It is critical that office staff are well educated in the signs and symptoms to look for in the event that a patient calls with concerns following filler injections.[7]

To date, there is no evidence-based, accepted standard of care for treating these patients; however, there are expert and consensus recommendations.[4,54] Injections should cease immediately if there are any concerns regarding serious adverse events. If there are visual symptoms, it is ideal to evaluate and document visual changes and confirm the diagnosis prior to any intervention, though this should not significantly delay interventions.[4,96] When considering vascular occlusion with impending skin necrosis, expedient injections of hyaluronidase should be performed at 10 to 20 units per 0.1 mL of HA filler injected up to several hundred units.[20,78,81] The hyaluronidase should be injected at the site of filler placement.[96] Repeated hyaluronidase injections can be performed hourly until resolution.[98]

Currently, it is uncertain whether the kinetics of retrobulbar hyaluronidase injection and subsequent transarterial passage can achieve the necessary local concentration of hyaluronidase and sustain it in order to dissolve a filler embolus in the ophthalmic-retinal artery system.[86,99] For patients with visual symptoms, injection of hyaluronidase can also be attempted at the supraorbital and supratrochlear notches, with the aim of cannulating the arteries and pushing the hyaluronidase retrograde to its required site of action.[4,83,96,100]

▶ CONCLUSIONS

Soft tissue augmentation is a valuable component of the cosmetic armamentarium. There are many different options available to provide optimal choices for particular clinical conditions. Filler products approved by regulatory bodies such as the US FDA are safe and effective at achieving the desired cosmetic outcomes. Injections should be performed by appropriately trained clinicians who have a strong understanding of facial anatomy. Furthermore, injectors should be acutely aware of possible adverse events and have an action plan in place, particularly for vascular occlusion and significant cutaneous necrosis.

REFERENCES

1. Imadojemu S, Sarwer DB, Percec I, et al. Influence of surgical and minimally invasive facial cosmetic procedures on psychosocial outcomes: a systematic review. *JAMA Dermatol.* 2013;149(11):1325-1333.
2. Surgeons ASoP. 2018 Plastic Surgery Statistics Report. https://www.plasticsurgery.org/documents/News/Statistics/2018/cosmetic-procedure-trends-2018.pdf.
3. Beauvais D, Ferneini EM. Complications and litigation associated with injectable facial fillers: a cross-sectional study. *J Oral Maxillofac Surg.* 2020;78(1):133-140.
4. Beleznay K, Carruthers JDA, Humphrey S, Carruthers A, Jones D. Update on avoiding and treating blindness from fillers: a recent review of the world literature. *Aesthet Surg J.* 2019;39(6):662-674.
5. Liu MH, Beynet DP, Gharavi NM. Overview of deep dermal fillers. *Facial Plast Surg.* 2019;35(3):224-229.
6. Alam M, Gladstone H, Kramer EM, et al. ASDS guidelines of care: injectable fillers. *Dermatol Surg.* 2008;34(suppl 1): S115-S148.

7. Alam M, Tung R. Injection technique in neurotoxins and fillers: indications, products, and outcomes. *J Am Acad Dermatol*. 2018;79(3):423-435.

8. Lee W, Hwang SG, Oh W, Kim CY, Lee JL, Yang EJ. Practical guidelines for hyaluronic acid soft-tissue filler use in facial rejuvenation. *Dermatol Surg*. 2020;46(1):41-49.

9. Guy GP, Berkowitz Z, Jones SE, et al. State indoor tanning laws and adolescent indoor tanning. *Am J Public Health*. 2014;104(4):e69-e74. doi:10.2015/AJPH.2013.301850.

10. Sundaram H, Voigts B, Beer K, Meland M. Comparison of the rheological properties of viscosity and elasticity in two categories of soft tissue fillers: calcium hydroxylapatite and hyaluronic acid. *Dermatol Surg*. 2010;36(suppl 3):1859-1865.

11. Rossi AM, Fitzgerald R, Humphrey S. Facial soft tissue augmentation in males: an anatomical and practical approach. *Dermatol Surg*. 2017;43(suppl 2):S131-S139.

12. Sundaram H, Fagien S. Cohesive polydensified matrix hyaluronic acid for fine lines. *Plast Reconstr Surg*. 2015;136(5 suppl):149S-163S.

13. Sundaram H, Cassuto D. Biophysical characteristics of hyaluronic acid soft-tissue fillers and their relevance to aesthetic applications. *Plast Reconstr Surg*. 2013;132(4 suppl 2):5S-21S.

14. Sundaram H, Rohrich RJ, Liew S, et al. Cohesivity of hyaluronic acid fillers: development and clinical implications of a novel assay, pilot validation with a five-point grading scale, and evaluation of six U.S. Food and Drug Administration-approved fillers. *Plast Reconstr Surg*. 2015;136(4):678-686.

15. Edsman KLM, Ohrlund A. Cohesion of hyaluronic acid fillers: correlation between cohesion and other physicochemical properties. *Dermatol Surg*. 2018;44(4):557-562.

16. Alam M, Tung R. Injection technique in neurotoxins and fillers: planning and basic technique. *J Am Acad Dermatol*. 2018;79(3):407-419.

17. Dayan S, Bruce S, Kilmer S, et al. Safety and effectiveness of the hyaluronic acid filler, HYC-24L, for lip and perioral augmentation. *Dermatol Surg*. 2015;41(suppl 1):S293-S301.

18. Vleggaar D, Fitzgerald R, Lorenc ZP, et al. Consensus recommendations on the use of injectable poly-L-lactic acid for facial and nonfacial volumization. *J Drugs Dermatol*. 2014;13(4 suppl):s44-s51.

19. Administration UFD. *Dermal Fillers Approved by the Center for Devices and Radiological Health*; 2018. Available at https://www.fda.gov/medical-devices/cosmetic-devices/dermal-fillers-approved-center-devices-and-radiological-health. Accessed October 9, 2019.

20. Carruthers A, Carruthers J. *Soft Tissue Augmentation*. 4th ed. Philadelphia, PA: Elsevier; 2018.

21. Hamilton RG, Strobos J, Adkinson NF Jr. Immunogenicity studies of cosmetically administered nonanimal-stabilized hyaluronic acid particles. *Dermatol Surg*. 2007;33(suppl 2):S176-S185.

22. Humphrey S, Carruthers J, Carruthers A. Clinical experience with 11,460 mL of a 20-mg/mL, smooth, highly cohesive, viscous hyaluronic acid filler. *Dermatol Surg*. 2015;41(9):1060-1067.

23. *Vitrase* [package insert]. Tampa, FL: Bausch & Lomb Inc; 2014.

24. *Amphadase* [package insert]. Rancho Cucamonga, CA: Amphastar Pharmaceuticals Inc; 2015.

25. *Hylenex* [package insert]. San Diego, CA: Halozyme Therapeutics Inc; 2016.

26. Lambros V. The use of hyaluronidase to reverse the effects of hyaluronic acid filler. *Plast Reconstr Surg*. 2004;114(1):277.

27. Summary of safety and effectiveness data. In: Administration USFaD, ed. *Poly-L-Lactic-Acid*. Available at https://www.accessdata.fda.gov/cdrh_docs/pdf3/p030050b.pdf. Accessed October 9, 2019.

28. Bartus C, William Hanke C, Daro-Kaftan E. A decade of experience with injectable poly-L-lactic acid: a focus on safety. *Dermatol Surg*. 2013;39(5):698-705.

29. Bassichis B, Blick G, Conant M, et al. Injectable poly-L-lactic acid for human immunodeficiency virus-associated facial lipoatrophy: cumulative year 2 interim analysis of an open-label study (FACES). *Dermatol Surg*. 2012;38(7 pt 2):1193-1205.

30. Wu DC, Goldman MP. The efficacy of massage in reducing nodule formation after poly-L-lactic acid administration for facial volume loss: a randomized, evaluator-blinded clinical trial. *Dermatol Surg*. 2016;42(11):1266-1272.

31. Busso M, Voigts R. An investigation of changes in physical properties of injectable calcium hydroxylapatite in a carrier gel when mixed with lidocaine and with lidocaine/epinephrine. *Dermatol Surg*. 2008;34(suppl 1):S16-S23; discussion S24.

32. Alam M, Havey J, Pace N, Pongprutthipan M, Yoo S. Large-particle calcium hydroxylapatite injection for correction of facial wrinkles and depressions. *J Am Acad Dermatol*. 2011;65(1):92-96.

33. Radiesse. In: Administration USFaD, ed. *Poly-L-Lactic-Acid*. Available at https://www.accessdata.fda.gov/cdrh_docs/pdf3/p030050b.pdf. Accessed October 9, 2019.

34. Silvers SL, Eviatar JA, Echavez MI, Pappas AL. Prospective, open-label, 18-month trial of calcium hydroxylapatite (Radiesse) for facial soft-tissue augmentation in patients with human immunodeficiency virus-associated lipoatrophy: one-year durability. *Plast Reconstr Surg*. 2006;118(3 suppl):34S-45S.

35. Alam M, Yoo SS. Technique for calcium hydroxylapatite injection for correction of nasolabial fold depressions. *J Am Acad Dermatol*. 2007;56(2):285-289.

36. Robinson DM. In vitro analysis of the degradation of calcium hydroxylapatite dermal filler: a proof-of-concept study. *Dermatol Surg*. 2018;44(suppl 1):S5-S9.

37. Rullan PP, Olson R, Lee KC. The use of intralesional sodium thiosulfate to dissolve facial nodules from calcium hydroxylapatite. *Dermatol Surg*. 2019.

38. Eremia S, Newman N. Long-term follow-up after autologous fat grafting: analysis of results from 116 patients followed at least 12 months after receiving the last of a minimum of two treatments. *Dermatol Surg.* 2000;26(12):1150-1158.

39. BellaFill instructions for use. In: Administration USFaD, ed. *BellaFill.* Available at https://www.accessdata.fda.gov/cdrh_docs/pdf2/P020012S009c.pdf. Accessed October 9, 2019.

40. Cohen S, Dover J, Monheit G, et al. Five-year safety and satisfaction study of PMMA-collagen in the correction of naso-labial folds. *Dermatol Surg.* 2015;41(suppl 1):S302-S313.

41. Karnik J, Baumann L, Bruce S, et al. A double-blind, randomized, multicenter, controlled trial of suspended polymeth-ylmethacrylate microspheres for the correction of atrophic facial acne scars. *J Am Acad Dermatol.* 2014;71(1):77-83.

42. Sundaram H, Carruthers J. *Glabella/central brown.* In: *Soft Tissue Augmentation.* 3rd ed. Elsevier; 2012.

43. Carruthers J, Carruthers A. Three-dimensional forehead reflation. *Dermatol Surg.* 2015;41(suppl 1):S321-S324.

44. Busso M, Howell DJ. Forehead recontouring using calcium hydroxylapatite. *Dermatol Surg.* 2010;36(suppl 3):1910-1913.

45. Viana GA, Osaki MH, Cariello AJ, Damasceno RW, Osaki TH. Treatment of the tear trough deformity with hyaluronic acid. *Aesthet Surg J.* 2011;31(2):225-231.

46. Kwak TI, Oh M, Kim JJ, Moon du G. The effects of penile girth enhancement using injectable hyaluronic acid gel, a filler. *J Sex Med.* 2011;8(12):3407-3413.

47. Casavantes L, Lemperle G, Morales P. Penile girth enhancement with polymethylmethacrylate-based soft tissue fillers. *J Sex Med.* 2016;13(9):1414-1422.

48. Hexsel D, Dal'Forno T, Caspary P, Hexsel CL. Soft-tissue augmentation with hyaluronic acid filler for labia majora and mons pubis. *Dermatol Surg.* 2016;42(7):911-914.

49. Farhadian JA, Bloom BS, Brauer JA. Male aesthetics: a review of facial anatomy and pertinent clinical implications. *J Drugs Dermatol.* 2015;14(9):1029-1034.

50. Moretti G, Ellis RA, Mescon H. Vascular patterns in the skin of the face. *J Invest Dermatol.* 1959;33:103-112.

51. Mayrovitz HN, Regan MB. Gender differences in facial skin blood perfusion during basal and heated conditions deter-mined by laser Doppler flowmetry. *Microvasc Res.* 1993;45(2):211-218.

52. Baker DC, Stefani WA, Chiu ES. Reducing the incidence of hematoma requiring surgical evacuation following male rhytidectomy: a 30-year review of 985 cases. *Plast Reconstr Surg.* 2005;116(7):1973-1985; discussion 1986-1977.

53. Alam M, Kakar R, Nodzenski M, et al. Multicenter prospective cohort study of the incidence of adverse events associated with cosmetic dermatologic procedures: lasers, energy devices, and injectable neurotoxins and fillers. *JAMA Dermatol.* 2015;151(3):271-277.

54. Signorini M, Liew S, Sundaram H, et al. Global aesthetics consensus: avoidance and management of complications from hyaluronic acid fillers-evidence- and opinion-based review and consensus recommendations. *Plast Reconstr Surg.* 2016;137(6):961e-971e.

55. DeLorenzi C. Complications of injectable fillers, part I. *Aesthet Surg J.* 2013;33(4):561-575.

56. DeLorenzi C. Complications of injectable fillers, part 2: vascular complications. *Aesthet Surg J.* 2014;34(4):584-600.

57. Leu S, Havey J, White LE, et al. Accelerated resolution of laser-induced bruising with topical 20% arnica: a rater-blinded randomized controlled trial. *Br J Dermatol.* 2010;163(3):557-563.

58. Mayo TT, Khan F, Hunt C, Fleming K, Markus R. Comparative study on bruise reduction treatments after bruise induc-tion using the pulsed dye laser. *Dermatol Surg.* 2013;39(10):1459-1464.

59. Cohen JL, Bhatia AC. The role of topical vitamin K oxide gel in the resolution of postprocedural purpura. *J Drugs Dermatol.* 2009;8(11):1020-1024.

60. Ho D, Jagdeo J, Waldorf HA. Is there a role for arnica and bromelain in prevention of post-procedure ecchymosis or edema? A systematic review of the literature. *Dermatol Surg.* 2016;42(4):445-463.

61. Karen JK, Hale EK, Geronemus RG. A simple solution to the common problem of ecchymosis. *Arch Dermatol.* 2010;146(1):94-95.

62. Brauer JA, Geronemus RG. Rapid resolution of post-face lift ecchymoses. *Plast Reconstr Surg.* 2013;132(6):1084e-1085e.

63. DeFatta RJ, Krishna S, Williams EF III. Pulsed-dye laser for treating ecchymoses after facial cosmetic procedures. *Arch Facial Plast Surg.* 2009;11(2):99-103.

64. Narurkar V. Post filler ecchymosis resolution with intense pulsed light. *J Drugs Dermatol.* 2018;17(11):1184-1185.

65. Jeong GJ, Kwon HJ, Park KY, Kim BJ. Pulsed-dye laser as a novel therapeutic approach for post-filler bruises. *Dermatol Ther.* 2018;31(6):e12721.

66. Dixit S, Lowe P, Fischer G, Lim A. Ice anaesthesia in procedural dermatology. *Australas J Dermatol.* 2013;54(4):273-276.

67. Nestor MS, Ablon GR, Stillman MA. The use of a contact cooling device to reduce pain and ecchymosis associated with dermal filler injections. *J Clin Aesthet Dermatol.* 2010;3(3):29-34.

68. Smith KC, Comite SL, Balasubramanian S, Carver A, Liu JF. Vibration anesthesia: a noninvasive method of reducing discomfort prior to dermatologic procedures. *Dermatol Online J.* 2004;10(2):1.

69. Cassuto D, Sundaram H. A problem-oriented approach to nodular complications from hyaluronic acid and calcium hydroxylapatite fillers: classification and recommendations for treatment. *Plast Reconstr Surg.* 2013;132(4 suppl 2):48S-58S.

70. Hong JY, Suh JH, Ko EJ, Im SI, Kim BJ, Kim MN. Chronic, intractable nodules after filler injection successfully treated with a bipolar radiofrequency device. *Dermatol Ther.* 2017;30(1).

71. Beleznay K, Carruthers JD, Carruthers A, Mummert ME, Humphrey S. Delayed-onset nodules secondary to a smooth cohesive 20 mg/mL hyaluronic acid filler: cause and management. *Dermatol Surg.* 2015;41(8):929-939.

72. King M. Management of Tyndall effect. *J Clin Aesthet Dermatol.* 2016;9(11):E6-E8.

73. Rodriguez LM, Martin SJ, Lask G. Targeted digital pressure to potentially minimize intravascular retrograde filler injections. *Dermatol Surg.* 2017;43(2):309-312.

74. Beleznay K, Carruthers JD, Humphrey S, Jones D. Avoiding and treating blindness from fillers: a review of the world literature. *Dermatol Surg.* 2015;41(10):1097-1117.

75. Carey W, Weinkle S. Retraction of the plunger on a syringe of hyaluronic acid before injection: are we safe? *Dermatol Surg.* 2015;41(suppl 1):S340-S346.

76. Carruthers JD, Fagien S, Rohrich RJ, Weinkle S, Carruthers A. Blindness caused by cosmetic filler injection: a review of cause and therapy. *Plast Reconstr Surg.* 2014;134(6):1197-1201.

77. Minkis K, Whittington A, Alam M. Dermatologic surgery emergencies: complications caused by occlusion and blood pressure. *J Am Acad Dermatol.* 2016;75(2):243-262.

78. Hirsch RJ, Cohen JL, Carruthers JD. Successful management of an unusual presentation of impending necrosis following a hyaluronic acid injection embolus and a proposed algorithm for management with hyaluronidase. *Dermatol Surg.* 2007;33(3):357-360.

79. Schanz S, Schippert W, Ulmer A, Rassner G, Fierlbeck G. Arterial embolization caused by injection of hyaluronic acid (Restylane). *Br J Dermatol.* 2002;146(5):928-929.

80. Administration UFD. *Unintentional Injection of Soft Tissue Filler Into Blood Vessels in the Face: FDA Safety Communication - Risk of Serious Patient Injury.* 2015. https://wayback.archive-it.org/7993/20170406123714/https://www.fda.gov/Safety/MedWatch/SafetyInformation/SafetyAlertsforHumanMedicalProducts/ucm448439.htm.

81. Cohen JL, Bicsman BS, Dayan SH, et al. Treatment of hyaluronic acid filler-induced impending necrosis with hyaluronidase: consensus recommendations. *Aesthet Surg J.* 2015;35(7):844-849.

82. von Bahr G. Multiple embolisms in the fundus of an eye after an injection in the scalp. *Acta Ophthalmol (Copenh).* 1963;41:85-91.

83. Goodman GJ, Clague MD. A rethink on hyaluronidase injection, intraarterial injection, and blindness: is there another option for treatment of retinal artery embolism caused by intraarterial injection of hyaluronic acid? *Dermatol Surg.* 2016;42(4):547-549.

84. Fagien S. Commentary on a rethink on hyaluronidase injection, intra-arterial injection and blindness. *Dermatol Surg.* 2016;42(4):549-552.

85. Tobalem S, Schutz JS, Chronopoulos A. Central retinal artery occlusion – rethinking retinal survival time. *BMC Ophthalmol.* 2018;18(1):101.

86. Zhu GZ, Sun ZS, Liao WX, et al. Efficacy of retrobulbar hyaluronidase injection for vision loss resulting from hyaluronic acid filler embolization. *Aesthet Surg J.* 2017;38(1):12-22.

87. Humzah MD, Ataullah S, Chiang C, Malhotra R, Goldberg R. The treatment of hyaluronic acid aesthetic interventional induced visual loss (AIIVL): a consensus on practical guidance. *J Cosmet Dermatol.* 2019;18(1):71-76.

88. Kleydman K, Cohen JL, Marmur E. Nitroglycerin: a review of its use in the treatment of vascular occlusion after soft tissue augmentation. *Dermatol Surg.* 2012;38(12):1889-1897.

89. Sito G, Manzoni V, Sommariva R. Vascular complications after facial filler injection: a literature review and meta-analysis. *J Clin Aesthet Dermatol.* 2019;12(6):E65-E72.

90. Ansari ZA, Choi CJ, Rong AJ, Erickson BP, Tse DT. Ocular and cerebral infarction from periocular filler injection. *Orbit.* 2019;38(4):322-324.

91. Hufschmidt K, Bronsard N, Foissac R, et al. The infraorbital artery: clinical relevance in esthetic medicine and identification of danger zones of the midface. *J Plast Reconstr Aesthet Surg.* 2019;72(1):131-136.

92. Jagdeo J, Hruza G. The Food and Drug administration safety communication on unintentional injection of soft-tissue filler into facial blood vessels: important points and perspectives. *Dermatol Surg.* 2015;41(12):1372-1374.

93. Liu L, Yin M, Liu S, Hu M, Zhang B. Facial filler causes stroke after development of cerebral fat embolism. *Lancet.* 2020;395(10222):449.

94. Lin YC, Chen WC, Liao WC, Hsia TC. Central retinal artery occlusion and brain infarctions after nasal filler injection. *QJM.* 2015;108(9):731-732.

95. He MS, Sheu MM, Huang ZL, Tsai CH, Tsai RK. Sudden bilateral vision loss and brain infarction following cosmetic hyaluronic acid injection. *JAMA Ophthalmol.* 2013;131(9):1234-1235.

96. Goodman GJ, Magnusson MR, Callan P, et al. A consensus on minimizing the risk of hyaluronic acid embolic visual loss and suggestions for immediate bedside management. *Aesthet Surg J.* 2019.

97. Sundaram H, Magnusson M, Papadopoulos T. Filler problems. In: Nahai F, Wojno T, eds. *Problems in Periorbital Surgery.* Stuttgart, Germany: Thieme; 2019:263-286.

98. DeLorenzi C. New high dose pulsed hyaluronidase protocol for hyaluronic acid filler vascular adverse events. *Aesthet Surg J.* 2017;37(7):814-825.

99. Papadopoulos T, Sundaram H, Magnusson M. Transarterial hyaluronidase: development of a pilot, real-time, in vivo model and the implications for treatment of visual loss from hyaluronic acid filler embolization. Paper presented at: Am Soc Aesthet Plast Surg Annual Meeting 2019; New Orleans, LA.

100. Tansatit T, Apinuntrum P, Phetudom T. An anatomic basis for treatment of retinal artery occlusions caused by hyaluronic acid injections: a cadaveric study. *Aesthet Plast Surg.* 2014;38(6):1131-1137.

Laser and Light Devices in Aesthetic Medicine

Jordan V. Wang, MD, MBE, MBA, and Nazanin Saedi, MD

Chapter Highlights

- The use of laser, light, and energy-based devices in aesthetic medicine has grown exponentially in recent years.
- Intense pulsed light is one of the most versatile and widely used devices in aesthetic dermatology, with applications for treatment of photoaging, telangiectasias, hair removal, and a variety of other skin conditions.
- Selective photothermolysis is the process by which laser therapy uses a particular wavelength of energy to target a specific structure within tissue.
- Aesthetic lasers include ablative and nonablative devices, both of which can be fractionated to decrease downtime.
- In addition to laser and light devices, energy devices utilizing radiofrequency, ultrasound, and microwave technologies have aesthetic applications.

The field of aesthetic medicine has continued to grow in recent years, especially as the technology behind laser, light, and energy-based devices has further developed. What were once considered revolutionary and pioneering procedures have evolved to become the mainstays of modern cosmetic treatment. In 2017, members of the American Society for Dermatologic Surgery (ASDS) performed nearly 3.3 million laser, light, and energy-based procedures, which was greatly increased from the 2 million procedures in 2012.[1] With the widespread adoption and routine use of these devices, aesthetic practitioners should be familiar with the technologies that are commonly utilized in the field. This chapter will provide an overview of the laser, light, and energy-based devices commonly used in aesthetic medicine.

▶ BACKGROUND

The use of laser technology in aesthetic medicine dates back to the 1960s when Theodore Maiman developed the first laser for clinical application. Several years later, Dr Leon Goldman demonstrated the use of lasers for several dermatologic applications, including tattoo removal and skin lesion destruction. In the 1980s, Drs R. Rox Anderson and John Parrish published the theory of selective photothermolysis, a process by which a wavelength of a particular energy can be used to selectively target and destroy a particular structure within the skin.[2,3] Since that time, the dermatologic armamentarium has exponentially expanded to include a myriad of laser, light, and energy-based devices with applications for use in aesthetic dermatology.

▶ INTENSE PULSED LIGHT

The intense pulsed light (IPL) device is one of the most commonly used and versatile devices in aesthetic medicine. The IPL technology utilizes a xenon flashlamp to emit an intense, broad-spectrum pulse of visible light, usually in the range of the electromagnetic spectrum of 400 to 1200 nm. Cooling of the epidermis with the contact method, aqueous gel, and/or exogenous forced chilled air is important to protect the overlying epidermis during treatment. In contrast to a laser which emits a single wavelength of energy, IPL can be used to treat numerous skin conditions due to the broad range of wavelengths emitted during therapy. However, this nonselectivity is the very reason why IPL is not typically a perfect treatment for any one specific skin disorder. Since IPL can improve a range of skin complaints, including telangiectasias and dyspigmentation, it is often used to treat cutaneous signs of photodamage (Figure 4.1). Studies have reported about 50% to 75% improvement in both the vascular and pigmented components with a relatively low and tolerable side effect profile.[4] Cutoff filters can also be utilized to target specific structures and chromophores, such as 550- or 560-nm filter for treatment of telangiectasias. Other common uses of IPL include photoepilation, or hair removal, acne vulgaris, rosacea, and melasma. Practitioners must ensure proper overlap of pulses in order to avoid "striping", which can manifest in the presence of untreated skin between the treated areas. Striping can be especially seen with single-pass treatment techniques; using multiple passes that

FIGURE 4.1   (A) Photodamage on the chest treated with one session of intense pulsed light using the 515 nm filter at the following settings: fluency 12 J/cm², pulse width 10 ms, cooling 18°C. (B) 4-wk follow-up. Notice mild "striping" as evident by well-demarcated treatment vs nontreatment areas.

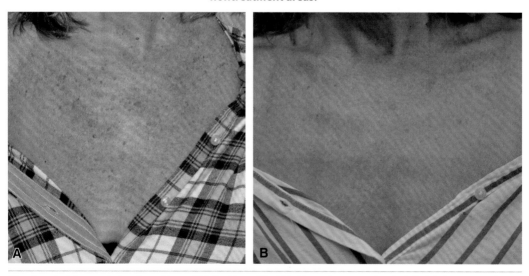

are oriented at different angles can help to ameliorate this risk. Caution should be used in darker skin types or tanned skin, as these patients are more likely to experience cutaneous burns and pigment alterations with IPL therapy. Patient comfort is typically achieved with contact cooling or topical anesthesia alone. For the majority of indications, a series of IPL treatments are needed to achieve the desired outcome. Treatments typically occur at 4 to 6 week intervals until optimal results are achieved, and touch-ups may be needed every few months thereafter.

❯ VASCULAR LESION LASERS

Vascular lesions are common complaints of aesthetic patients. Such concerns can include background erythema, telangiectasias, poikiloderma of Civatte, small leg veins, and port wine stains. Traditionally, the pulsed dye laser (PDL) has been the prototypical laser for these concerns (Figure 4.2). However, other lasers can be used, including the 532-nm potassium titanyl phosphate (KTP) laser, the 755-nm alexandrite laser, and the 1064-nm neodymium:yttrium-aluminum-garnet (Nd:YAG) laser.

The PDL was first developed to treat capillary malformations and port wine stains, but its use has expanded to the treatment of vascular lesions of various etiologies. The initial lasers emitted a 577-nm light; modern devices emit 585 or 595 nm to allow for deeper tissue penetration (up to 1.2 mm). Treatment parameters can be adjusted to elicit specific responses according to the desired posttreatment downtime and clinical efficacy. For example, shorter pulse durations can cause purpura from intravascular coagulation, but may also be more effective for treating lesions. In contrast, longer pulse durations can offer shorter downtime, but may require multiple treatments to achieve the desired clinical outcome. The addition of pulse stacking can also help to improve clinical efficacy.[5] Practitioners must ensure proper overlap of pulses in order to avoid "footprinting", which appears as a honeycomb-like pattern in the presence of untreated skin between the treated circles. Recently, a 585-nm light has been developed with a diode laser, in order to avoid dye kits, and in combination with a scanning handpiece.[6]

The KTP laser was originally created by passing the light of a 1064-nm Nd:YAG laser through a KTP crystal, which doubles the frequency and halves the wavelength.[7] The resultant wavelength is absorbed competitively by melanin, oxyhemoglobin, and tattoo

FIGURE 4.2 Port wine stain before (A) and after (B) multiple treatments with pulsed dye laser.

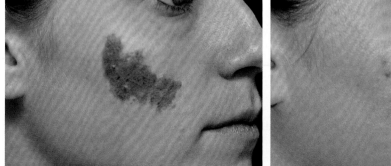
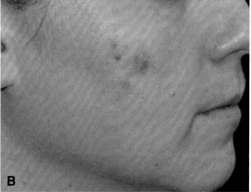

(Reprinted with permission from Chung KC. *Grabb and Smith's Plastic Surgery*. 8th ed. Philadelphia, PA: Wolters Kluwer; 2019.)

pigment. Therefore, postprocedural dyspigmentation can be a side effect, especially when treating skin of color or tanned individuals. For many KTP lasers, a chilled sapphire plate or glass window is utilized in order to provide cooling to the skin surface and to protect from epidermal injury. The small beam diameter often induces fewer side effects than the PDL, including bruising, swelling, pain, and erythema. While long-pulsed PDL was shown to achieve better clearance of facial telangiectasias, patients often preferred multiple treatments with the KTP due to its favorable side effect profile.[8]

The Nd:YAG laser is another laser commonly used to treat vascular lesions, due to its deeper penetration and decreased affinity for melanin. However, the 1064-nm wavelength has significantly less hemoglobin absorption than the PDL and KTP lasers, which makes higher fluences or multiple treatments often necessary. The deeper penetration allows for treatment of larger caliber vessels, which are typically darker in color and anatomically deeper within tissue. Examples of appropriate targets include venous lakes on the lips and perialar telangiectasias. The limited absorption by epidermal melanin makes the Nd:YAG safe in darker skin tones, whereas other wavelengths may result in posttreatment pigment alteration in these individuals. When using higher fluences and longer pulse durations, practitioners must be cautious of the potential for volumetric heating and collateral damage to adjacent tissue. This makes the need for cooling even more important in order to protect the epidermis from thermal injury and scarring and to control patient discomfort.

▶ PIGMENTED LESION LASERS

With the widespread adoption of quality-switching, or Q-switch (QS), lasers in the 1980s, the treatment of pigmented skin lesions was revolutionized. These lasers quickly became the standard treatment and remain so even several decades later. With selective photothermolysis, sufficient energy must be delivered to the target chromophore with a pulse duration that is less than or equal to its thermal relaxation time. A strong burst of energy delivered within this small amount of time causes rapid expansion and contraction of the target with subsequent mechanical fragmentation of pigment particles through a photoacoustic effect. The particles of pigment are then released into the extracellular space and eliminated through the lymphatic system.

QS nanosecond lasers provided the ability to appropriately target melanosomes for destruction. QS lasers have traditionally been an effective treatment for lightening lentigines. In medium dark skin tones, lower fluences should be used in order to reduce the risk of postinflammatory hyper- or hypopigmentation. QS 1064-nm Nd:YAG can also be utilized for darker skin tones. The intended treatment end point is immediate graying or whitening from rapid heating of the target chromophore. The lentigines then darken over several days before lightening or fading away. The treatment of café-au-lait macules is typified by mixed results, and patients must therefore be counseled appropriately. Lesions may initially fade, but typically recur in time. Despite medical and laser advancements, melasma remains a challenging pigmentary disorder to treat with only modest results. While laser therapy may lighten the pigmentation associated with melasma, difficulty remains in achieving long-term remission even with concomitant strict photoprotection and topical lightening agents. Additional larger studies may focus on combining laser treatments for melasma with kojic acid, bakuchiol, and oral, intradermal, and topical tranexamic acid formulations.

Recently, picosecond (PS) lasers have been developed and broadly commercialized for the treatment of pigmented lesions and tattoos. These lasers deliver energy in the picosecond range, which is one-trillionth of a second. Although PS lasers have been available for several years, their prohibitive costs represented a major roadblock to their widespread adoption. The field is just now experiencing an influx of scientific studies in the medical literature demonstrating their clinical utility.[9] PS lasers have been shown to be effective for the treatment of various pigmented lesions and disorders, including solar lentigines, nevus of Ota, melasma, and café-au-lait macules.[9-13]

▶ LASER TATTOO REMOVAL

Laser tattoo removal procedures have experienced a recent rise in demand. In 2017, about 85,000 laser, light, and energy-based tattoo removal procedures were performed by ASDS members alone.[1] With improved technology and increasing knowledge of the treatment of tattoo pigments, clinical outcomes have continued to improve. The first step in treating tattoos is to properly evaluate the pigment as different pigments preferentially absorb specific wavelengths of light. Therefore, the goal of optimizing treatment is to specifically target the correct color. A rapid rise in temperature of the targeted chromophore leads to a pressure wave that exceeds the tensile strength of the pigment particle, causing it to shatter into smaller fragments. Short pulse durations allow for photoacoustic and photomechanical destruction of pigment while avoiding significant collateral thermal damage. In comparison to melanin, tattoo pigments have a significantly shorter thermal relaxation time, so shorter pulse durations, especially in the picosecond range, may prove to be more efficacious.[14,15]

For many years, QS nanosecond lasers were considered the standard of care for tattoo removal.[16] The most common wavelengths of laser devices for tattoo removal are 1064, 532, 694, and 755 nm.[17-19] The 1064-nm Nd:YAG laser can treat black, dark blue, and brown tattoos, while the frequency doubled 532 nm can treat brown, red, orange, and yellow tattoos. The 755-nm alexandrite laser can effectively treat black, blue, and green colors, while the 694-nm ruby laser can remove black, blue, green, and purple. Some colors are known to offer variable results, including purple, green, yellow, and red. Flesh-colored pigments are notoriously difficult to treat. A common phenomenon that can occur with their treatment is paradoxical darkening immediately after a single laser pulse. This is caused by a shift from an oxidized to a reduced state in the tattoo pigment.

The recent development and commercialization of PS lasers have reportedly led to improved treatment outcomes for tattoo removal[9] (Figure 4.3). Even historically stubborn tattoo pigments have been demonstrated to have improved responses. This technology takes advantage of the short thermal relaxation time of tattoo pigments by delivering energy in shorter durations than the traditional QS nanosecond lasers. With PS lasers, lower fluences can be used with a smaller number of overall treatments for most

FIGURE 4.3   Homemade tattoo before (A) and after (B) laser removal.

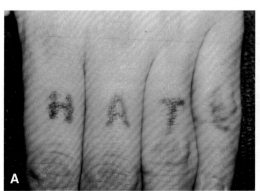
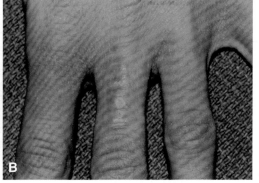

(Reprinted with permission from Hall JC, Hall JB. *Sauer's Manual of Skin Diseases*. 11th ed. Philadelphia, PA: Wolters Kluwer; 2017.)

tattoos.[20-22] However, a recent study showed no difference in clinical outcomes between the QS and PS lasers, despite less pain with PS.[23] Larger randomized and controlled studies are still needed to determine the role of PS in laser tattoo removal.

The use of topical perfluorodecalin has also been studied to improve laser tattoo removal. It has been approved by the US Food and Drug Administration for use with various wavelengths of QS and PS lasers. Perfluorodecalin is available as an infused patch that provides epidermal protection from thermal injury. It also reduces the optical scattering of light in order to allow for deeper tissue penetration of the laser. With this patch, multiple passes can be tolerated in a single treatment session, which has resulted in a more rapid tattoo clearance and increased satisfaction.[24,25]

▶ LASER HAIR REMOVAL

Unwanted or excess facial and body hair is a common concern of patients. While complaints have traditionally originated from female patients, men also represent an important segment. Excessive hair growth may be a marker of endocrine disorders, hormonal imbalances, and medication side effects, and practitioners should remember to assess patients for such potential causes prior to performing any photoepilation procedures. Patients may have attempted temporary modalities prior to consultation, such as shaving, plucking, waxing, and chemical depilatories, and laser devices can offer a more effective, reliable, and durable solution for hair removal.

The concept of photoepilation revolves around the selective delivery of energy to the bulge of the hair follicle. This heats the target area in an effort to cause destruction of the follicular stem cells. Nonselective injury to surrounding tissue can also be minimized. The hair shaft, outer root sheath of the infundibulum, and hair bulb matrix are also melanin targets. The long-pulsed 755-nm alexandrite, long-pulsed 694-nm ruby, long-pulsed 1064-nm Nd:YAG, long-pulsed 810-nm diode, and IPL can each be used to reach the appropriate target.[26]

Thick and darker hairs are easier targets for photoepilation, whereas thin and lighter hairs are more difficult. The skin tone of the patient also affects efficacy and side effect profile. Lighter skin tones can allow for improved targeting of melanin associated with the hair follicle instead of competing with that of the adjacent or overlying epidermis. For this reason, tanned patients should not be treated in order to reduce the risks for burns, scars, and dyspigmentation. Sufficient epidermal cooling is important to protect unintended targets from excessive heat. The 1064-nm Nd:YAG laser can be used in darker phenotypes due to its reduced epidermal melanin absorption.[27] However, higher energies may be required, which can cause increased pain and reduced efficacy.

Since the target chromophore is the melanin in the hair, patients should be instructed to avoid waxing, plucking, and threading prior to being treated. Shaving should be done before the procedure to sustain the target in the dermis and remove the overlying hair on top of the skin, which can cause unwanted heat and injury to the epidermis. The treatment endpoint is perifollicular edema. Graying of the epidermis is an ominous sign of nonspecific heat injury, which can indicate subsequent blistering and necrosis. A typical treatment course requires multiple treatments, such as 3 to 8 treatments at 4- to 10-week intervals. At 6-month follow-up, 70% to 90% hair reduction has been demonstrated.[28]

Since laser hair removal was the most commonly performed procedure in litigation cases related to injury secondary to cutaneous laser surgery, significant caution should be exercised by practitioners.[29] Safety and efficacy are operator-dependent, based on knowledge, training, and experience with using the device. One of the most important parameters is pulse duration, which should align with the thermal relaxation time of the hair follicle (10-100 ms).[30] Greater pulse widths may cause unwanted thermal injury and potentially lead to scarring. Patients should also be warned about the risk for paradoxical hypertrichosis, which is not uncommon and has been reported in 0.6% to 10% of patients treated with the diode and alexandrite lasers and also the IPL.[31-33] While the exact mechanism is still unknown, risk factors include darker skin tone, darker and thicker hair, and hormonal imbalance. If encountered, patients should be reassured, as continued treatments have been effective in reducing the unwanted hair growth.

▶ ABLATIVE RESURFACING LASERS

Ablative resurfacing lasers were once the gold standard for facial rejuvenation. The 10,600-nm carbon dioxide (CO_2) laser represented the prototype that was initially used. This laser offered nonspecific treatment by targeting water in the skin, leading to controlled vaporization when delivered with an appropriate threshold. Subsequently, the 2940-nm erbium-doped:yttrium-aluminum-garnet (Er:YAG) laser was utilized and it provided more efficient absorption by water-containing tissues. This produced less thermal injury to the surrounding treated tissue, which led to improved healing, erythema, and dyspigmentation. However, because of the prolonged downtime due to the need for complete re-epithelialization, risk for permanent dyspigmentation, and increased risk for infection during the healing period, fully ablative laser treatments have become less popular with patients.

Fractional photothermolysis, introduced in 2004, has changed the way that ablative resurfacing is performed.[34] Instead of treating the entire epidermis, fractional lasers treat only a portion of the epidermis through microscopic thermal injury, creating microscopic treatment zones (MTZ) (Figure 4.4). The parameters of the MTZ can be controlled, such as the density, depth, and width. Each cylinder of damaged skin is surrounded by normal unaffected skin, which acts as a healing reservoir for the microwounds. This allows for a relatively safe treatment of previously difficult to treat areas using fully ablative

FIGURE 4.4 **Comparison of continuous (complete) coverage and fractionated coverage with laser.**

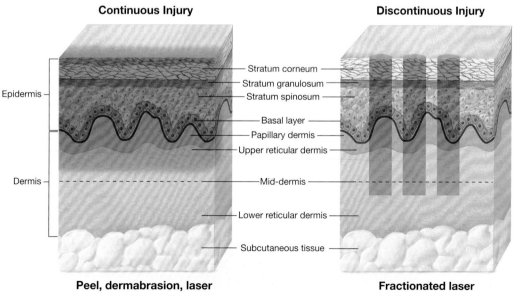

(Reprinted with permission from Chung KC. *Grabb and Smith's Plastic Surgery*. 7th ed. Philadelphia, PA: Wolters Kluwer; 2014.)

resurfacing methods. The 10,600-nm CO_2 laser, 2940-nm Er:YAG laser, and 2790-nm yttrium-scandium-gallium-garnet (YSGG) laser are available as fractionated ablative devices, which have wavelengths that are absorbed by the water in tissue. The YSGG laser allows for more collateral thermal injury than the Er:YAG laser, but less than the CO_2 laser, due to its intermediate absorption coefficient of water.

With its areas of normal untreated skin, fractional ablative resurfacing offers more rapid healing times compared to traditional ablative lasers. Following treatment with the fractional ablative laser, punctate bleeding and serosanguinous drainage are the expectation (Figure 4.5). These then dry into a thin crust, while the erythema improves over a period of several days. However, mild erythema and edema may persist for several weeks in some patients. A postprocedural topical corticosteroid can be used to help ameliorate some of these expected side effects. It is important to note that the neck and chest represent underprivileged areas, which cannot tolerate high energies and densities due to its thinner dermis with less abundant adnexal structures.[35] Aggressive treatment can lead to clinical scarring. Each area of treatment should be evaluated individually when selecting treatment parameters (Figure 4.6).

▶ NONABLATIVE AESTHETIC LASERS

Nonablative laser therapy was developed as a means to reduce downtime during photorejuvenation procedures. In nonablative treatment, thermal energy is used to create a controlled injury within the dermis, allowing for neocollagenesis, while maintaining an intact and functional epidermis. Although treatments are well tolerated, clinical outcomes are modest when compared to conventional ablative resurfacing treatments.

Nonablative fractional resurfacing (NAFR) utilizes narrow beams of energy that target water in the tissue to induce thermal damage in fractionated columns without affecting the tissue adjacent to the MTZ's. The microscopic epidermal necrotic debris (MEND) overlying the MTZ contains various cellular components, which are slowly extruded over a period of 1 to 2 weeks. Despite visible necrosis of the epidermis and dermis in the MTZ's, the stratum corneum remains histologically and functionally intact (Figure 4.7). Various

FIGURE 4.5   Laser skin resurfacing. Treatment of perioral wrinkles and dyspigmentation with fractional CO_2 laser. Immediately after treatment with punctate bleeding from microscopic treatment zones.

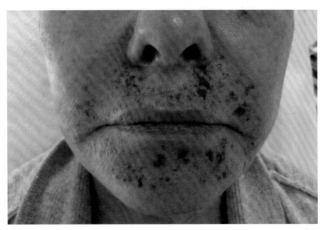

(Reprinted with permission from Chung KC. *Grabb and Smith's Plastic Surgery*. 7th ed. Philadelphia, PA: Wolters Kluwer; 2014.)

FIGURE 4.6   Cribriform scarring after resurfacing procedure.

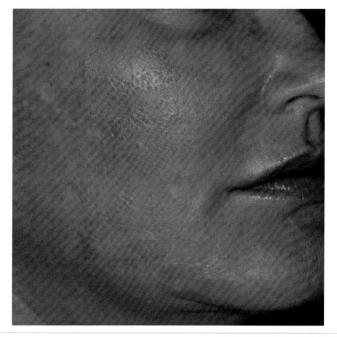

(Reprinted with permission from Krakowski AC, Shumaker PR. *The Scar Book*. 1st ed. Philadelphia, PA: Wolters Kluwer; 2018.)

wavelengths have been utilized, including 1550 and 1927 nm, and depths up to 1.5 mm can be obtained. NAFR has been studied to treat numerous skin ailments, including photoaging of facial and nonfacial surfaces, acne scars, traumatic scars, striae distensae, dyspigmentation, and actinic keratoses. The significant versatility of NAFR devices makes them popular among laser practitioners (Figure 4.8).

In contrast to ablative treatment, nonablative fractional lasers cause little to no downtime, and the associated erythema and edema are expected to resolve within 1 to 2 days of treatment. It is important for the practitioner to avoid bulk heating of the tissue in order to avoid any potential complications, which can include scarring. Repeatedly treating the same areas, especially without allowing for sufficient time to pass for cooling, can induce full thickness skin loss and unintended tissue damage.

▶ SKIN-TIGHTENING DEVICES

Medical devices utilizing radiofrequency (RF) and ultrasound energies have become popular treatment options for those seeking skin tightening with decreased downtime compared to more invasive surgical procedures. Because of this rise in demand, significant research and resources have gone into developing devices based on this technology.

RF can be used as a modality to heat tissue at selected depths and areas by controlling the frequency and delivery design. The depth of penetration is inversely proportional to the frequency. These devices generate heat as a result of tissue resistance to the movement of electrons within the RF field. The localized heat injury serves to stimulate neocollagenesis and neoelastogenesis, which lead to clinical tightening of the skin and improvements of sagging. Electron microscopy has demonstrated increased diameter of collagen fibers following treatment.[36] It can additionally be used to heat adipose tissue during procedures for purposes of body contouring.

FIGURE 4.7   (A) Histology after 1550-nm nonablative fractional laser treatment showing dermal coagulation but no corridors. (B) Histology after Er:YAG 2940-nm ablative fractional laser treatment showing open channels creating a pathway for topical penetration of drugs, cells, and cosmeceuticals into the dermal compartment.

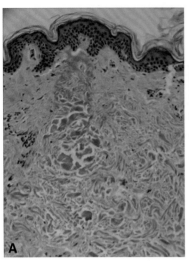 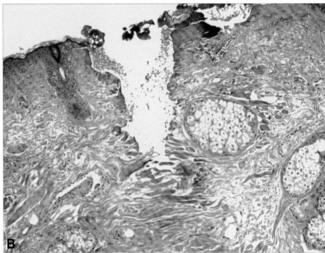

(Reprinted with permission from Krakowski AC, Shumaker PR. *The Scar Book*. 1st ed. Philadelphia, PA: Wolters Kluwer; 2018.)

RF devices can be monopolar, bipolar, or unipolar. Monopolar devices utilize a grounding plate. The energy is delivered through the skin, into the patient's body, and then subsequently to the grounding plate. In comparison, bipolar devices use two electrodes, which are typically on the handpiece. The RF energy travels between the alternating positive and negative poles, and the distance between them determines the depth of penetration. Recently, RF has also been combined with microneedling, where the tips of the needles serve to deliver the RF energy. This allows for deeper effects in the dermis in addition to the conventional epidermal resurfacing of microneedling.

With the advent of real-time monitoring systems and built-in safety mechanisms, RF devices have become a relatively safe treatment option. Practitioners can adjust the heating power according to real-time measurements in order to avoid overheating or bulk heating of the target tissue, which can lead to blistering and necrosis. Precise and even treatment can more easily be achieved. The most common side effects are typically transient erythema and edema. The newer generation of devices has been well tolerated by patients.

Ultrasound energy is another technology used for skin tightening/lifting and body contouring. Focused ultrasound can be delivered focally deep into the target tissue, sparing the over- and underlying structures. The ultrasound field vibrates the tissue, which in turn creates friction between the molecules and generation of heat. When skin tightening is the desired outcome, the dermis or muscular fascia is the targeted tissue. When body contouring/fat reduction is desired, adipose tissue is the target. Available devices employ high-intensity focused ultrasound. Lower frequency probes are associated with deeper tissue effect than higher frequency probes. Localized hyperthermia directly causes collagen contraction and lysis of adipocytes and also triggers a reparative process and neocollagenesis. Treatments are generally well tolerated with mild intraprocedural pain paired with transient erythema and swelling. The main advantage of this technology is deeper penetration of the energy without allowing for significant injury to the epidermis.

FIGURE 4.8   **Improvement of dyschromia. Fractional nonablative therapy with low energy low density 1927-nm laser was used with 7 mJ fluence at 10% density.**

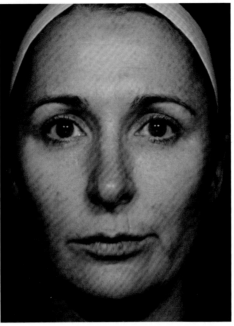

(Reprinted with permission from Chung KC, Thorne CH, Sinno S. *Operative Techniques in Facial Aesthetic Surgery.* 1st ed. Philadelphia, PA: Wolters Kluwer; 2020.)

▶ DEVICE THERAPY FOR HYPERHIDROSIS

Clinical hyperhidrosis can be a challenging disorder for patients and physicians alike, due to its profound effect on quality of life and the difficulty to effectively treat. It is not uncommon for patients to fail topical therapy (e.g., aluminum chloride), intradermal therapy (e.g., botulinum toxin), and oral therapy (e.g., glycopyrrolate). In 2011, the US Food and Drug Administration approved the miraDry® system (Miramar Labs, Sunnyvale, CA) for the treatment of axillary hyperhidrosis. The miraDry® device delivers controlled microwave energy beneath axillary skin, heating sweat glands and inducing thermolysis. The microwaves induce physical rotation of dipole molecules, which in turn creates heat. The top layer of skin is cooled for protection, creating an interface where heat is restricted to the small zone where sweat glands are located. Multiple treatments are often required. Outcomes were demonstrated to be durable at 1 and 2 years following treatment.[37,38] Common side effects include erythema, swelling, tenderness, and numbness. While significant adverse events are rare, scarring and brachial plexus injury have been reported.[39]

▶ CONCLUSION

The aesthetic field is home to numerous laser, light, and energy-based devices. In recent years, the continuous improvement and rapid expansion of medical device technology has only served to further increase this number. While many devices have demonstrated significant clinical utility, others are still relatively new, and their roles are yet to be determined. Consumer demand for procedures that utilize medical devices is expected to continue on an upward trajectory in the near future. Aesthetic practitioners should be familiar with the various devices that are currently available and appreciate which can be used for the treatment of particular skin disorders. Sufficient and adequate training with laser, light, and energy-based devices is necessary in order to deliver safe and effective patient care.

REFERENCES

1. American Society for Dermatologic Surgery. *ASDS Survey on Dermatologic Procedures*. 2018. https://www.asds.net/portals/0/PDF/procedure-survey-results-presentation-2017.pdf. Accessed May 2019.
2. Wheeland RG. History of lasers in dermatology. *Clin Dermatol*. 1995;13(1):3-10.
3. Anderson RR, Parrish JA. Selective photothermolysis: precise microsurgery by selective absorption of pulsed radiation. *Science*. 1983;220(4596):524-527.
4. Goldman MP, Weiss RA. Treatment of poikiloderma of Civatte on the neck with an intense pulsed light source. *Plast Reconstr Surg*. 2001;107(6):1376-1381.
5. Rohrer TE, Chatrath V, Iyengar V. Does pulse stacking improve the results of treatment with variable-pulse pulsed-dye lasers? *Dermatol Surg*. 2004;30(2 pt 1):163-167.
6. Correia E, Wang JV, Saedi N. Recalcitrant facial port-wine stain successfully responding to 585 nm diode laser. *Skinmed*. 2020, in press.
7. Keller GS. KTP laser offers advances in minimally invasive plastic surgery. *Clin Laser Mon*. 1992;10(9):141-144.
8. West TB, Alster TS. Comparison of the long-pulse dye (590-595 nm) and KTP (532 nm) lasers in the treatment of facial and leg telangiectasias. *Dermatol Surg*. 1998;24(2):221-226.
9. Torbeck RL, Schilling L, Khorasani H, Dover JS, Arndt KA, Saedi N. Evolution of the picosecond laser: a review of literature. *Dermatol Surg*. 2019;45(2):183-194.
10. Kung KY, Shek SY, Yeung CK, Chan HH. Evaluation of the safety and efficacy of the dual wavelength picosecond laser for the treatment of benign pigmented lesions in Asians. *Lasers Surg Med*. 2019;51(1):14-22.
11. Chan MWM, Shek SY, Yeung CK, Chan HH. A prospective study in the treatment of lentigines in Asian skin using 532 nm picosecond Nd:YAG laser. *Lasers Surg Med*. 2019;51:767-773.
12. Sakio R, Ohshiro T, Sasaki K, Ohshiro T. Usefulness of picosecond pulse alexandrite laser treatment for nevus of Ota. *Laser Ther*. 2018;27(4):251-255.
13. Artzi O, Mehrabi JN, Koren A, Niv R, Lapidoth M, Levi A. Picosecond 532-nm neodymium-doped yttrium aluminium garnet laser-a novel and promising modality for the treatment of café-au-lait macules. *Lasers Med Sci*. 2018;33(4):693-697.
14. Ho DD, London R, Zimmerman GB, Young DA. Laser-tattoo removal – A study of the mechanism and the optimal treatment strategy via computer simulations. *Lasers Surg Med*. 2002;30(5):389-397.
15. Zachary CB, Rofagha R. Laser therapy. In: Bolognia J, Jorizzo J, Schaffer J, eds. *Dermatology*. 3rd ed. Philadelphia, PA: Elsevier Saunders; 2012:2261-2282.
16. Kent KM, Graber EM. Laser tattoo removal: a review. *Dermatol Surg*. 2012;38(1):1-13.
17. Sardana K, Ranjan R, Ghunawat S. Optimising laser tattoo removal. *J Cutan Aesthet Surg*. 2015;8(1):16-24.
18. Luebberding S, Alexiades-Armenakas M. New tattoo approaches in dermatology. *Dermatol Clin*. 2014;32(1):91-96.
19. Bernstein EF. Laser tattoo removal. *Semin Plast Surg*. 2007;21(3):175-192.
20. Herd RM, Alora MB, Smoller B, Arndt KA, Dover JS. A clinical and histologic prospective controlled comparative study of the picosecond titanium:sapphire (795 nm) laser versus the Q-switched alexandrite (752 nm) laser for removing tattoo pigment. *J Am Acad Dermatol*. 1999;40(4):603-606.
21. Ross V, Naseef G, Lin G, et al. Comparison of responses of tattoos to picosecond and nanosecond Q-switched neodymium:YAG lasers. *Arch Dermatol*. 1998;134(2):167-171.
22. Lorgeou A, Perrillat Y, Gral N, Lagrange S, Lacour JP, Passeron T. Comparison of two picosecond lasers to a nanosecond laser for treating tattoos: a prospective randomized study on 49 patients. *J Eur Acad Dermatol Venereol*. 2018;32(2):265-270.
23. Pinto F, Große-Büning S, Karsai S, et al. Neodymium-doped yttrium aluminium garnet (Nd:YAG) 1064-nm picosecond laser vs. Nd:YAG 1064-nm nanosecond laser in tattoo removal: a randomized controlled single-blind clinical trial. *Br J Dermatol*. 2017;176(2):457-464.
24. Biesman BS, O'Neil MP, Costner C. Rapid, high-fluence multi-pass q-switched laser treatment of tattoos with a transparent perfluorodecalin-infused patch: a pilot study. *Lasers Surg Med*. 2015;47(8):613-618.
25. Biesman BS, Costner C. Evaluation of a transparent perfluorodecalin-infused patch as an adjunct to laser-assisted tattoo removal: a pivotal trial. *Lasers Surg Med*. 2017;49(4):335-340.
26. Dierickx CC. Hair removal by lasers and intense pulsed light sources. *Dermatol Clin*. 2002;20(1):135-146.
27. Alster TS, Bryan H, Williams CM. Long-pulsed Nd:YAG laser-assisted hair removal in pigmented skin: a clinical and histological evaluation. *Arch Dermatol*. 2001;137(7):885-889.
28. Lepselter J, Elman M. Biological and clinical aspects in laser hair removal. *J Dermatolog Treat*. 2004;15(2):72-83.
29. Jalian HR, Jalian CA, Avram MM. Increased risk of litigation associated with laser surgery by nonphysician operators. *JAMA Dermatol*. 2014;150(4):407-411.

30. van Gemert MJ, Welch AJ. Time constants in thermal laser medicine. *Lasers Surg Med.* 1989;9(4):405-421.

31. Willey A, Torrontegui J, Azpiazu J, Landa N. Hair stimulation following laser and intense pulsed light photo-epilation: review of 543 cases and ways to manage it. *Lasers Surg Med.* 2007;39(4):297-301.

32. Alajlan A, Shapiro J, Rivers JK, MacDonald N, Wiggin J, Lui H. Paradoxical hypertrichosis after laser epilation. *J Am Acad Dermatol.* 2005;53(1):85-88.

33. Desai S, Mahmoud BH, Bhatia AC, Hamzavi IH. Paradoxical hypertrichosis after laser therapy: a review. *Dermatol Surg.* 2010;36(3):291-298.

34. Manstein D, Herron GS, Sink RK, Tanner H, Anderson RR. Fractional photothermolysis: a new concept for cutaneous remodeling using microscopic patterns of thermal injury. *Lasers Surg Med.* 2004;34(5):426-438.

35. Fife DJ, Fitzpatrick RE, Zachary CB. Complications of fractional CO2 laser resurfacing: four cases. *Lasers Surg Med.* 2009;41(3):179-184.

36. Kist D, Burns AJ, Sanner R, Counters J, Zelickson B. Ultrastructural evaluation of multiple pass low energy versus single pass high energy radio-frequency treatment. *Lasers Surg Med.* 2006;38(2):150-154.

37. Hong HC, Lupin M, O'Shaughnessy KF. Clinical evaluation of a microwave device for treating axillary hyperhidrosis. *Dermatol Surg.* 2012;38(5):728-735.

38. Lupin M, Hong HC, O'Shaughnessy KF. Long-term efficacy and quality of life assessment for treatment of axillary hyperhidrosis with a microwave device. *Dermatol Surg.* 2014;40(7):805-807.

39. Puffer RC, Bishop AT, Spinner RJ, Shin AY. Bilateral brachial plexus injury after MiraDry® procedure for axillary hyperhidrosis: a case report. *World Neurosurg* 2019;124:370-372.

5

Chemical Peels

Frankie G. Rholdon, MD

Chapter Highlights

- Chemical peels are traditionally categorized as being superficial (epidermal), medium-depth (papillary dermis), and deep (reticular dermis).
- Selection of the type of chemical peel depends upon the patient's expectations, desired outcome, and downtime available.
- Pretreatment with a topical retinoid can assure even penetration of the peeling agent.
- Care should be taken during the treatment to prevent ocular injury, such as the use of petrolatum at the medium and lateral canthi, avoiding the passing of peeling solutions over the patient, and by having eyewash solution readily available at all times during the procedure.
- Common superficial chemical peels include glycolic acid, salicylic acid, and Jessner solution.
- Common medium-depth chemical peels combine 35% trichloroacetic acid with either Jessner solution, 70% glycolic acid, or solid carbon dioxide.
- Phenol peels are the most common deep chemical peels.

Chemical peeling (chemoexfoliation) is the application of a chemical agent to the skin to cause controlled destruction of portions of the epidermis and possibly dermis. This results in exfoliation and removal of superficial lesions, as well as regeneration and remodeling of epidermal and dermal tissues. Chemical peeling to improve aesthetics has evolved throughout history, beginning with the ancient Egyptians using animal oils, salt, alabaster, and sour milk. The active ingredient in sour milk is lactic acid, an alpha hydroxy acid, which is still used in chemical peeling today. Dermatologists have been utilizing modern peeling techniques since the late 1800s. Large advances came with P.G. Unna's descriptions of salicylic acid (SA), resorcinol, phenol, and trichloroacetic acid (TCA) in 1882. Deep chemical peeling was refined in the 1960s and 1970s by Drs Thomas Baker and Harold Gordon using a saponated formula of phenol and croton oil. Medium-depth chemical peeling was pioneered by Drs Harold Brody, Gary Monheit, and William Coleman in the 1980s.[1] These peeling techniques have been optimized, and many commercially available proprietary formulations are now available. Dermatologists performed 434,000 chemical peel procedures in 2017,[2] compared to 425,000 in 2016.[3] Society's desire for a more youthful appearance is driving an increase in the demand for chemical peeling.

The goal of chemical peeling is to remove a uniform thickness of skin to eliminate damaged or unwanted cells and to stimulate rejuvenation through wound healing. Caustic agents used in chemical peeling cause exfoliation through keratocoagulation, denaturation of proteins, and/or disruption of intercellular adhesion. Removal of the epidermis improves pigmentation and texture and destroys unwanted epidermal growths. The wounding also causes the release of pro-inflammatory cytokines and chemokines, activating the inflammatory cascade. This targeted inflammation stimulates neocollagenesis and neoelastinogenesis, reorganization of dermal connective tissue, and regeneration of keratinocytes. This results in epidermal and dermal thickening which can improve the clinical appearance of rhytides and acne scarring. The depth of tissue injury correlates with the amount of tissue remodeling and therefore chemical peels are traditionally categorized by depth of wounding into superficial, medium, and deep chemical peels (Table 5.1).

Superficial chemical peels involve injury to varying levels of the epidermis. Medium-depth peels penetrate the full thickness of epidermis and into the papillary dermis. Deep chemical peels wound into the reticular dermis. The depth of a chemical peel can be influenced by several factors including the type of chemical used, chemical concentration, mode of application, number of applications, and amount of time the chemical is active on the skin. The depth of injury directly correlates with healing time, risk of complication, and cosmetic outcome.

▶ PREOPERATIVE (TABLE 5.2)

History/Physical Examination

Patient consultation is vital to a successful procedure and should begin by assessing the patient's goals and motivation. There are several patient factors that will impact the success of the treatment, including unrealistic expectations, inability to tolerate the procedure or accommodate downtime, and inability to avoid the sun. A targeted medical history should include pregnancy and breastfeeding status, any previous facial resurfacing procedures, smoking status, recent facial surgeries, previous radiation in the treatment area, history of abnormal scar formation or pigmentation, isotretinoin therapy in the previous 6 months, and history of hepatic, renal, or cardiac disease (relative to deep peeling only). Physical exam involves evaluation of areas of patient concern, degree of photoaging, Fitzpatrick skin type (Table 5.3), as well as identifying any contraindications such as active infection, uncontrolled dermatitis, open wounds, or abnormal scars.

Counseling

Proper patient counseling is essential in both outcome and patient satisfaction (Table 5.4). Patient goals and expectations should be communicated and aligned with the chosen procedure. The provider should ensure that the patient understands the expected outcome and limitations of the treatment. Detailed information regarding the preparation required prior to the procedure, as well as the procedure technique,

TABLE 5.1   Chemical Peel Types

	Superficial Peel	Medium-Depth Peel	Deep Peel
Depth of injury	• Epidermis	• Papillary to upper reticular dermis	• Mid reticular dermis
Indications	• Pigmentation abnormalities • Acne • Undesirable superficial skin texture (not including rhytides or scarring)	• Pigmentation abnormalities • Superficial rhytides • Superficial scarring • Superficial epidermal growths	• Pigmentation abnormalities • Superficial to deep rhytides • Scarring • Superficial epidermal growths
Contraindications	• Active infection • Open wounds • Uncontrolled dermatitis • History of abnormal scarring • Unrealistic patient expectations • Inability of the patient to tolerate the procedure and recovery • Patient inability to avoid sun exposure	• Active infection • Open wounds • Uncontrolled dermatitis • History of abnormal scarring • Unrealistic patient expectations • Inability of the patient to tolerate the procedure and recovery • Patient inability to avoid sun exposure • Previous, recent (<6 mo) facial undermining surgery in the treatment area • Isotretinoin in the previous 6 mo • History of facial radiation in the treatment area • Smoking (may interfere with healing) • Fitzpatrick skin types IV-VI	• Active infection • Open wounds • Uncontrolled dermatitis • History of abnormal scarring • Unrealistic patient expectations • Inability of the patient to tolerate the procedure and recovery • Patient inability to avoid sun exposure • Previous, recent (<6 mo) facial undermining surgery in the treatment area • Isotretinoin in the previous 6 mo • History of facial radiation in the treatment area • Smoking (may interfere with healing) • Fitzpatrick skin types IV-VI • History of cardiac or hepatorenal disease if application is more than one cosmetic unit
Agents	• Salicylic acid • Glycolic acid • Jessner solution • Tretinoin • Glycolic acid • Lactic acid • TCA 10%-35% • Mandelic acid • Pyruvic acid • Others	• TCA 50% as single frost • Solid CO_2 followed by 35% TCA • Jessner solution followed by 35% TCA • Glycolic acid solutions applied and washed off, followed by 35% TCA • Full strength phenol, USP 88%	• Phenol-croton oil peels

(Continued)

TABLE 5.1   Chemical Peel Types (Continued)

	Superficial Peel	**Medium-Depth Peel**	**Deep Peel**
Complications	• Post inflammatory pigment alteration • Prolonged erythema • Infection (bacterial, fungal, viral) • Reactivation of HSV • Allergic reaction • Increased skin sensitivity	• Post inflammatory pigment alteration • Prolonged erythema • Infection (bacterial, fungal, viral) • Reactivation of HSV • Allergic reaction • Increased skin sensitivity • Acneiform eruption • Milia formation • Scarring	• Post inflammatory pigment alteration • Prolonged erythema • Infection (bacterial, fungal, viral) • Reactivation of HSV • Allergic reaction • Increased skin sensitivity • Acneiform eruption • Milia formation • Scarring • Cardiotoxicity/ arrhythmia (due to systemic absorption of phenol) • Hepatotoxicity • Nephrotoxicity

expected discomfort, anticipated downtime, aftercare protocol, and potential complications, must be reviewed with the patient in detail. The patient should understand normal healing and be educated on potential adverse events to enable early identification and intervention in the case of complications. After the patient is educated and given the opportunity to ask questions, written documentation of informed consent is obtained.

TABLE 5.2   Preoperative

1. History.
    a. History of abnormal scar formation, including keloids.
    b. Pregnant or lactating.
    c. Previous facial surgical procedures, dermabrasion, or chemical peels.
    d. Tobacco use.
    e. Previous radiation exposure.
    f. Determine patient's subjective areas of concern, goals, and exceptions.
2. Physical exam.
    a. Fitzpatrick skin type (Table 5.3).
    b. Assess degree of photoaging and goals of treatment to determine chemical peel type.
    c. Presence of active infection (especially HSV).
3. Prescribe antiviral prophylaxis (if indicated).
4. Prepare the skin with tretinoin and sun protection prior to the scheduled procedure.
5. Obtain patient consent.
6. Take patient photographs.
7. Hyperkeratotic lesions may be removed prior to chemical peeling.
8. Cleanse and degrease the face appropriately using cleansers, acetone, alcohol, or a combination.
9. Ensure proper eyewash equipment is readily accessible in case of accidental ocular exposure of peeling solution.

TABLE 5.3   Fitzpatrick Skin Types

I	Always burns, never tans
II	Always burns, tans minimally
III	Burns moderately, tans gradually
IV	Burns minimally, always tans uniformly
V	Rarely burns, tans easily
VI	Never burns, deeply pigmented

TABLE 5.4   Medium-Depth Chemical Peel Patient Instructions

Pretreatment instructions:
- You should not have this treatment if you are pregnant or if you have taken isotretinoin (Accutane) within the previous 6 mo.
- Discontinue topical retinoids or retinol 1 d prior to the treatment.
- Avoid excessive sun exposure at least 2 wk prior to the procedure.
- Avoid microdermabrasion, waxing, aggressive exfoliation, or any other treatments that may be irritating to the skin for at least 1 wk prior to the procedure.
- Your provider may recommend antiviral medication prior to the treatment to help prevent fever blisters from occurring after the procedure. If so, take as instructed.

What to expect during your treatment:
- Arrive with the treatment area clean, free of makeup and lotions and clean shaven.
- A medical staff member will take photographs prior to your treatment to track the results.
- The skin will be prepped for the chemical peel with alcohol and acetone.
- The physician will rub the skin with solid CO_2 (dry ice). This is cold and can sting in some areas.
- As the peeling solution is applied to the skin, you may experience tingling, a heat sensation, stinging or burning. This is temporary and will last about 5-10 min.
- Cold compresses will then be applied to cool the skin and provide comfort.
- A soothing ointment will then be applied to the skin.
- Your skin will appear white with an underlying pink/red coloration. The white color will fade in 1-2 h.

Posttreatment instructions:
- After 24 h, cleanse the face with a gentle facial cleanser twice daily. Avoid scrubbing.
- Apply a thin layer of white petrolatum immediately after cleansing the face. Reapply as needed for itchy, tight skin.
- Facial swelling will occur on post peel days 1-4. The swelling will be worse in the morning and improve throughout the day.
- Peeling will begin on day 3 or 4 and continue until day 9 or 10.
- Avoid scrubbing, picking, or peeling the skin during the healing process.
- Avoid sun exposure during the healing process. Once the peeling is completed, wear sunscreen daily and protect from sun for at least 6 mo.
- Once the peeling is complete and the skin no longer feels sensitive, resume skin care regimen as instructed by physician.
- You should not have pain, worsening redness, or oozing during this process. If these occur, call the office.

Preprocedure Treatment

To ensure optimal outcomes, a pretreatment skin care regimen is recommended for at least 4 weeks prior to the chemical peel. Patient compliance with the pretreatment regimen primes the skin for uniform penetration of the peeling agent, reduces healing time, ensures tolerability and compliance to topical agents, and decreases the risk of complications. Any infection, dermatitis, or inflammation of the skin within the treatment area should be addressed and treated appropriately. The patient should be advised to aggressively photoprotect the treatment area with daily application of broad-spectrum sunscreen and sun protective behaviors (UV protective clothing, hats, avoidance of excessive sun, etc.). It is not recommended to have facial hair in the treatment area; the patient should be instructed to shave the area 12 to 24 hours prior to the scheduled procedure if necessary. The patient should also be instructed to arrive on the day of the procedure with clean skin and not wearing contact lenses.

Topical vitamin A preparations are recommended prior to the planned procedure. Retinoids act on the upper papillary dermis by increasing type I collagen production and decreasing collagen destruction by matrix metalloproteinases. They have also been shown to efface rhytides through epidermal hyperplasia, compaction of the stratum corneum, and thickening of the granular cell layer of the epidermis.[4] Tretinoin, or all-*trans*-retinoic-acid, is a first-generation naturally occurring retinoid and is the most extensively studied in aesthetic medicine. The preoperative use of topical tretinoin decreases healing time after a chemical peel.[5] It is recommended to apply tretinoin cream 0.05% or 0.1% daily for 4 weeks prior to chemical peeling and discontinue use 24 hours before the scheduled procedure. Although not studied prior to chemical peeling, tazarotene is a synthetic retinoid that has shown to improve the cosmetic appearance of photoaging. Tazarotene 0.05% cream was shown to be equivalent to tretinoin 0.05% cream in the treatment of the mottled hyperpigmentation and fine rhytides of photodamaged skin.[6] In the case of retinoid sensitivity, patients may use topical adapalene. Adapalene is a synthetic third-generation retinoid with a lower incidence of retinoid dermatitis. Although studies comparing tretinoin to retinol are lacking, it is generally believed that retinols are not as clinically effective antiaging products as prescription retinoids.

Pigmentation is a common indication for chemical peeling. Topical preparations are frequently used to decrease skin pigmentation both before and after chemical peeling. Hydroquinone, the most commonly used agent, decreases pigment production through the inhibition of tyrosinase, the rate limiting enzyme in melanin synthesis. Although research involving the use of topical hydroquinone prior to chemical peels is insufficient, it is commonly used when pigmentation is the indication for chemical peeling.

Reactivation of the herpes simplex virus (HSV) is a known complication of chemical peeling. Herpetic infections following chemical peeling lead to increased morbidity, delayed reepithelialization, and scarring. This risk of reactivation correlates with the depth of wounding. It is recommended to assess the patient's history of orolabial herpes preoperatively. In superficial peeling, pretreatment with antiviral prophylaxis is optional and should be considered in patients with a history of recurrent HSV outbreaks. Prophylactic antiviral therapy should be initiated prior to all medium and deep chemical peel procedures, regardless of patient history. Valacyclovir at a dose of 500 mg twice daily beginning the morning of the procedure was found to be an effective prophylaxis against HSV reactivation.[7] In the study, the treatment was continued for 14 days, but it is generally believed safe to discontinue once reepithelialization is complete.

Isotretinoin (13-*cis*-retinoic acid) is a metabolite of vitamin A that is FDA-approved for the treatment of severe and nodulocystic acne. The package insert advises against performing cosmetic procedures, including chemical peels, within 6 months of therapy due to risk of scarring.[8] These recommendations were based on sporadic adverse events. A systematic review of the literature provided a consensus recommendation that there is insufficient evidence to recommend delaying superficial chemicals in patients treated with isotretinoin.[9] The American Society for Dermatologic Surgery Guidelines Task Force released consensus recommendations regarding the safety of cosmetic procedures after isotretinoin use in 2017, stating that "superficial peels can be safely administered to patients taking isotretinoin within 6 months after isotretinoin therapy." There was no recommendation on the use of medium or deep chemical peeling due to insufficient data.[10] It is therefore recommended to delay medium and deep-depth chemical peeling to at least 6 months after isotretinoin therapy.

Botulinum toxin type A is available as an injection for the treatment of dynamic facial rhytides, with well-established safety and efficacy. Pretreatment of glabellar, forehead, and periocular rhytides with botulinum toxin should be considered prior to chemical peeling. This is not only an adjuvant treatment of facial rhytides, but also may improve the cosmetic outcome of the subsequent chemical peel. A key factor in scar formation is the tension that acts on the wound during the healing phase. By blocking acetylcholine neurotransmitter release at the neuromuscular junction, botulinum toxin inhibits muscle tension at the site of the healing wound. Botulinum toxin pretreatment has shown to improve the cosmetic appearance of scar formation following surgical procedures on the face and neck[11] as well as improve the hyperdynamic facial lines following laser resurfacing.[12] If rhytid improvement is a goal of the chemical peel, pretreatment with botulinum toxin should be discussed with the patient in the preoperative period.

Superficial and medium-depth peels are generally tolerable and do not require anesthesia. The patient should be evaluated prior to the procedure regarding anxiety and pain tolerance. For chemical peels with more discomfort, such as the medium-depth peels and higher concentration TCA peels, an anxiolytic medication given 30 minutes prior to the procedure is optional. If this medication is prescribed, the patient should not drive to or from the procedure.

Photographic Documentation

The treatment area should be photographed prior to the chemical peel procedure. Ensure that the area is clean and free of makeup. Distractions should be minimized; therefore, it is recommended to use a headband to position hair away from the face and to remove jewelry. Photos should be standardized using consistent positioning and lighting. The photographs are part of the medical record, require Health Insurance Portability and Accountability Act (HIPAA)-compliant storage, and should be used for patient care as part of the medical record. If identifiable photographs are to be used for publications or advertising, written patient consent is necessary.

▶ OPERATIVE (TABLE 5.5)

Prior to beginning the chemical peel, all necessary supplies (Table 5.6) should be present and readily accessible. Care should be taken to ensure that the correct chemical peeling agent and concentration were selected and labeled accurately. The patients should wash their face with a gentle skin cleanser and position hair away from the treatment area using a headband or cap. For facial peeling, position the patient reclined at 30° to 45° angle with eyes closed. Alcohol and/or acetone on a gauze are used to clean and degrease the treatment area. A fan can be helpful to protect the patient from the noxious fumes.

TABLE 5.5   Operative (Superficial and Medium-Depth Peels)

1. Patient preparation.
   a. Ensure the treatment area is clean.
   b. Position hair away from the treatment area using headband or cap.
   c. Position the patient (for facial peeling at 30°-45° angle with eyes closed is recommended).
   d. Ensure an eyewash bottle of normal saline is readily accessible.
2. Clean and degrease the skin with alcohol and/or acetone on a gauze.
3. Protect any areas of concern with petroleum jelly as needed.
4. Check the solution labeling to ensure correct agent and concentration prior to transfer into the small glass container.
5. Apply the peeling solution.
   a. Apply the chemical quickly using appropriate instrument (cotton-tipped applicators, sable brush, gauze).
   b. Prevent lines of demarcation with a light application at the border of the treatment area.
   c. Number of applications and end points vary by chemical peel.
6. Termination of the chemoablation (varies by chemical peel).
   a. Glycolic acid: neutralizes with dilute sodium bicarbonate solution.
   b. Lactic acid.
   c. Mandelic acid.
   d. Pyruvic acid.
   e. TCA is self-neutralizing; however, cool water compresses can be used once depth of ablation is achieved to prevent unwanted deeper injury.
7. Apply cold compresses for patient comfort.
8. Apply emollient and physical sunblock.

To avoid accidental spillage, the peeling solution should never be passed over the patient. Special care is taken to avoid drips or spills near the eye area, and the patient's eyes should remain closed for the procedure. An eyewash bottle of normal saline should be present in the procedure room at all times in case of accidental exposure. It is optional to protect vulnerable areas with the application of white petrolatum. The medial canthus and nasojugal folds can pool peeling solution resulting in deeper than desired wounding. The medial and lateral canthi can also be protected with petrolatum to prevent tears from

TABLE 5.6   Peeling Supplies

Correctly labeled peeling agents, including concentrations
Gentle skin cleanser
Alcohol and acetone
Cold water
Eyewash bottle filled with normal saline
Small glass container to hold the peeling solution
Fan for patient comfort
Gloves
Gauze
Cotton-tipped applicators
Disposable waterproof lap bibs
Tool to apply peeling solution (sable brush, gauze, cotton-tipped applicators)
Timer (for alpha hydroxy acid peels)

interacting with the peeling solution. This can result in premature neutralization of peeling solution or "wicking" of peeling solution into the eyes. Clean gauze or cotton-tipped applicators should also be used to prevent complications from tearing.

The application of the chemical peeling agent varies by peel type (see below). The agent can be applied with brushes, gauze, or cotton-tipped applicators. Generally, for superficial and medium-depth chemical peels, the chemical is applied to the skin quickly following cosmetic subunits. When treating the entire face, the sequence most commonly followed is forehead, cheeks, nose, chin, lower eyelids, and perioral area. Some chemical peels require neutralization. Once the peel is complete, cool compresses are often employed for patient comfort. Physical block sunscreens and/or a bland ointment can be applied after the procedure.

▶ POSTOPERATIVE (TABLE 5.7)

The goal of postoperative care is to promote proper wound healing. This will minimize complications and assist in early recovery. The post-peel period includes erythema, edema, and exfoliation, and is often referred to as "downtime." The severity of symptoms and length of the recovery period correlate with the depth of wounding. The recovery period for a superficial chemical peel ranges from 1 to 7 days, medium-depth peels 7 to 10 days, and deep peels 10 to 14 days. During this time, clear instructions must be given to the patients to ensure proper care. The treatment area should be washed twice daily with a gentle skin cleanser. Scrubbing, intentional exfoliation, or peeling of the skin should be avoided. A bland emollient should be applied immediately after washing and reapplied as necessary. Sun avoidance is of paramount importance following a chemical peel. In the case of unavoidable sun exposure, a physical sunblock can be applied. All other skin care practices and topical preparations should be avoided until the recovery period is complete. The feeling of "tight skin" and mild itching are common in the postoperative period; cool compresses and bland emollients can be used for patient comfort during this time. Severe itching, worsening redness, discharge, or pain are not part of normal healing and often signal a complication. If these occur, the provider must evaluate the patient promptly to ensure early intervention. Once the peeling has resolved and the skin is no longer sensitive, a post-peel skin care regimen can be started. An appropriate maintenance program is essential to maintain the results of chemical peeling.

▶ SUPERFICIAL CHEMICAL PEELS

Superficial depth peeling is achieved with injury to the epidermis only, ranging from mild exfoliation of the corneal cell layer to full thickness chemoexfoliation of the epidermis to the basal cell layer. The goal is to treat conditions of the epidermis including

TABLE 5.7   Postoperative Care (Superficial and Medium-Depth Peels)
• Cleanse the face with a gentle facial cleanser twice daily.
• Apply a thin layer of white petrolatum immediately after cleansing the face and reapply as needed.
• Avoid scrubbing, picking, or peeling the skin during the healing process.
• Avoid sun exposure during the healing process. Once the peeling is completed, apply sunscreen daily and protect from sun exposure.
• Once the peeling is complete and the skin no longer feels sensitive, patient may resume skin care regimen.
• Instruct the patient to notify the physician if they experience pain, worsening redness, discharge, or pustule formation during the healing process, as this could indicate an infectious process.

pigmentation (melasma, post-inflammatory pigment alteration, lentigines, ephelides), superficial texture, and acne (comedones, inflammatory acne, acne excoriae) while minimizing downtime.

Superficial chemical peeling is the most common type of peel performed due to its many advantages including low cost, minimal downtime, favorable safety profile, minimal discomfort, and versatility in all Fitzpatrick skin types and various body sites. Commonly used on the face, superficial peels can also be performed on areas of the body including dorsal hands, arms, neck, chest, and back. Deeper peels are generally contraindicated on the body due to increased risk of scarring. Superficial chemical peels are indicated for the treatment of pigmentary abnormalities (melasma, post-inflammatory pigment alteration (PIPA), ephelides, and lentigines), acne (comedones, inflammatory acne, acne excoriae), and superficial textural abnormalities. There are several limitations due to the shallow depth of wounding, as this method is ineffective for the treatment of full thickness epidermal lesions (macular seborrheic keratoses and actinic keratoses), rhytides, and scars. Repeat chemical peels are often necessary to achieve the desired cosmetic outcome, even when treating appropriate indications. Complications are generally limited (Table 5.1) and can include PIPA, prolonged erythema, infection and increased sensitivity to wind, sun, and temperature changes. Improperly performed chemical peels can include more serious complications such as scarring.

Peeling agents are numerous and include alpha hydroxy acids (AHAs) (lactic acid, glycolic acid, mandelic acid), beta hydroxy acids (salicylic acid), trichloroacetic acid 10% to 35%, tretinoin, and pyruvic acid. Jessner solution (JS) is a commonly used chemical peel containing a combination of chemicals including lactic acid, SA, and resorcinol. There are also many commercially available chemical peels containing proprietary combinations of various chemicals.

Alpha Hydroxy Acids (AHAs)

AHAs are carboxylic acids naturally found in fruits, vegetables, and sour milk. These were among the first chemicals used in aesthetic peeling in recorded history. Application of these to the skin causes exfoliation through reduction in desmosomes and tonofilament aggregation.[13]

The most popular AHA used in chemical peeling is glycolic acid (GA). GA peels are commercially available as free acids, partially neutralized (higher pH), buffered, or esterified solutions, in various concentrations ranging from 20% to 70%. The pH is determined by the free acid content. The factors affecting degree of peeling include concentration, pH, vehicle formulation, conditions of delivery, amount of acid applied, and duration of time the acid remains on the skin, which is most important. The multiple factors influencing GA peels make standardization of protocols and outcomes difficult. Generally, a GA peel of 30% to 50% for 1 to 3 minutes will produce minimal exfoliation. A peel of 50% to 70% for 1 to 4 minutes will produce light exfoliation, treating conditions such as acne or melasma.[14] Application of 70% for 3 to 7 minutes will produce greater peeling and is used to treat photoaging, skin texture, and solar lentigines. When using GA peels, one should begin with lower concentrations with short contact times and slowly increase with subsequent treatments, as indicated every 2 to 4 weeks.

When preparing the skin for a GA peel, one should not aggressively degrease the skin as recommended with other chemical peels. A gentle skin cleansing and single wipe with acetone or alcohol is sufficient. Scrubbing of the skin can result in uneven or unpredictable outcomes. The acid is applied using a large cotton-tipped applicator, gauze, or cotton ball to cover the treatment area swiftly, and a timer is set. Once the predetermined amount of time has passed, the peel is neutralized with water-soaked gauze. The patient can then rinse the area with water to ensure complete neutralization and removal of any remaining acid.

Salicylic Acid (SA)

SA is a lipophilic beta hydroxy acid. When applied to the skin, it decreases corneocyte adhesion and promotes exfoliation. As a derivative of aspirin (acetylsalicylic acid), SA also exhibits anti-inflammatory properties. In chemical peeling, SA is typically used in concentrations of 20% to 30% in an ethyl alcohol or polyethylene glycol vehicle to treat pigmentary abnormalities, comedonal and inflammatory acne, and rosacea. Formulation in a polyethylene glycol vehicle decreases systemic absorption and has shown to have minimal stinging and posttreatment hyperpigmentation.[15] The lipophilic nature of SA allows for penetration into the follicular unit and comedones. This quality accounts for SA peels efficacy in the treatment of acne vulgaris. Findings from a study comparing serial 30% SA peels to serial JS peels in the treatment of acne found that SA was superior at reducing comedonal acne and equal to JS at improving inflammatory lesions.[16] SA peels are very well tolerated and have an established safety profile in all Fitzpatrick skin types. Higher concentrations over large body surface areas pose a risk of systemic absorption causing salicylism. For this reason, SA peels are cautioned during pregnancy.

SA is applied to the skin using cotton-tipped applicators, gauze, or a brush. The patient may experience burning or stinging, which subsides rapidly, as SA has anesthetic properties. Evaporation of the vehicle leaves a white precipitate on the skin surface, allowing for easy evaluation of uniform application. The peel is self-limited and does not require neutralization or timing. After about 3 to 5 minutes, the treatment area is rinsed with tap water. Post-peel erythema and edema are minimal. Desquamation usually begins 2 to 3 days after the peel and lasts up to 7 days. Repeat peeling every 2 to 4 weeks is common to achieve aesthetic goals.

Trichloroacetic Acid (TCA)

TCA has been a staple in chemical peeling since the publication of Monash experiments in 1945.[1] It is a derivative of acetic acid, which when applied to the skin causes coagulation of proteins. TCA solution used in chemical peeling is created by mixing 100% anhydrous TCA crystals with distilled water. The concentration is calculated in weight/volume.[17] The solution is clear and colorless without precipitate. It is not sensitive to light and does not require refrigeration.[17] The acid will destroy plastic containers made of polycarbonate or low-density polyethylene tetrathalate and should therefore be poured from the master bottle into a small glass container, such as a shot glass.[18] TCA as a chemical peel does not require neutralization, as serum from the cutaneous vessels neutralizes the solution.

TCA 10% to 35% is used to accomplish superficial chemical peeling. The concentration correlates directly with the depth of penetration.[19] TCA 35% can reach the papillary dermis with multiple applications and is therefore considered a medium-depth peel by some. Penetration of the acid is significantly impaired by oils on the skin. It is therefore imperative to completely degrease the skin with alcohol and/or acetone on an abrasive gauze to ensure even penetration of the peeling solution. The acid is typically applied using a damp gauze or cotton-tipped applicators. TCA causes protein denaturation resulting in a white discoloration of the skin known as "frosting" (Figure 5.1). There are three levels of frosting: Level I is a light reticular frost over an erythematous background, Level II frost is a confluent white frost with scant erythema showing through, and Level III is opaque white without erythema. Because TCA penetration is slow, it is recommended to wait 5 minutes to assess the frosting end point before applying more solution to areas of need.[18] Although neutralization is not necessary, cold water compresses can be applied once the desired end point/frosting is achieved to prevent further penetration and assist with patient comfort.

FIGURE 5.1   Level II frost seen after 35% TCA application.

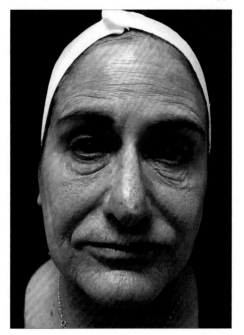

Jessner Solution (JS)

JS consists of 14% resorcinol, 14% SA, and 14% lactic acid in 95% ethanol (Table 5.8). Employed since the 1900s,[1] each component has specific effects on the skin. SA is a lipophilic compound which removes intercellular lipids causing disruption of corneocyte adhesion. This effect causes exfoliation and also enhances penetration of other agents. Lactic acid is an AHA, which diminishes corneocyte adhesion, resulting in desquamation. Resorcinol is structurally and chemically similar to phenol. It disrupts the weak hydrogen bonds of epidermal keratin. Due to the irritating and potentially allergic quality of resorcinol, a "modified Jessner's solution" was created, which replaced resorcinol with citric acid (Table 5.8).

JS is clear, faintly amber colored, sensitive to both light and air, and stable at room temperature. It is applied to the skin most commonly using a sable hair brush in two to three coats with an interval of 3 to 4 minutes each. The patient experiences burning upon application. White precipitation occurs on the skin with evaporation of the ethanol, resulting in a pseudo-frost. Exfoliation will typically last for 5 to 10 days depending on the amount of solution applied, pressure used, and number of coats. Peeling can be repeated at 4-week

TABLE 5.8 Composition of Jessner and Modified Jessner Solution	
Jessner Solution	**Modified Jessner Solution**
14% Lactic acid	17% Lactic acid
14% Salicylic acid	17% Salicylic acid
14% Resorcinol	8% Citric acid
In 95% ethanol	In 95% ethanol

intervals if necessary. It is recommended to begin conservatively and increase as needed with subsequent treatments.[18] JS can also be used in combination with TCA, resulting in a medium-depth peel (see medium-depth peels below).

▶ MEDIUM-DEPTH CHEMICAL PEELS

Medium-depth peeling involves injuring the skin to the level of the papillary or upper reticular dermis. This complete destruction of the epidermis leads to improvement in pigmentation abnormalities (melasma, PIPA, lentigines, and ephelides) and epidermal growths (macular seborrheic keratoses and actinic keratoses) (Figure 5.2). Penetration into the papillary dermis stimulates collagen growth, thereby improving superficial rhytides and scarring. The first medium-depth chemical peeling agent described was TCA 50%, which was unpredictable. Uneven penetration leads to erosions, PIPA, and scarring. Combination peels offer a more predictable and safer approach to medium-depth chemical peeling. With combination peels, the initial physical or chemical treatment of the skin causes disruption of the epidermis allowing for deeper, even penetration of the subsequent application of 35% TCA. The first combination peel was described by Harold Brody in 1986, combining solid carbon dioxide (CO_2) followed by 35% TCA. This is the deepest of the medium-depth chemical peels and is referred to as the "Brody peel."[20] Gary Monheit described using JS followed by 35% TCA, referred to as the "Monheit peel" in 1989.[21] The "Coleman peel" uses GA 70% followed by 35% TCA.[22] The results of a medium-depth peel can last for months to years depending on individual patient factors. A repeat peeling procedure is generally not recommended within 6 months.

The Brody Peel

CO_2 slush was commonly used in the 1980s as a physical modality to wound the epidermis, promoting exfoliation in the treatment of acne. This practice involves rubbing the skin with solid CO_2 ($-78.5°C$) dipped in 3:1 solution of acetone to alcohol allowing the dry ice to move freely over the skin and facilitate cooling of the skin surface. When used with chemical peeling, this decrease in skin temperature produces microepidermal

FIGURE 5.2   Before (A) and 1 month post medium-depth chemical peel (B) using solid carbon dioxide followed by 35% TCA.

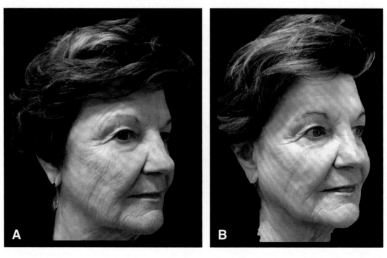

vesiculobullous formation, allowing deeper penetration of the subsequent TCA application. The pressure and amount of time the CO_2 is in contact with the skin (3-15 seconds) can be varied to facilitate deeper wounding of the skin. When CO_2 application is firm for 8 to 15 seconds, the wound depth can reach 0.62 mm, making it the deepest of the medium-depth chemical peels. As with all TCA peels, thorough skin cleansing and degreasing is essential for even penetration of the peeling solution. The application of TCA is most commonly described in reverse order for this peel, beginning with the lower eyelids and vermillion border using a damp cotton-tipped applicator. This is followed by application to the cheeks, chin, and forehead using a damp gauze. Once adequate frosting has occurred, ice packs are placed for patient comfort. The intense stinging will subside in 5 to 9 minutes. Once the patient is comfortable, the ice packs can be removed and a petroleum-based ointment is applied. Significant facial edema occurs in the first few days; however, discomfort is mild. The peeling usually begins on post-peel day 3 or 4 and is complete by day 10 (Figure 5.3).[20]

FIGURE 5.3 **Normal healing process following a medium-depth chemical peel using solid CO2 followed by TCA 35%. (A) Before, (B) day 1, (C) day 2, (D) day 3, (E) day 4, (F) day 5, (G) day 6, (H) day 7, (I) day 8, (J) day 10. The patient experiences significant facial edema on post peel days 1-3 and exfoliation on days 3-10**

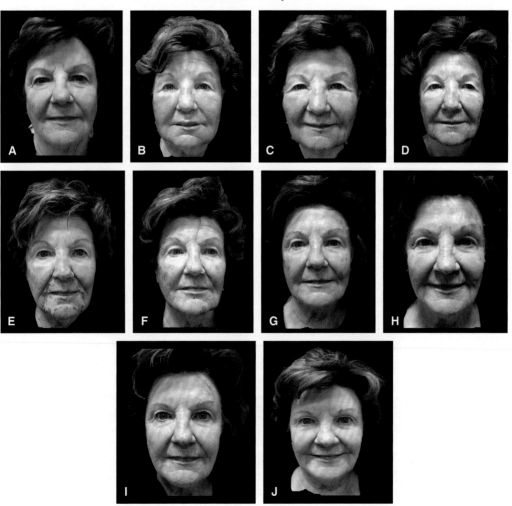

(Courtesy of Hema Sundaram, MD.)

▶ THE MONHEIT PEEL

First described in 1989, this combination medium-depth peel includes use of JS followed by 35% TCA. The JS acts as a keratolytic agent to further the absorption and penetration of the subsequent TCA peel. The procedure is usually performed with mild preoperative sedation and nonsteroidal anti-inflammatory agents. Thorough cleansing and degreasing are necessary for even penetration of the peeling solutions. The JS is first applied evenly using damp cotton-tipped applicators or a gauze. The application begins with the forehead and proceeds to the cheeks, nose, chin, and lastly the lower eyelids. One or two coats is required to achieve a light reticular frost. The frost achieved with JS is much lighter than that of TCA. Once the desired end point is achieved, 35% TCA is applied in the same manner. The white frost from the TCA application usually takes 30 seconds to 2 minutes. A Level II frost is desired. Uniform application of the peeling solution should result in even frosting; however, after 3 to 4 minutes, any incomplete areas can be retreated. The TCA should be reapplied to areas of need only. Once the desired end point is achieved, cool water or saline compresses are applied for 5 to 10 minutes until the patient is comfortable. Postoperative edema is expected for 2 to 4 days and desquamation will last for 7 to 10 days.[21]

The Coleman Peel

William Coleman III described a combination peel using 70% GA followed by 35% TCA. According to histologic studies, this peel produces the most superficial wounding of the medium-depth peels.[21] Aggressive degreasing is not needed prior to this procedure. After the face is washed with a gentle cleanser and dried, 70% GA is applied to the entire face with a thick cotton swab (such as a rectal swab). After 2 minutes, the peeling solution is neutralized with tap water. The face is patted dry and 35% TCA is applied using cotton-tipped applicators or gauze pads. Once the desired Level II frosting is achieved, cool compresses are applied until the patient is comfortable. Postoperative course is similar to those of the other medium-depth chemical peels.[22]

▶ DEEP CHEMICAL PEELS

Deep-depth peeling involves wounding to the reticular dermis and is indicated for the treatment of deeper rhytides and scarring. Phenol (carbolic acid) is currently the only chemical used to facilitate deep chemical peeling. Phenol causes keratocoagulation of the epidermis and dermis. When used alone (phenol 88%) in chemical peeling, the epidermal keratocoagulation limits further penetration, resulting in a medium-depth chemical peel. Croton oil is an epidermolytic agent, allowing for deeper penetration of the phenol when added to the formulation. This produces a deep chemical peel. The traditional deep chemical peel was first described by Baker and Gordon[23] and is still in use today. The formula (Table 5.9) is a combination of phenol, distilled water, Septisol©, and croton oil.[24] Septisol© is the emulsifying agent in all phenol-croton oil peel formulations described in the literature. This detergent contains triclosan, which has been banned by the US Food and Drug Administration, making Septisol© no longer commercially available. Clinical trials to replace the emulsifying agent with another detergent are ongoing.[24]

Complications are more common with deep chemical peeling, including cardiotoxicity, prolonged erythema, scarring, hypopigmentation, and infection. Deep chemical peeling is usually reserved for Fitzpatrick skin types I-III due to risk of pigmentation abnormalities. Appropriate antibacterial, antiviral, and yeast prophylaxis should be instituted based on

TABLE 5.9   Baker-Gordon Peel Formula

Phenol	49.3%	3 mL (phenol 88%)
Croton oil	2.1%	3 drops
Water		2 mL
Septisol©		8 drops

the peel and patient history. Phenol is rapidly absorbed through the skin. It is metabolized by the liver and renally excreted. Cardiotoxicity is a well-established systemic effect of phenol. Evaluation of liver function, renal function, and a baseline electrocardiogram (EKG) is indicated prior to performing a phenol peel. Arrhythmias are the most common cardiac abnormality seen.[25] This is more common in patients on medications known to cause QT interval prolongation, such as antihypertensives and antidepressants. Cardiac safety is a concern for procedures involving more than one cosmetic unit. A cosmetic unit is considered <0.5% body surface area (equivalent to the size of a palm without fingers). The face is divided into the following cosmetic units: forehead, perioral, periocular, nose, right cheek, and left cheek. To minimize the risk of phenol cardiotoxicity, the following precautions should be taken: hydration (oral for single cosmetic unit or intravenous for multiple cosmetic units), safety pauses of 10 to 15 minutes between cosmetic units, and continuous EKG monitoring.[24] Phenol is also irritating to the respiratory tract; therefore, proper room ventilation and provider masks are recommended.[26] Neoprene gloves are to be worn, as phenol may penetrate through latex and nitrile.[24]

Phenol has analgesic properties, but deep chemical peels require additional anesthesia. Numerous variations of preoperative, intraoperative, and postoperative analgesia are employed. These include nonsteroidal anti-inflammatories, opioids, benzodiazepines, regional nerve blocks, and field blocks. For full-face deep chemical peels, analgesics are often used in combination under the instruction of an anesthesiologist or nurse anesthetist.[26]

Phenol-croton oil peels are varied based on croton oil concentration, phenol concentration, use of occlusion, pressure used, number of strokes,[24] and number of consecutive days of treatment.[26] Recently, modified phenol formulas with croton oil in the range of 0.1% to 1.1% were described by Hetter. The lower croton oil concentrations (below 1%) have a decreased risk of pigmentation abnormalities and delayed healing.[27] Preoperative care, intraoperative technique, and postoperative care are complex and require specialized training through a residency training program or supervised hands-on continuing medical education.[24]

Segmental peels are commonly employed to optimize outcomes. The face is divided into six cosmetic units: forehead, periocular, perioral, nose, left cheek, and right cheek. These cosmetic units can be treated separately. For example, the perioral area can be treated with a deep peel to address severe rhytides while the rest of the face is treated with a medium-depth peel to address finer rhytides and photoaging.

TCA concentrations above 35% are only used for focal treatment of individual lesions, since scarring and pigmentary complications are common when used over large areas. TCA (>80%) can be used focally to treat specific skin conditions including rhinophyma, xanthelasma,[28] earlobe tears,[29] and ice pick acne scars.[30]

TCA used to treat acne scarring with a method known as chemical reconstruction of skin scars (CROSS) was first described by Lee et al. in 2002.[30] This technique utilizes a sharpened wooden stick or toothpick to apply 65% to 100% TCA focally into ice pick or boxcar acne scarring, as well as dilated pores (Figure 5.4). CROSS is safe in all Fitzpatrick skin types and does not require HSV prophylaxis. Aftercare is minimal, requiring twice

FIGURE 5.4   TCA CROSS application for the treatment of ice pick acne scarring.

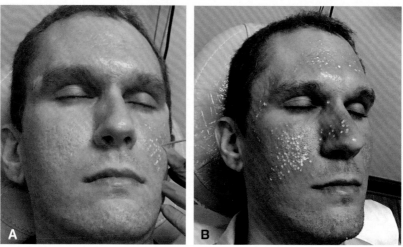

daily gentle skin cleansing, emollients, and sun protection. Healing is rapid, with only 5 to 7 days of downtime. Repeat treatments are necessary, as the degree of improvement is proportional to the number of CROSS treatments. Most cases require 3 to 6 courses with intervals of 4 to 6 weeks.

TCA 90% has also been reported for incomplete earlobe cleft repair (Figure 5.5). TCA is applied inside the earlobe cleft until frosting develops. No neutralization is needed. The ear lobule is then covered with micropore tape until complete cicatricial adhesion of the cleft occurs. Weekly treatments of TCA are repeated until all epidermis in the cleft is removed by TCA, allowing complete adhesion of the edges of the cleft. An average of 3.8 treatments were needed for complete repair. A linear inversion of the repaired cleft is common and can be treated with another application of TCA 90% to the linear indentation. The procedure is generally well tolerated.[29]

FIGURE 5.5   Incomplete ear lobe cleft defect before (A) and 6 weeks after (B) three treatments of TCA 90%.

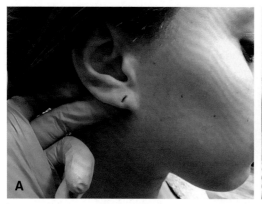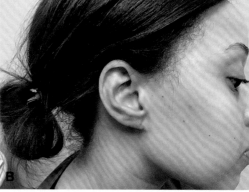

▶ BODY PEELING

Chemical peeling has traditionally been limited to the face, as non-facial areas are unpredictable and have higher complication rates. Compared to the face, non-facial skin has fewer hair follicles, sebaceous glands, and dermal vessels, which translates to decreased healing capacity. It is therefore recommended to limit chemical peeling of non-facial skin to superficial chemical peels only. Serial treatments are often times necessary to reach the aesthetic goal.

TCA 20% to 25% is commonly used to treat photoaging of the hands, arms, neck, chest, and upper back. It is recommended to treat the area with tretinoin for at least 4 weeks prior to the chemical peel. This will decrease healing time as well as decrease the time needed to achieve the end point of a frost.[18] A Level I or Level II frost is desired. These peels can be repeated every 14 to 60 days, once the erythema has completely resolved.

When treating macular seborrheic keratoses on the upper extremities, a 25% or 35% TCA is applied focally to the keratoses. Once frosting appears (usually 3-5 minutes), the entire area is treated with a lighter 20% to 25% TCA peel. This will provide a more uniform appearance of the skin.[18]

Kim and William Cook reported over 3000 cases using GA followed by TCA on non-facial skin.[31] Referred to as the "Cook Body Peel", potential treatment areas include arms, hands, chest, neck, back, and legs. First 70% GA gel is applied to the treatment area using a gauze, immediately followed by TCA 40% in the same manner. The desired end point is Level I frost (stippled frosting on an erythematous background). Once the end point is met, the peel is neutralized with a copious amount of 10% sodium bicarbonate solution. It is important to use GA gel and not solution, as the gel acts as barrier to the subsequent TCA. Use of GA solution could result in deeper penetration and scar formation.

▶ COMPLICATIONS

Pain

Pain and burning are expected during chemical peels. The intensity varies between patients and increases with the depth of the chemical peel. Some medium-depth and all deep chemical peels require analgesia to alleviate patient discomfort during the procedure. The patient should be pain-free at the conclusion of the chemical peel. There should not be postoperative pain except for the 8 to 12 hours after a deep chemical peel. If the patient experiences pain during the healing process, they should be evaluated for infection or contact dermatitis.

Ocular Injuries

Inadvertent ocular contact with the peeling solution can result in pain, possible scarring, and vision impairment. To avoid contact with the eyes, the patient's head should be positioned at a 30° to 45° angle and the peeling solution should never be passed over the patient's eyes. Care should also be taken to drain excess peeling solution from the cotton-tipped applicator or gauze to avoid dripping during application. Peeling solution can also be 'wicked' into the eyes through contact with tears. It is recommended to have an assistant blot any patient tears with a clean cotton-tipped applicator or gauze to avoid this. If ocular exposure occurs, an eyewash bottle of saline must be immediately available for flushing. In the case of phenol, mineral oil should be used for ocular flushing.

Cicatricial ectropion of the lower eyelid has been reported with deep chemical peeling. Predisposing factors include a history of blepharoplasty and senile lid laxity.[25] This usually resolves spontaneously within several months. Treatment includes adequate ocular moisturization and gentle massage of the lower eyelid skin.

Pruritus

Pruritus is common with exfoliation and reepithelialization. It is an expected part of the healing process and usually resolves within 1 to 4 weeks. Extreme pruritus can be a sign of allergic contact dermatitis and should be evaluated. Treatment includes oral antihistamines, topical emollients, and mild topical steroids.

Infection

Due to the disruption of the body's physical defense system, infections are possible. Bacterial, viral, and candidal infections can occur with chemical peeling. Bacterial infections are most commonly caused by *Staphylococcus*, *Streptococcus*, or *Pseudomonas* species.[32] The patient can present with pain, postponed wound healing, pustules, ulceration, discharge, or crusting. If a bacterial infection is suspected, a culture should be taken for identification and sensitivity and empiric antibiotics begun. Some physicians recommend dilute 0.5% acetic acid compresses three times daily or antimicrobial cleansers to prevent infections; however, research is lacking.

Reactivation of HSV is a well-established complication of chemical peeling. Antiviral prophylaxis should be considered in patients undergoing superficial chemical peeling with a history of recurrent orolabial HSV and always given in medium-depth and deep chemical peeling. HSV infection typically presents with pain and ulcerations. If suspected, a swab should be sent for HSV PCR and valacyclovir therapy started immediately. Scarring is possible following HSV reactivation.

Candidal infections can present with worsening erythema, pustules, pain, and pruritus. Treatment consists of oral fluconazole.

Toxic shock syndrome (TSS) has been reported with the use of an occluded phenol-croton oil peel. Symptoms of TSS include fever, hypotension, vomiting, diarrhea, myalgias, and rash. Immediate hospital admission, IV fluids, and appropriate antibiotic therapy are indicated if TSS is suspected.

Allergic Reactions

Allergic contact dermatitis (ACD) can occur with peeling solutions (resorcinol, SA, kojic acid, and lactic acid) as well as topical preparations used in aftercare, such as lanolin, neomycin, and additives (fragrances or preservatives). ACD typically takes 48 hours to develop and is characterized by intense pruritus, erythema, swelling, and vesicles (sometimes). Allergic reactions should be treated with avoidance of the allergen, antihistamines, and steroids (topical or systemic depending on severity of reaction).

Persistent Erythema

Erythema is common with all types of chemical peeling. It usually resolves in 3 to 5 days following superficial peels, 15 to 30 days following medium-depth peels, and 60 to 90 days following deep peels.[25] Erythema lasting beyond the expected timeframes should be evaluated. Some causes include infection, contact dermatitis (including retinoid dermatitis), and preexisting skin conditions (rosacea, atopic dermatitis). Prolonged erythema can also be a sign of impending scarring. Treatments include sun protection, topical steroids, and light treatments (intense pulsed light, pulsed dye laser, or KTP laser).

Pigmentary Changes

Pigmentary complications are more common in Fitzpatrick skin types IV-VI. In general, a chemical peel will result in a decrease in pigmentation. The margin of the chemical peel may result in a demarcation line due to the desired end point of pigmentary improvement immediately adjacent to the untreated skin. This can be avoided by feathering the peeling solution at the borders of the chemical peel.

Hypopigmentation commonly occurs following chemical peels due to removal of the melanin-containing epidermal cells, as well as melanocytes in medium-depth and deep chemical peels. This is usually temporary. Deep chemical peels using higher amounts of croton oil are at higher risk for permanent hypopigmentation.

Hyperpigmentation is the most common complication of chemical peeling. Risk factors include skin types III-VI, sun exposure, and use of exogenous hormones.[25] Treatment includes aggressive sun protection with daily use of physical sunscreen and sun avoidance, along with topical inhibitors of melanogenesis (hydroquinone, kojic acid, ascorbic acid, and azelaic acid). Superficial chemical peels (AHA or SA) can also be used to treat hyperpigmentation.

Milia

Milia are small follicular inclusion cysts that can occur 1 to 3 months after a chemical peel. They are usually temporary and can be treated with topical retinoids and extraction if the patient desires.

Acneiform Eruptions

Follicular inflammatory papules can occur soon after a peel. This can be due to the chemical peel itself or the use of comedogenic emollients. Oral anti-inflammatory antibiotics (tetracycline class) can be helpful.

Scarring

Scars are a rare but extremely undesirable complication of chemical peeling. High risk areas include the neck and body, as there are fewer pilosebaceous units to facilitate reepithelialization. Although uncommon, scarring with medium-depth and deep chemical peels is more common in areas of increased movement (jawline and perioral area).[18] Persistent erythema can predict scarring early, allowing for early intervention. Treatment includes topical steroids, intralesional steroids, silicone sheeting, vascular lasers, and resurfacing lasers.

▶ SUMMARY

Chemical peeling has demonstrated excellent clinical success and safety with treatment of the appropriate indication using an ideal technique. The level of wounding by the application of the chemical solution dictates recovery time, outcome, and potential complications.

Proper preoperative counseling is essential to minimizing risk, optimizing outcome, and patient satisfaction. The physician should be familiar with the chosen chemical to ensure that the operative technique is appropriate. Complications can be minimized by preparing the skin preoperatively, choosing the correct procedure, using proper application technique, and performing appropriate aftercare. The physician should be familiar with potential complications in order to recognize and treat them promptly. The use of chemical peeling to improve aesthetics has been practiced for centuries and will remain an essential part of the cosmetic surgeon's armamentarium.

REFERENCES

1. Brody HJ, Monheit GD, Resnik SS, Alt TH. A history of chemical peeling. *Dermatol Surg.* 2000;26:405-409.
2. *ASDS Procedure Survey 2017. American Society for Dermatologic Surgery 2018 Annual Report. 2018.* Available at www.asds.net/portals/0/pdf/annual-report-2018.pdf.
3. *American Society of Dermatologic Surgery procedure Survey 2016.* 2017 Available at https://www.asds.net/skin-experts/news-room/press-releases/asds-survey-nearly-105-million-treatments-performed in 2016.
4. Buchanan PJ, Gilman RH. Retinoids:literature review and suggested algorithm for use prior to facial resurfacing procedures. *J Cutan Aesthet Surg.* 2016;9(3):139-144.
5. Hevia O, Nemeth AJ, Taylor JR. Tretinoin accelerates healing after TCA peel. *Arch Dermatol.* 1991;127(5):678-682.
6. Kanye S, Leyden JJ, Lowe NJ, et al. Tazarotene cream for the treatment of facial photodamage. *Arch Dermatol.* 2001;137:1597-1604.
7. Gilbert S, McBurney E. Use of valacyclovir for herpes simplex virus-1 (HSV-1) prophylaxis after facial resurfacing: a randomized clinical trial of dosing regimens. *Dermatol Surg.* 2000;26:50-54.
8. Food and Drug Administration. *Accutane© Isotretinoin Capsules.* 1982. Availabe at https://www.accessdata.fda.gov/drugsatfda_docs/label/2008/018662s059lbl.pdf. Accessed. August 19, 2019.
9. Spring LK, Krakowski AC, Alan M, et al. Isotretinoin and timing of procedural interventions. A systemic review with consensus recommendations. *JAMA Dermatol.* 2017;153:802-809.
10. Waldman A, Bolton D, Arendt KA, et al. ASDS guidelines task force: consensus recommendations regarding the safety of lasers, dermabrasion, chemical peels, energy devices, and skin surgery during and after isotretinoin use. *Dermatol Surg.* 2017;43:1249-1262.
11. Hu L, Zou Y, Chang SJ, Qui Y. Effects of botulinum toxin on improving facial surgical scars: a prospective, split-scar, double-blind, randomized controlled trial. *Plast Recontr Surg.* 2018;141:646-650.
12. Zimbler MS, Holds JB, Lokoska MS, Glaser DA, Prendiville S. Effect of Botulinum toxin pretreatment on laser resurfacing results. *Arch Facial Plast Surg.* 2001;3:165-169.
13. Zakopoulou N, Kontochristopoulos G. Superficial chemical peels. *J Cos Dermatol.* 2006;5:246-253.
14. Moy LS, Murat H, Moy RL. Glycolic acid peels for the treatment of wrinkles and photoaging. *J Dermatol Surg Oncol.* 1993;19:243-246.
15. Dainichi T, Ueda S, Imayama S, et al. Excellent clinical results with a new preparation for chemical peeling in acne: 30% salicylic acid in polyethylene glycol vehicle. *Dermatol Surg.* 2008;34:891-899.
16. Dayal S, Amrani A, Shahu P, et al. Jessner's solution vs 30% salicylic acid peels: a comparative study of the efficacy and safety in mild to moderate acne vulgaris. 2016;16:42-51.
17. Bridenstine JB, Dolezal JF. Standardizing chemical peel solution formulations to avoid mishaps. *J Dermatol Surg Oncol.* 1994;20:813-816.
18. Brody HJ. *Chemical Peeling and Resurfacing.* Atlanta, GA: Emory University Digital Library Publications; 2008.
19. Lee KC, Wambier CG, Soon SL. Basic chemical peeling-superfical and medium-depth peels. *JAMA Dermatol.* 2019;81:313-324.
20. Brody HJ, Hailey CW. Medium-depth chemical peeling of the skin:a variation of superficial chemosurgery. *J Dermatol Surg Oncol.* 1986;12:1268-1275.
21. Monheit GD. The Jessner's + TCA peel:a medium-depth chemical peel. *J Dermatol Surg Oncol.* 1989;15:945-950.
22. Coleman WP III, Durrell JM. The glycolic acid trichloroacetic acid peel. *J Dermatol Surg Oncol.* 1994;20:76-80.
23. Baker TJ. The ablation of rhytides by chemical means. A preliminary report. *J Fla Med Assoc.* 1961;48:451-454.
24. Wambier CG, Lee KC, Soon SL, et al. Advanced chemical peels: phenol-croton oil peel. *J Am Acad Dermatol.* 2019;81(2)327-336. doi:10.1016/j.jaad.2018.11.060.
25. Costa IMC, Damasceno PS, Costa MC, et al. Review in peeling complications. *J Cosmet Dermatol.* 2017;16:319-326.
26. Rullan PP, Lemon J, Rullan J. The 2-day phenol chemabrasion for deep wrinkles and acne scars: a presentation of face and neck peels. *Am J Cosmet Surg.* 2004;21:15-26.
27. Hetter GP. An examination of the phenol-croton oil peel:part IV. Face peel results with different concentrations of phenol and croton oil. *Plast Reconstr Surg.* 2000;105:1061-1083.
28. Hague M, Ramesh V. Evaluation of three different strengths of trichloroacetic acid in xanthelasma palpebrarum. *J Dermatolog Treat.* 2006;17:48-50.

29. De Mendonca MC, de Oliver's AR, Araujo JM, et al. Nonsurgical technique for incomplete earlobe cleft repair. *Dermatol Surg.* 2009;35:446-450.
30. Lee JB, Chung WG, Kwahck H, et al. Focal treatment of acne scars with trichloroacetic acid:chemical reconstruction of skin scars method. *Dermatol Surg.* 2002;28:1017-1021.
31. Cook KK, Cook WR. Chemical peel of nonfacial skin using glycolic acid gel augmented with TCA and neutralized based on visual staging. *Dermatol Surg.* 2000;26:994-999.
32. Brody HJ. Complications of chemical peeling. *J Dermatol Surg Oncol.* 1989;15:1010-1019.

Hair Loss: Established Treatments and Emerging Therapies

Marc Avram, MD, and Nikhil Shyam, MD

Chapter Highlights

- Hair loss affects a significant number of men and women and has a profound effect on the quality of life.
- Androgenetic alopecia is the most common cause of hair loss and can be treated with topical, oral, or light therapy.
- Platelet-rich plasma is an emerging therapy for alopecia, although optimal preparations and protocols remain to be elucidated.
- Hair transplantation is another option for patients with hair loss, refractory to other therapies.

air loss, or alopecia, affects a significant proportion of the world's population and can have numerous psychological and social consequences. Alopecia is known to be associated with depression, introversion, and lower self-esteem. While there are several different types of hair loss, they are broadly categorized into two forms: nonscarring (preservation of hair follicles) and scarring (loss of follicular ostia). The most common type of hair loss is androgenetic alopecia (AGA) and affects 80% of men and 50% of women in the course of their lifetime.[1-3]

▶ ANDROGENETIC ALOPECIA

AGA is an androgen-dependent loss of hair that occurs in genetically predisposed men and women. Androgens, specifically dihydrotestosterone (DHT), have been shown to play an important role in the progression of AGA. Testosterone is converted to DHT by the type II isoenzyme of 5-alpha reductase that is expressed in the dermal papillae of hair follicles. Elevated levels of DHT result in many of the classic features of AGA including miniaturization of terminal hairs to vellus-like hairs and a prolonged telogen phase with shortening of the anagen growth phase.[4-6] Several androgen receptor polymorphisms have been noted, highlighting a polygenetic condition as well as an autosomal dominant inheritance.[7,8] Several studies have also reported single-nucleotide polymorphisms at different genomic loci associated with hair loss, including the AR/ EDA2R locus and 20p11 locus.[9] Clinically, men and women often exhibit different patterns of hair loss that have been described as male pattern hair loss (MPHL) and female pattern hair loss (FPHL), respectively. However, overlap in terms of distribution of hair loss may occur as well.

Male Pattern Hair Loss

Androgen-dependent hair loss is well established in men and typically presents with gradual thinning of hairs in the vertex scalp along with recession of the frontotemporal hairline. Typically, the occipital and parietal scalp remain unaffected. Classically, the Hamilton-Norwood scale (Figure 6.1) is utilized to describe the severity of MPHL.

Diagnosis is usually made through clinical history and physical exam with notable decreased density of hairs in the bitemporal and vertex scalp with prominent sparing of occipital and parietal areas.

Female Pattern Hair Loss

The role of androgens in the progression of FPHL is less well established. However, there is a strong genetic predisposition with 40% to 54% of patients reporting family history of pattern hair loss. The frequency of FPHL increases with age with 12% of women reporting symptoms by age 29%, 25% by 49 years, and >50% by 79 years.[10]

While FPHL and MPHL share a similar pathology resulting in progressive follicular miniaturization of terminal to vellus hairs and decreased anagen growth phase, the etiology of FPHL remains unclear. Interestingly, unlike MPHL, miniaturization in FPHL is not uniform and intense with relatively few areas of complete alopecia. While androgens are a primary driver of MPHL, many women with FPHL do not have elevated androgens. However, a genetic predisposition may exist whereby normal circulating levels of androgens act on follicular receptors that are highly sensitized. In addition, androgen-independent pathways may also exist that have yet to be elucidated.[11-13]

Polycystic ovarian syndrome and metabolic syndrome are the two most commonly associated comorbidities noted with FPHL. The association of decreased iron levels and thyroid disorders has also been associated with FPHL. Some studies have shown that antiandrogen therapy is more efficacious in patients with ferritin levels >40 μg/L.[14,15]

The diagnosis of FPHL is largely based on clinical history and physical exam. Details including when the hair loss started, whether it was gradual or sudden onset, and any associated physical, mental, or emotional stressors within the prior 3 to 6 months of hair loss are important to rule out acute and chronic telogen effluvium. Details regarding possible signs of hyperandrogenism including hirsutism, menstrual irregularities, acne, infertility, and ovarian abnormalities should be ascertained as positive findings and may necessitate laboratory workup. The physical exam is usually notable for widening of the central part with diffuse reduction in hair density over the frontal scalp (Figure 6.2). If there is any question regarding the diagnosis of hair loss, a scalp biopsy can provide valuable information.

FIGURE 6.1   The Hamilton-Norwood scale of male pattern hair loss.

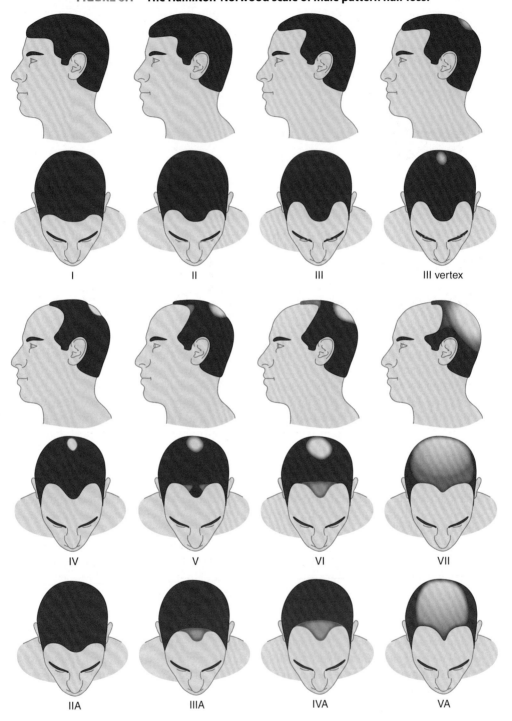

FIGURE 6.2   Ludwig scale classification of female pattern hair loss.

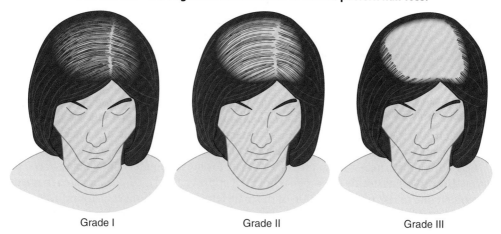

Grade I   Grade II   Grade III

▶ ESTABLISHED TREATMENTS OF ANDROGENETIC ALOPECIA

First-Line Treatments

Currently, the only US Food and Drug Administration (FDA)-approved drugs for pattern alopecia are minoxidil for men and women and finasteride for men alone. The only FDA-cleared device is low-level light therapy, also known as photobiomodulation therapy (PBMT). A recent meta-analysis on the treatment for AGA published in the *Journal of the American Academy of Dermatology* in 2017 supported these findings.[16]

Minoxidil

Minoxidil is a potent vasodilator that was initially approved for hypertension by the FDA in 1979. The topical formulations of 2% and 5% were eventually approved for the treatment of AGA in men in 1988 and 1991, respectively. In 1991, the FDA approved 2% minoxidil for FPHL and most recently approved 5% minoxidil foam for once daily application in 2014.

Minoxidil is a prodrug that is converted to minoxidil sulfate by sulfotransferase enzymes in the outer root sheath of hair follicles. It functions through opening potassium channels and stimulates hair growth by increasing the anagen phase of the hair cycle. It also improves perifollicular angiogenesis. The recommended treatment dose is 1 mL of the 2% solution twice daily to the affected areas (males can use the 5% solution as well) or 1 mL of the 5% foam once daily to affected areas. A minimum period of 12 months of treatment is required to determine efficacy. Clinically, approximately 40% of patients show significant improvement after 3 to 6 months of treatment. However, response is only sustained with continuous treatment and cessation of medication may induce telogen effluvium within 4 to 6 months. In addition, patients may experience transient shedding during the first few months of treatment. While generally well tolerated, few patients may develop an allergic or irritant contact dermatitis, which is related to propylene glycol that is present in the solution formulation but not the foam.

Finasteride

In terms of systemic treatment, finasteride is the only FDA-approved medication for the treatment of AGA in men and was approved in 1997. Finasteride inhibits the type II 5-alpha reductase enzyme thereby preventing the conversion of testosterone to the more potent DHT. Clinically, the drug is administered orally at a dose of 1 mg daily for the treatment of MPHL. Studies have shown that consistent use of the medication for 5 years may decrease hair loss by about 50% to 90% with notable increases in hair diameter and growth rate.[17] Hair regrowth is more likely in those who are younger and have milder hair loss. However, similar to minoxidil, the efficacy of finasteride is dependent on its continued use. Importantly, while clinical improvement may be seen as early as 3 months, consistent use of the medication for 6 to 12 months is necessary in order to evaluate for nonresponders (20%-30%).

The use of finasteride in women is not FDA approved and is contraindicated in pregnant women due to risk of feminization of the male fetus. While Shum et al. found 1.25 mg/day of finasteride improves FPHL in women with hyperandrogenism, there was no improvement in those without elevated androgens.[18] Additionally, Price et al. showed that 1 mg/day of finasteride taken for 12 months was ineffective in postmenopausal women with FPHL.[19] While some clinicians prescribe 1 to 5 mg of finasteride daily in postmenopausal women, its efficacy is highly variable. Larger, randomized controlled studies are required to determine the dosage and efficacy of finasteride in FPHL.

Post-Finasteride Syndrome

While finasteride is FDA approved for men and treatment is generally well tolerated, several side effects have been reported. These most commonly include decreased libido, erectile dysfunction, and decreased ejaculate volume that occur in approximately 1% to 4% of men. Prostate-specific antigen (PSA) levels may be reduced by approximately 50% during treatment due to decrease in DHT levels. This could mask an early diagnosis of prostate cancer and a baseline PSA is recommended in men older than 50 years prior to treatment initiation.[20,21] Other reported adverse events include gynecomastia, impotence, anxiety, depression, and memory disturbances. While these side effects generally resolve following cessation of the medication, there are growing reports of persistence of many of these symptoms post discontinuation in what has been referred to as a "post-finasteride syndrome." The most frequent symptoms reported include sexual dysfunction and psychological impairments including depression. Recent evidence suggests that finasteride may affect the metabolism of steroids in the brain and induce γ-aminobutyric acid imbalances, which could account for the symptoms noted in post-finasteride syndrome.[22] However, further research is required to understand this syndrome as well as potential risk factors for patients who may develop these symptoms. Prior to initiation of finasteride, it is important all patients are informed of the risks regarding post-finasteride syndrome in addition to a low risk of gynecomastia, reversible sexual side effects, and the effect finasteride has on PSA and prostate cancer.

Photobiomodulation Therapy

PBMT, also known as low-level light therapy or low-level laser therapy, is a relatively new FDA-cleared treatment for AGA but has its origins in the 1960s. Dr Endre Mester first noted the beneficial effects of accelerated hair growth in mice following use of a low-power 694-nm ruby laser in 1967.[23] The initial skepticism due to lack of studies with PBMT has gradually dissipated over the last decade with more evidence demonstrating its efficacy in the treatment of hair loss.

The FDA first cleared a PBMT device for the treatment of AGA in males in 2007. Subsequently, the direct-consumer market for hair loss devices has grown rapidly with an increasing number of FDA-cleared PBMT devices including combs, headbands, caps, and helmets. These devices are cost-effective and have an excellent safety profile.

Currently, there are 29 FDA-cleared devices for the treatment of AGA in men and women (Fitzpatrick I-IV) with 13 of these devices commercially available for home-use treatment. All PBMT devices contain either diode lasers or light-emitting diodes (LEDs) which emit light continuously or in short, rapid pulses. Compared with lasers, LED devices may be more appealing as they are easier and safer to use with less risk of burns, as they emit noncoherent light. They can also deliver energy to a wider area of the scalp and are less expensive. Most devices use wavelengths between 650 and 700 nm and contain anywhere between 7 and 272 diode lasers/LEDs conferring a total power output between 35 and 1360 mW.[24] The specifics of each FDA-cleared device for home-use is listed in Table 6.1.

There are no head-to-head studies comparing the efficacy between various PBMT devices. Patient preference is most important when selecting the appropriate device

TABLE 6.1 FDA-Cleared Lasers for Home Use

PBMT Device	Device Design	Light Parameters	Treatment Regimen	Approximate Retail Price
HairMax Prima 7 Laser Comb	Comb	7 LDs; 655 + 10 nm CW	15 min; 3 times a week	$295
HairMax Ultima 9 Laser Comb	Comb	9 LDs; 655 + 10 nm CW	15 min; 3 times a week	$395
HairMax Ultima 12 Laser Comb	Comb	12 LDs; 655 + 10 nm CW	8 min; 3 times a week	$495
NutraStim Laser Hair Comb	Comb	12 LDs; 655 + 10 nm CW	8 min; 3 times a week	$279
Theradome LH80 PRO	Helmet	80 LDs; 678 + 8 nm CW	20 min; 2 times a week	$895
iRestore Hair Growth System	Helmet	21 LDs; 650 + 10 nm CW 30 LEDs; 660 + 5 nm PE	25 min; every other day	$595
iGrow Hair Growth System	Helmet	21 LDs; 655 nm CW 30 LEDs; 655 nm PE	25 min; every other day	$695
Capillus82 Laser Cap	Sports cap	82 LDs;	30 min; 3-4 times a week	$799
Capillus202 Laser Cap	Sports cap	202 LDs; 650 nm PE	30 min; 3-4 times a week	$1999
Capillus272 Pro Laser Cap	Sports cap	272 LDs; 650 nm PE	30 min; 3-4 times a week	$3000
LaserCap LCPRO	Sports cap	224 LDs; 650 nm PE	36 min; every other day	$3000
HairMax LaserBand 41	Headband; moved by user every 30 s	41 LDs; 655 + 10 nm CW	3 min; 3 times a week	$595
HairMax LaserBand 82	Headband; moved by user every 30 s	82 LDs; 655 + 10 nm CW	90 s; 3 times a week	$795

CW, continuous wave; LD, laser diodes; LED, light-emitting diodes; PE, pulsed emission.
From Dodd EM, Winter MA, Hordinsky MK, Sadick NS, Farah RS. Photobiomodulation therapy for androgenetic alopecia: A clinician's guide to home-use devices cleared by the Federal Drug Administration. *J Cosmet Laser Ther.* 2018;20(3):159-167. Adapted by permission of Taylor & Francis Ltd, www.tandfonline.com.

including design, ease of use, and affordability. Office-based PBMT devices such as Capillus272™ OfficePro (Capillus LLC, Miami, FL) and the Sunetics Clinical Laser (Sunetics International Marketing Group LLC, Dallas, TX) are useful for patients who may not wish to purchase a device or who feel uncomfortable operating an at-home device.

Mechanism of Action

Photobiomodulation involves the use of low-energy light to induce a photochemical reaction at the cellular level. While the precise mechanisms underlying the therapeutic benefits of PBMT are still being elucidated, several theories have been proposed. PBMT stimulates mitochondrial signaling through activation of photoreceptors localized to the mitochondrial respiratory chain, specifically cytochrome C oxidase. Nitric oxide is known to inhibit cellular respiration and PBMT serves to release this inhibition thereby enhancing mitochondrial respiration. The subsequent increase in ATP results in increased production of growth factors, extracellular matrix deposition, and cell proliferation including hair growth. Photobiomodulation prolongs the anagen growth phase, increases existing hair diameter, and reverses miniaturization in AGA.

Interestingly, photobiomodulation exhibits the concept of hormesis with respect to activation of the mitochondrial respiratory chain. At low doses, PMBT stimulates the mitochondria but at a certain threshold, high doses may result in respiratory overdrive resulting in apoptosis. This could account for variability in treatment results and underscores the concept that more powerful devices or longer treatment sessions may not necessarily provide better results.

Efficacy and Side Effects

Patients with mild to moderate hair loss are most likely to benefit from PBMT but evidence is lacking for its use in the management of AGA. The efficacy of PBMT is comparable to minoxidil and up to 80% of patients report satisfaction with their results. Response to treatment may take between 12 and 16 weeks. Similar to minoxidil and finasteride, efficacy is dependent upon continuous use of the device. Importantly, PBMT empowers patients with a treatment option at home for their hair loss.

Contraindications for PBMT include pregnancy and breastfeeding primarily due to lack of any studies in these groups. Side effects are rare and most commonly include xerosis (5.1%), pruritus (2.5%), and scalp tenderness (1.3%). Irritation, redness, mild urticaria, and warm sensation have also been reported. While there is currently no evidence of toxicity or carcinogenesis, caution should be taken when using PBMT in areas of prior cancers (such as melanoma and nonmelanoma skin cancers on the scalp). Additionally, there are no reports of any ocular injury from any of the FDA-cleared devices, but patients should be counseled to avoid contact with eyes given the theoretical risk of damage to the retina from light exposure.[24]

Further studies are required to determine the optimal parameters for each PBMT device including power settings, wavelengths, and frequency of use for the treatment of AGA.

Second-Line Treatments for Androgenetic Alopecia

Spironolactone

Spironolactone is the most commonly used off-label antiandrogenic medication for the treatment of FPHL and hirsutism. It is a structural antagonist of aldosterone and also a potassium-sparing diuretic. It acts through competitive blockade of the androgen receptors as well as inhibition of ovarian androgen production. While published studies supporting the efficacy of spironolactone are limited, recommended treatment dosages range between 100 and 200 mg daily. While most patients tolerate the medication well, possible side effects include hypotension, electrolyte abnormalities (especially in the setting of renal disease), menstrual irregularities, breast tenderness, fatigue, and urticaria. Owing to its antiandrogenic effects, the medication may result in feminization of the male fetus and should be avoided in pregnancy and lactation.

Emerging Treatment for Androgenetic Alopecia

Platelet-Rich Plasma

Recently, platelet-rich plasma (PRP) has garnered significant interest in the treatment of alopecia. PRP is a plasma fraction that contains a greater concentration of platelets relative to whole blood, typically three- to sevenfold increased. Platelets contain alpha granules and upon their activation, secrete numerous growth factors (Table 6.2).

PRP may induce perifollicular angiogenesis, stimulate the proliferation of dermal papillary cells, and prolong the anagen growth phase, thereby offering an attractive option in the treatment of AGA. However, the precise mechanism by which PRP promotes hair growth remains under active investigation.

While there are numerous commercial and manual PRP processing techniques, the fundamental method remains the same. Typically, 10 to 60 mL of whole blood is collected from the patient on the day of treatment. Anticoagulants, like acid citrate dextrose or sodium citrate, are added to prevent coagulation and premature secretion of the alpha granules. The blood is then centrifuged to separate cell types based on specific gravity. Following centrifugation, three layers are noted (Figure 6.3): a top layer of plasma containing mostly platelets and few white blood cells (WBCs), a central buffy coat layer dense in WBCs, and a bottom layer of red blood cells (RBCs).

For the production of pure PRP (P-PRP) (Figure 6.4), only the most superficial buffy coat is collected with the lower portion of plasma. When leukocyte-rich PRP (L-PRP) is desired, the entire buffy coat is collected with the lower plasma layer. A second spin is sometimes performed to further concentrate the platelets. Finally, calcium gluconate, calcium chloride, or thrombin can be added prior to administration for activation of PRP (autologous activated PRP; AA-PRP). Active growth factor secretion begins within 10 minutes of activation. Alternatively, nonactivated PRP (autologous nonactivated PRP; NA-PRP) utilizes host dermal collagen and thrombin as endogenous activators.

TABLE 6.2	Major Growth Factors Within Platelet Alpha Granules
Platelet-derived growth factor (PDGF)	Promotes angiogenesis; mitogen for mesenchymal cells; upregulates the Erk pathway involved in cell proliferation and differentiation
Epidermal growth factor (EGF)	Stimulates differentiation of epithelial cells; upregulates the ERK pathway involved in cell proliferation and differentiation
Transforming growth factor beta	Promotes proliferation and differentiation of mesenchymal cells; promotes collagen synthesis
Fibroblast growth factor	Stimulates and regulates mitoses of mesenchymal cells; stimulates cell differentiation
Insulin-like growth factor 1	Stimulates proliferation and differentiation of mesenchymal cells; promotes collagen synthesis; induces and prolongs anagen growth phase
Vascular endothelial growth factor	Promotes angiogenesis; differentiation of endothelial cells; increases permeability of endothelial cells

FIGURE 6.3   Layers of blood after centrifugation.

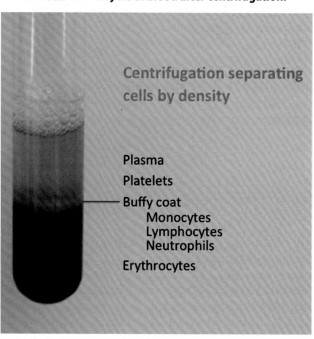

(Reprinted from Hessler MJ, Shyam N. Platelet-rich plasma and its utility in medical dermatology: a systematic review. *J Am Acad Dermatol.* 2019;81(3):834-846. Copyright © 2019 American Academy of Dermatology, Inc. With permission.)

Magalon et al. (2016) proposed four parameters for reporting PRP processing in hopes of creating a standardized protocol. Collectively, this is referred to as DEPA: dose, efficiency, purity, and activation. The dose is calculated by multiplying the platelet concentration in PRP by the obtained volume of PRP (measured in billions or millions of platelets).

FIGURE 6.4   Pure platelet-rich plasma (PRP) versus leukocyte-rich PRP in a single-spin (softspin) technique or a two-spin technique.

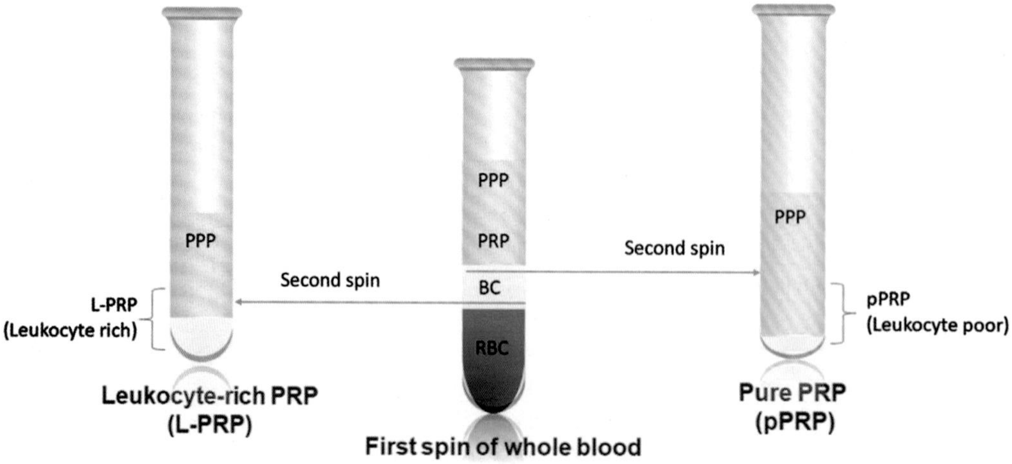

(Reprinted from Hessler MJ, Shyam N. Platelet-rich plasma and its utility in medical dermatology: a systematic review. *J Am Acad Dermatol.* 2019;81(3):834-846. Copyright © 2019 American Academy of Dermatology, Inc. With permission.)

The efficiency is the percentage of platelets recovered in the PRP from whole blood. Purity refers to the composition of platelets, WBCs, and RBCs in the final PRP preparation. Activation denotes the agent used to activate PRP.[25] The most optimal PRP collection technique that yields the greatest clinical results remains to be defined.

PRP is generally considered safe with minimal side effects and few contraindications as noted below (Table 6.3).

PRP as Monotherapy in Androgenetic Alopecia

There have been numerous studies evaluating the use of both AA-PRP and NA-PRP in the treatment of AGA. While single injections of NA-PRP appear to lack efficacy, a recent study by Kachhawa et al. (2017) showed promising results with leukocyte-rich, NA-PRP when used as a series of treatments. Specifically, patients reported subjective improvements in hair quality when PRP injections were performed serially every 3 weeks for a total of six sessions. Patients with milder AGA experienced better results compared to patients with more advanced alopecia. Patients reported subjective increases in hair quality/thickness and 55% reported increased hair density.[26]

Several studies have evaluated PRP following activation with calcium gluconate or calcium chloride. Gentile et al. (2017) treated 20 males with AGA every 30 days for three total injections.[27] At 3 months, the PRP group showed a significantly greater increase in mean hair count and terminal hair density compared to placebo. Patients were followed for 16 months, the longest documented follow-up time published to date. Histologically, PRP-treated skin showed increases in epidermal thickness and numbers of follicles, higher Ki67 in basal keratinocytes and hair follicular bulge cells, and an increase in perifollicular vasculature, compared to baseline. At 12 months, disease relapse was observed in 20% of patients requiring retreatment at 16 months.

Alves and Grimalt (2016) treated 22 patients with AA-PRP in a series of three monthly injections. Compared to control, patients treated with PRP showed an increase in mean total hair density at both 3 and 6 months.[28] Tawfik et al. (2018) evaluated activated L-PRP in 30 females with FPHL in weekly treatments for four consecutive weeks. Patients were followed up at 6 months and folliscope measurements noted a significant increase in both hair density and hair thickness in the PRP-treated scalp compared to placebo. At 6 months, hair pull test improved in 83% of PRP-treated areas and patients reported an overall high satisfaction with a mean rating of 7.0 of 10.[29]

PRP as Adjunct Treatment for Androgenetic Alopecia

Given the benefit of PRP as monotherapy in the treatment of AGA, several studies have focused on the utility of PRP in conjunction with existing treatment options, such as minoxidil or finasteride. Importantly, many patients with AGA fail these first-line treatments and PRP may present a valuable adjunct in this population.

TABLE 6.3   Contraindications to PRP

Absolute Contraindication	Relative Contraindication
• Critical thrombocytopenia • Platelet dysfunction • Hemodynamic instability • Sepsis • Local infection at the site of platelet-rich plasma administration • Patient unwilling to accept risk	• NSAID use within 48 h • Glucocorticoid injection at the treatment site within 1 mo • Systemic glucocorticoid use within 2 wk • Tobacco use • Recent illness or fever • Cancer, especially bone or hematolymphoid • Anemia to hemoglobin <10 gm/dL • Thrombocytopenia to <105 platelets/µL

Alves and Grimalt (2017) performed a randomized, double blind, placebo-controlled, split-scalp study of 24 subjects (11 males; 13 females) who received three monthly treatments of intralesional nonactivated-PRP to one-half of the scalp and saline to the other half. These patients were randomized to either concomitant topical 5% minoxidil twice a day or oral finasteride 1 mg daily. At 6 months, significantly greater increases in mean hair count, hair density, and terminal hair density were documented with PRP compared to saline. Notably, the PRP/minoxidil combination produced significantly greater improvement in mean hair count, hair density, anagen to telogen percentages, and mean anagen/telogen ratio compared to PRP/finasteride combination therapy.[30]

Proposed Treatment Protocol for Androgenetic Alopecia

The current evidence of PRP for the treatment of AGA is promising. Numerous studies have noted benefits utilizing a wide range of outcome measures including photography, mean hair count and density, anagen to telogen ratio, hair pull test, and patient satisfaction surveys. While PRP may be utilized as monotherapy, its optimal efficacy lies as combination treatment with other first-line therapies such as minoxidil and/or finasteride.

In the current literature, there is wide variability in the preparation of PRP—utilizing commercial versus manual techniques, single versus double spin centrifugations, AA-PRP versus NA-PRP, variable platelet concentrations, injection volumes ranging between 2 and 12 mL, and variability in depth of injection (dermal versus subdermal). Based on the review of current literature, most positive studies utilize mean platelet concentrations of three to sixfold the mean platelet concentration of whole blood with monthly treatment sessions for 3 to 4 months. While results are noted with both dermal and subdermal injections, there is less pain with the latter as well as increased diffusion possibly minimizing the number of required injections per treatment area. While most studies do not follow patients' clinical course beyond 6 months, Gkini et al. (2014) noted reduction in hair density at 6 and 12 months. In addition, Gentile et al. (2015) noted relapse at 16 months. This is congruent with the current clinical practice of administering maintenance injections 3 to 6 months post the initial series of 3 to 4 monthly treatments. Subsequent treatment should be performed on an individual basis given lack of current clinical data. PRP is well tolerated with only transient erythema or pain noted at the time of injection with resolution within 24 hours.

▶ HAIR TRANSPLANTATION

Hair transplantation is an outpatient, local anesthetic, surgical treatment option for women and men with thinning hair. With advancements over the last two decades, patients can expect consistently naturally appearing transplanted hair compared to the past (Figure 6.5).

This is because of an evolution in technique from "plugs" containing 10 to 20 hair follicles harvested from the donor region in the occipital scalp to exclusively utilizing natural 1 to 4 follicular units that grow on the scalp harvested either via a donor ellipse or by a follicular unit extraction (FUE) (Figure 6.6).

Candidate selection and surgical technique are vital to the success of the procedure.

Candidate Selection

As with all surgical procedures, candidate selection is the key to success for hair transplantation. Patients must have adequate donor density in their posterior scalp to donate to fill thinning areas in their frontal scalp. The higher the donor density (follicular units per cm^2), the more the hair available to transplant. If a patient has poor donor density, there is minimal impact a transplant can provide for a patient.

FIGURE 6.5   (A) Pre and (B) post hair transplantation utilizing follicular units to restore a natural hairline appearance.

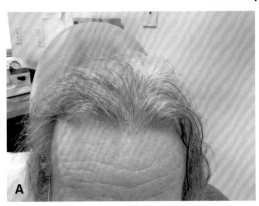
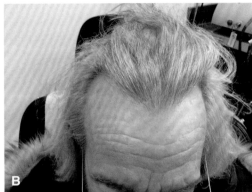

For all patients, both FUE (robotic or nonrobotic) and elliptical donor harvesting are reviewed. Both elliptical donor harvesting and FUE remain state-of-the-art donor harvesting techniques and should be discussed with patients as options. Both create individual follicular units that when placed in recipient area will create natural appearing transplanted hair. For FUE, a patient's donor hair needs to be trimmed to 1 mm for harvesting whether performed manually or with the robot. For many men with shorter hairstyles, this a minor inconvenience. They overwhelmingly choose robotic FUE to avoid a linear scar that could be visible with their shorter hairstyle and due to the minimally invasive nature of this technique, where sutures are not needed. For most women and some men, trimming their hair to 1 mm is a major practical limit to pursuing FUE. They opt for elliptical donor harvesting that leaves a linear scar and will be camouflaged by their hair.

MPHL and FPHL are chronic conditions with ongoing hair loss throughout life. The rate and extent of hair loss varies from person to person but it always continues. This is

FIGURE 6.6   Magnified image showing transplantation of natural follicular units ranging from one to four hairs.

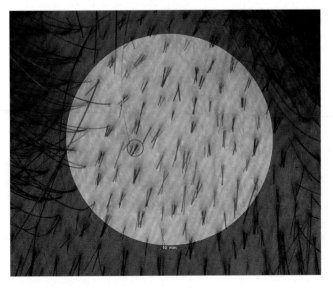

a vital concept to review with all patients. The physician must plan for optimal short- and long-term cosmetic results. A discussion of medical therapy to maintain existing hair is done for all patients. Clearly, minimizing future loss through medical therapy allows maximum cosmetic impact from a hair transplant. A combination of successful medical therapy plus surgery will create the most perceived density from a procedure. The physician should always plan a procedure assuming a patient *may* want to stop medical therapy in the future and should consider how that would impact the cosmetic appearance of the transplant. The frontal scalp for men and women has the greatest cosmetic impact with the least long-term cosmetic risk for most patients.

Preoperative and postoperative wound care and activities should be reviewed with patients (Table 6.4).

Patients should understand the finite amount of donor hair, the ongoing nature of MPHL and FPHL, and how that will impact the density and cosmetic appearance of their hair over time. The ability to place hair where it will look natural in both the short and long term is also essential when determining whether a patient is a candidate for hair transplantation. As with all elective procedures, if a patient does not understand the limitations of the procedure, it should not be performed.

Operative Technique

Elliptical Donor Harvesting

The optimal donor area is the mid occipital scalp for both men and women. This region is the highest density with the lowest chance to naturally thin in the future. The donor region is trimmed to 1 mm. The hair above it is taped up so that after the procedure, it will cover the sutures.

The patient is placed in the prone position and anesthetized with lidocaine with epinephrine. The length and width depend on the number of follicles needed to transplant into the frontal scalp. Once the ellipse is removed, the wound is closed with a single layer of staples or sutures, which are removed 7 to 10 days postoperatively.

Robotic Follicular Unit Extraction Operative Technique

It is mandatory with robotic hair transplantation that the hair in the donor region is trimmed to 1 mm before the procedure is performed. The hair is trimmed to 1 mm by the surgical assistants using a moustache trimmer (Figure 6.7).

TABLE 6.4   Preoperative and Postoperative Instructions

Preoperative Instructions	Postoperative Instructions
• Review consent and written instructions sent to patient before the procedure. Anything unclear contact the office. • Day of procedure eat/drink normally. • Written consent/verbal postoperative instructions reviewed. • Area to be transplanted marked and photographed. • MD reviews procedure with patient.	• Resume regular activities immediately. • Avoid heavy exercise 5-7 d postoperatively. • Prednisone 40 mg daily for 3 d. • Pain medication first 12-24 h. • Overnight dressing removed next day. • Shower day after surgery. Avoid picking scabs off. Let time/shower remove scabs over 5-8 d. • Emollients to the donor region twice daily for 5-10 days. • Transplanted hair begins to grow 3-6 mo. • Full hair growth 9-18 mo.

Longer hair will prevent the robot from working at maximum efficiency. The optical scanner of the robot used to identify and harvest follicular units needs to see pigment in hair follicles to function. Patients with gray, blond, or red hair have the hair follicles dyed black by the assistants after being trimmed. This is of no practical cosmetic impact since the hair is only 1 mm in length. The patient lies in the prone position while the donor region is anesthetized. Once completed, the patient moves to the robot for donor harvesting. The patient sits in the chair designed for the robot with their head leaning forward and with their chin touching the top of their chest. This allows the robot to see and harvest the grafts optimally. A 3 cm × 3 cm grid is placed into the anesthetized area on the posterior scalp. This grid has fiducial markers to guide the robot to harvest follicular units within that grid. The robot calibrates and removes 90 to 110 follicular units from each grid (Figure 6.8).

Depending on the number of follicular units needed for the procedure, 5 to 20 grids are used per procedure. The robot uses two punches—one sharp to cut through the dermis followed by one "dull" punch that then fires deeper into the superficial subcutaneous tissue to loosen an individual follicles unit from the skin. The robot has an algorithm that will not allow it to deplete a region on the scalp. The robot will not harvest grafts closer than 1.6 mm between follicular units.

Once the grafts have been created by the robot, a surgical assistant removes the follicular units and places them into a holding solution until they are placed into the recipient site (Figure 6.9).

It is vital that the hairs do not desiccate. If they desiccate, they will not grow.

After the last follicular units are removed from the donor region, a temporary pressure dressing is applied to the scalp. The patient may get up, stretch, and take a break, possibly checking their messages or having a snack. After the break, the patient returns to the room for placement of grafts into the recipient zone.

FIGURE 6.7   The donor area is trimmed to 1 mm when utilizing the follicular unit extraction technique.

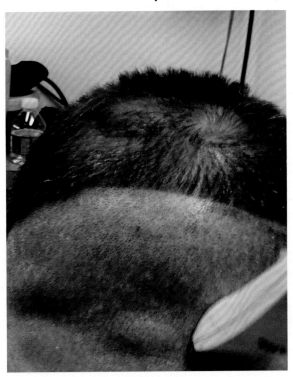

FIGURE 6.8   A 3 cm × 3 cm grid serves as a fiducial marker to guide robotic harvesting of follicular units within that grid.

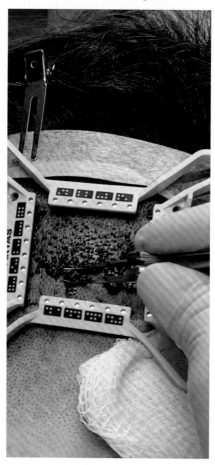

Creating Recipient Sites and Placing Grafts

The robot is able to create recipient sites and place grafts as well as harvest follicular units from the donor region. There are several practical impediments that make creating recipient sites and placing grafts with a robot less popular than donor harvesting. These include:

1. Needing to trim hair in the frontal scalp to 1 mm to make recipient sites and place grafts.
2. Slower speeds than a trained staff in placing grafts.
3. Less flexibility in creating custom hairlines than with a traditional #19-#21 gauge needle.

Many men will trim their posterior scalp for FUE but many will be reluctant to trim their entire scalp to 1 mm for harvesting, site making, and graft placement. If there was a clear advantage in quality or speed, some would be willing to comply but there is no clear advantage over a trained physician and surgical team in making sites and placing grafts manually with the current technology. For physicians without experience in making sites or without an experienced surgical team, the robot can be helpful but offers no clear advantage for their patients.

Recipient sites created manually are done so with a variety of different needles ranging in size from #19 to #21 gauge. Sites are created at 30° to 40° angles parallel to existing hair

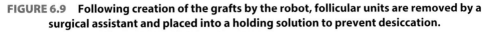

FIGURE 6.9   **Following creation of the grafts by the robot, follicular units are removed by a surgical assistant and placed into a holding solution to prevent desiccation.**

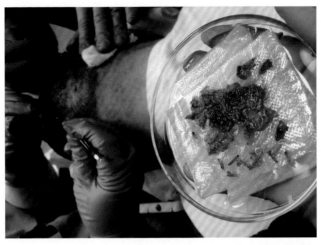

follicles. Many physicians use magnified polarized LED lights for clarity and to assist in making recipient sites without transecting existing hair follicles (Figure 6.10).

The surgical team then places the grafts using microvascular forceps.

Postsurgical Wound Care

Once the last graft is placed either robotically or by the surgical team, an overnight dressing is placed. The dressing is to protect the grafts while they heal overnight. Patients can resume regular activities immediately but are told to avoid strenuous exercise for 7 days. Patients are given a short course of oral steroids to prevent frontal edema and a few pills of a mild pain medication. Unless medically indicated, antibiotics are not prescribed. The day after the procedure, the dressing is removed by the patient and they can shower. Patients are then instructed to apply emollients to the donor region for 5 to 7 days. Patients can resume full sports and strenuous physical activities 1 week after the procedure. Postsurgical perifollicular hemorrhagic crusting dissipates within 6 to 8 days with a daily shower. The transplanted hair enters a telogen resting phase 3 to 6 months post surgery. The hair follicles begin to grow 3 to 9 months post surgery and have a cosmetic impact for patients 9 to 14 months postsurgery.

Robotic Versus Manual Techniques

Over the past two decades, men and women have been able to expect consistently natural appearing transplanted hair. This is due to the use of individual follicular units as opposed to larger grafts used in the past. The challenge for physicians performing contemporary hair transplant surgery is the ability to harvest and place hundreds to thousands of hair follicles during a procedure. To accomplish this, a team of trained surgical assistants is required to efficiently perform the procedure. Elliptical donor harvesting and FUE whether performed robotically or nonrobotically are state-of-the-art techniques for donor harvesting. For physicians not performing hair transplantation regularly, creating hundreds or thousands of follicular units from an ellipse is challenging. The robot is able to perform much of the work a trained surgical team would have done in the past. For some physicians this has been a revolutionary new tool. The challenges that remain include appropriate candidate selection, realistic expectations, successful medical therapy to maintain existing hair, and planning a procedure for both potential short- and long-term future hair loss. Furthermore, the robot is a state-of-the-art instrument but does not have the judgment and artistic ability of an experienced hair transplant surgeon.

FIGURE 6.10   Recipient sites are created manually under magnification at angles parallel to existing hair follicles.

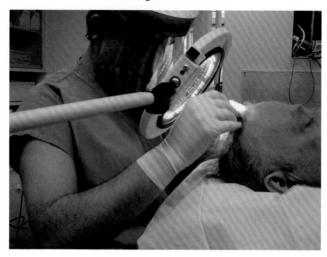

PRP and Hair Transplantation

Recently, there have been two studies that explored the utility of PRP in combination with FUE hair transplant surgery. Growth factors in PRP may serve as both an optimal follicular graft preservation solution as well as stimulating the receptor area prior to follicle implantation.

Suruchi Garg (2016) performed a single-blind, prospective randomized study on 40 patients undergoing FUE. Nonactivated, leukocyte-rich PRP (NA-L-PRP) was injected in the dermis and subcutaneous scalp of patients in the PRP group immediately following creation of slits in the recipient area. Control groups were injected with normal saline. Evaluation was performed at 2, 4, and 8 weeks as well as 3 and 6 months. At 6 months, all 20 subjects in the PRP group had >75% hair regrowth compared to only four patients in the control group. Compared to controls, the PRP group demonstrated faster time to achieving high density of hairs, reduced catagen loss of transplanted hairs, faster postsurgical healing, and activation of dormant follicles. Patients in the PRP group also noted increased hair lengths compared to the control group.[31]

Most recently, Navarro et al. (2018) evaluated 30 hair transplant patients (19 male, 11 female) where 15 patients received FUE surgery in combination with PRP compared to conventional FUE surgery alone. The combination group underwent treatment of the receptor sites with injections of 3 to 4 cm^3 of activated, pure PRP (AA-P-PRP). In addition, during the harvesting phase, follicular transfer units were immersed in AA-P-PRP with the formation of a fibrin clot around the grafts as a preservation biomaterial for three hours prior to implantation. Patients with combination treatment showed faster postsurgical crust healing and hair fixation compared to the control group (9 ± 1 days versus 18 ± 5 days, respectively). The PRP-treated group showed reduced postsurgical follicle loss compared to controls. In addition, the postsurgical inflammation period was also significantly reduced including scalp pain, itching, and redness resulting in a faster postoperative recovery period. Importantly, no adverse events were noted in any treatment groups.[32]

▶ SUMMARY

There have been significant advances in the treatment of AGA in the past few decades. Hair transplantation remains the most definitive treatment for androgenetic hair loss.

With new emerging treatments such as PRP and photobiomodulation, it is likely that combination treatment will become the cornerstone of therapy for pattern hair loss.

REFERENCES

1. Cash TF. The psychological effects of androgenetic alopecia in men. *J Am Acad Dermatol.* 1993;26(6):926-931.
2. Cash TF, Price VH, Savin RC. Psychological effects of androgenetic alopecia on women: comparisons with balding men and with female control subjects. *J Am Acad Dermatol.* 1993;29(4):568-575.
3. Drupa Shankar DS, Chakravarthi M, Shilpakar R. Male androgenetic alopecia: population-based study in 1005 subjects. *Int J Trichology.* 2009;1(2):131-133.
4. Braun-Falco O, Plewig G, Wolff HH, Landthaler M. *Braun-Falco's Dermatology.* 3rd ed. Berlin, Heidelberg: Springer-Verlag Berlin Heidelberg; 2009.
5. Batrinos ML. The endocrinology of baldness. *Hormones (Athens).* 2014;13:197-212.
6. Sawaya ME, Price VH. Different levels of 5α-reductase type I and II, aromatase, and androgen receptor in hair follicles of women and men with androgenetic alopecia. *J Invest Dermatol.* 1997;109:296-300.
7. Heilmann S, Kiefer AK, Fricker N, et al. Androgenetic alopecia: identification of four genetic risk loci and evidence for the contribution of WNT signaling to its etiology. *J Invest Dermatol.* 2013;133:1489-1496.
8. Hagenaars SP, Hill WD, Harris SE, et al. Genetic prediction of male pattern baldness. *Plos Genet.* 2017;13:e1006594.
9. Cobb JE, Zaloumis SG, Scurrah KJ, et al. Evidence for two independent functional variants for androgenetic alopecia around the androgen receptor gene. *Exp Dermatol.* 2010;19:1026-1028.
10. Birch MP, Lalla SC, Messenger AG. Female pattern hair loss. *Clin Exp Dermatol.* 2002;27:383-388.
11. Herskovitz I, Tosti A. Female pattern hair loss. *Int J Endocrinol Metab.* 2013;11(4):e9860.
12. Redler S, Messenger AG, Betz RC. Genetics and other factors in the aetiology of female pattern hair loss. *Exp Dermatol.* 2017;26:510-517.
13. Orme S, Cullen DR, Messenger AG. Diffuse female hair loss: are androgens necessary? *Br J Dermatol.* 1999;141:521-523.
14. Ramos PM, Miot HA. Female pattern hair loss: a clinical and pathophysiological review. *Bras Dermatol.* 2015;90(4):529-543.
15. El Sayed MH, Abdallah MA, Aly DG, Khater NH. Association of metabolic syndrome with female pattern hair loss in women: a case-control study. *Int J Dermatol.* 2016;55:1131-1137.
16. Adil A, Godwin M. The effectiveness of treatments for androgenetic alopecia: a systematic review and meta-analysis. *J Am Acad Dermatol.* 2017;7(1):136-141.
17. Kaufman KD. Long-term (5-year) multinational experience with finasteride 1 mg in the treatment of men with androgenetic alopecia. *Eur J Dermatol.* 2002;12:38-49.
18. Shum KW, Cullen DR, Messenger AG. Hair loss in women with hyperandrogenism: four cases responding to finasteride. *J Am Acad Dermatol.* 2002;47:733-739.
19. Price VH, Roberts JL, Hordinsky M, Olsen EA, Savin R, Bergfeld W. Lack of efficacy of finasteride in post-menopausal women with androgenetic alopecia. *J Am Acad Dermatol.* 2000;43:768-776.
20. D'Amico AV, Roehrborn CG. Effect of 1 mg/day finasteride on concentrations of serum prostate-specific antigen in men with androgenic alopecia: a randomised controlled trial. *Lancet Oncol.* 2007;8:21-25.
21. Guess HA, Gormley GJ, Stoner E, Oeserling JE. The effect of finasteride on prostate specific antigen: review of available data. *J Urol.* 1992;155:3-9.
22. Motofei IG, Rowland DL, Tampa M, et al. Finasteride and androgenetic alopecia; from therapeutic options to medical implications. *J Dermatol Treat.* 2020;31:415-421. doi:10.1080/09546634.2019.1595507.
23. Mester E, Szende B, Tota JG. Effect of laser on hair growth of mice. *Kiserl Orvostud.* 1967;19:628-631.
24. Dodd EM, Winter MA, Hordinsky MK, Sadick NS, Farah RS. Photobiomodulation therapy for androgenetic alopecia: a clinician's guide to home-use devices cleared by the Federal. *Drug Adm.* 2018;20(3):159-167.
25. Magalon J, Chateau AL, Betrand B, et al. DEPA classification: a proposal for standardizing PRP use and a retrospective application of available devices. *BMJ Open Sport Exerc Med.* 2016;2(1):e000060.
26. Kachhawa D, Vats G, Sonare D, Rao P, Khuraiya S, Kataiya R. A spilt head study of efficacy of placebo versus platelet-rich plasma injections in the treatment of androgenic alopecia. *J Cutan Aesthet Surg.* 2017;10:86-89.
27. Gentile P, Garcovich S, Bielli A, Scioli MG, Orlandi A, Cervellia V. The effect of platelet-rich plasma in hair regrowth: a randomized placebo controlled trial. *Stem Cell Transl Med.* 2015;4:1317-1323.
28. Alves R, Grimalt R. Randomized placebo-controlled, double-blind, half-head study to assess the efficacy of platelet-rich plasma on the treatment of androgenetic alopecia. *Dermatol Surg.* 2016;42:491-497.
29. Tawfik AA, Osman MAR. The effect of autologous activated platelet-rich plasma injection on female pattern hair loss: a randomized placebo-controlled study. *J Cosmet Dermatol.* 2018;17:47-53.
30. Alves R, Grimalt R. Platelet-rich plasma in combination with 5% minoxidil topical solution and 1 mg oral finasteride for the treatment of androgenetic alopecia. *Dermatol Surg.* 2017;44:1.
31. Garg S. Outcome of intra-operative injected platelet-rich plasma therapy during follicular unit extraction hair transplant: a prospective randomized study in forty patients. *J Cutan Aesthet Surg.* 2016;9(3):157-164.
32. Navarro RM, Pino A, Martinez-Andres A, et al. The effect of plasma rich in growth factors combined with follicular unit extraction surgery for the treatment of hair loss: a pilot study. *J Cosmet Dermatol.* 2018;17(5):862-873.

Treatment of Excess Fat

Ethan C. Levin, MD, Jessica B. Dietert, MD, and
Eva A. Hurst, MD

Chapter Highlights

- Tumescent liposuction has revolutionized the ability to offer in-office fat reduction therapy.
- Further modifications such as laser-assisted liposuction may result in increased skin tightening and improved aesthetic results.
- Adipocyte sensitivity to low temperatures results in selective apotposis during cryolipolysis.
- Radiofrequency and high-intensity focused ultrasound devices have also emerged as noninvasive technologies for fat reduction.
- Deoxycholic acid is an injectable therapy for treatment of localized submental fat.

▶ LIPOSUCTION

Liposuction was developed in Europe during the late 1970s as a localized fat-removal technique. It was first performed in the United States in 1982 by otolaryngologist Dr Norman Martin. However, up to this point in time, the procedure was performed using general anesthesia or IV sedation. It was not until 1987, when dermatologist Jeffrey Klein first described the tumescent technique, that liposuction was performed exclusively using local anesthesia.[1] This development greatly increased the safety and tolerability of liposuction. In subsequent years, pioneers in the field reported low overall complications across thousands of cases treated with up to 55 mg/kg total dose of lidocaine.[2-5]

▶ TUMESCENT TECHNIQUE FOR LOCAL ANESTHESIA

The term tumescent describes the firm and swollen quality of tissue when infiltrated with large volumes of fluid. The technique allows for significant amounts of dilute lidocaine, epinephrine, and sodium bicarbonate solution to be delivered to the skin and subcutaneous tissues. By diluting the concentration of anesthetic, systemic absorption is slowed.[4,5] The large volume of interstitial fluid creates a local tissue reservoir, which prolongs the duration of action and reduces the need for postoperative narcotics. Another benefit of tumescence is that it physically lifts the targeted fat, creating a hydrodissection effect. This enables a uniform, precise removal during aspiration.

Prior to the use of epinephrine in the anesthetic solution, the amount of whole blood in the liposuction aspirate approached half of the volume. This is reduced to 1% to 3% when epinephrine is used. As a result, there is decreased bruising, decreased postoperative pain, and a vastly reduced need for intraoperative fluid replacement.

As with other locally injected anesthetics, sodium bicarbonate is added to reduce discomfort on infiltration. Unbuffered lidocaine has a pH of 3.5 to 5.5, which can result in significant burning and stinging when infused into the skin. Adding bicarbonate raises the pH to a physiologic range, minimizing these side effects.

While the principles of tumescence can apply to many anesthetics, lidocaine is the most commonly used and has the greatest safety record.[4,6-10] According to the full prescribing information, the maximum recommended dose of lidocaine is 7 mg/kg in adults. In general, a total dose of 500 mg should not be exceeded.[11] However, up to 35 to 55 mg/kg can be safely used in tumescent anesthesia.[4,5] The pharmacokinetics can be explained by the effect of concentration gradient on the rate of diffusion.

Lidocaine is a hydrophobic molecule that diffuses quickly across cell membranes. Blood levels correlate with signs of systemic toxicity. The amount of lidocaine that moves from the infiltrated tissue into the vascular space is proportional to the concentration gradient. In other words, higher concentrations of lidocaine lead to higher blood levels and increased risk of toxicity. In a study of almost 10,000 nerve blocks, all eight toxicity events were attributed to inadvertent intravascular injection.[12] In mice studies, the higher the concentration injected subcutaneously, the lower the lethal dose (Table 7.1).[13] Thus, dilute concentrations allow for the use of a higher total dose of lidocaine.

Lidocaine is metabolized by the cytochrome P450 system in the liver. Those patients with a history of liver disease or abnormal liver function may be at increased risk for lidocaine toxicity. Medications which are known to inhibit the cytochrome P450 system should be reviewed. If these medications cannot be safely discontinued, the maximum dose of lidocaine should be adjusted. Initial manifestations of lidocaine toxicity include circumoral paresthesias, lightheadedness, and euphoria. As lidocaine levels increase, symptoms progress to include nausea, vomiting, blurred vision, seizures, and cardiac and respiratory depression (Table 7.2).

In tumescent anesthesia, the concentration of lidocaine ranges from 0.05% to 0.15%. The lowest, 0.05%, results in the greatest tumescence and is the dose recommended in Klein's seminal study.[4] However, some authors note that higher concentrations of 0.1% or 0.15% provide better anesthesia for sensitive sites such as the inner thighs, stomach, flanks and breasts. One strategy to maximize the efficiency of each treatment is to infiltrate with 0.05% lidocaine solution and keep 0.1% solution on hand during the session for any areas that require additional anesthetic for patient comfort. The recipe for tumescent lidocaine solution, sample dosing volumes, and a maximum dose calculation is shown in Tables 7.3, 7.4, and 7.5, respectively.

TABLE 7.1   Effect of Lidocaine Dilution on Fatal Toxicity in Mice After Subcutaneous Injection[13]

Lidocaine Concentration (%)	LD$_{50}$ of Lidocaine in Mice (gm/kg)
0.5	1.07
1.0	0.72
2.0	0.59
4.0	0.42

TABLE 7.2   Lidocaine Levels and Toxicity[4]

3-6 µg/mL	Subjective toxicity • Lightheadedness, euphoria • Digital and circumoral paresthesias • Restlessness, drowsiness
5-9	Objective toxicity • Nausea, vomiting, tremors, blurred vision • Tinnitus, confusion, excitement, psychosis • Fasiculations
8-12	Seizures, cardiorespiratory depression
12	Coma
20	Respiratory arrest
26	Cardiac arrest

TABLE 7.3   Recipe for Tumescent Lidocaine Solution (Lidocaine 0.05%, Epinephrine 1:1,000,000)[4]

Lidocaine	500 mg (50 mL of 1% Lidocaine Solution)
Epinephrine	1 mg (1 mg of 1:1000 epinephrine solution)
Sodium bicarbonate	12.5 mEq (12.5 mL of 8.4% NaH_2CO_3 solution)
Normal saline	1000 mL of 0.9% NaCl solution

The resultant solution is lidocaine (0.047%), epinephrine (1:1,063,500), and sodium bicarbonate 11.8 mEq/L in 1063.6 mL of saline 0.84%.

TABLE 7.4   Tumescent Lidocaine Solution Approximate Volumes by Anatomic Site[4]

Abdomen, Upper, and Lower	500-2000 mL
Hip	400-1000
Thigh, lateral and medial	600-1200
Knee	200-500
Male breast	400-1200
Submental chin	100-200
Upper arms	500-1200

TABLE 7.5   Maximum Dosage Calculation for Tumescent Lidocaine 0.05% Solution in a 70 kg Patient

(55 mg/kg) (70 kg) = 3850 mg
(3850 mg)/(0.5 mg/mL[a]) = 7700 mL

[a]1% lidocaine solution is 10 mg/mL; 0.05% lidocaine solution is 0.5 mg/mL.

Maximum anesthetic dosing limits the amount of liposuction that can be done in a given tumescent treatment session. When more than one treatment session is needed to maintain safe dosing levels, we recommended 1 month interval between treatments. However, some surgeons treat additional sites within several days. In order to maximize the efficiency of each treatment, it is important to aspirate within 10 to 30 minutes after infiltration. While the lidocaine's onset is almost instantaneous, epinephrine takes longer to reach the therapeutic threshold. Blanching of the overlying skin is a visible clue that vasoconstriction has occurred. Waiting too long after infiltration diminishes the efficacy of the lidocaine and increases the chance that more anesthetic will be needed.

Prilocaine does not have an indication for tumescent anesthesia in the United States, but it is used in Germany and other European countries. Limited clinical data show it to be effective and well tolerated.[14-16] In comparison to lidocaine, prilocaine has less cardiotoxicity and more rapid excretion. Some surgeons advocate for use of a combination of lidocaine and prilocaine when large volumes of tumescent anesthesia are needed in order to reduce the risk of side effects.[14] One disadvantage of prilocaine is that it results in the dose-dependent formation of methemoglobin. However, this has not proven to be clinically significant in causing any adverse events while used during tumescent liposuction.[16] There are no data for other anesthetics, including bupivacaine, for use in tumescent anesthesia during liposuction.

Patient Selection and Preoperative Counseling

Appropriate surgical candidates for liposuction are generally in good health and at or near ideal body weight. Localized areas of excessive fat deposits can be targeted. Patients should understand that liposuction is not an appropriate treatment for generalized obesity.

A thorough medical history is obtained with particular attention given to history of clotting disorders, liver disease, and allergy to lidocaine. Medications are reviewed and adjustments made to those that inhibit cytochrome P450.

A physical exam is performed. During this time, the provider will formulate a plan with the patient based on priority areas to treat and anticipated volume of tumescent anesthesia. Preoperative photographs are obtained. If indicated by history, review of systems, or extent of planned treatment, preoperative laboratory studies can be performed including complete blood count with differential, basic metabolic panel, liver function tests, prothrombin time, and partial thromboplastin time. Hepatitis and HIV screening may also be done.

Once the treatment plan has been agreed upon with the patient, expectations for the treatment and postoperative period are reviewed. Patients are instructed to wear dark, loose fitting clothing. They can eat breakfast and medications normally on the day of surgery. Supplements that cause increased risk for bleeding or those that inhibit lidocaine metabolism are stopped. While there is no data to support this recommendation, most surgeons prescribe antibiotics beginning the evening before the procedure and extending for 5 to 7 days after. We prefer a first-generation cephalosporin. Trimethoprim/sulfamethoxazole or doxycycline are appropriate substitutes if there is a contraindication or a patient history of methicillin-resistant *Staphylococcus aureus*. To help with pain control and patient comfort, lorazepam can be given before the procedure.

Surgical Equipment

There are three types of devices used to administer tumescent anesthesia: infusion pumps, syringes, and cuffs. Powered pumps are the most practical way to deliver high volumes of

FIGURE 7.1   Powered pump (Wells Johnson Company, Tucscon, AZ) with tubing and 22-gauge spinal needle for administering tumescent anesthesia.

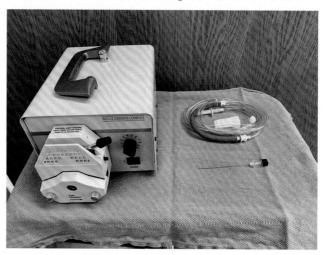

solution (Figure 7.1). Syringes may be preferred for small areas requiring more control. Pressure cuffs are a third option. They are inexpensive and do not require power to operate.

All of these devices are connected to needles or cannulas to deliver the anesthetic solution into the tissues. While cannulas allow for faster infusion time, needles are preferred for tough or fibrous areas. Twenty or twenty-two gauge, three-and-one-half inch spinal needles are a good choice because of their length and flexibility (Figure 7.2). Due to their blunt tips, cannulas are more comfortable for patients during repositioning. They often have multiple ports at the distal end, which enables a larger area to be infiltrated and decreases the need for repositioning. When withdrawing the cannula, back-pressure events can cause the anesthetic solution to spray out of the ports that are no longer inside the patient. To prevent this from happening, a stopcock is used or the distal end of the infusion tubing is kinked before withdrawal of the cannula.

Once the treatment areas have been adequately tumesced with anesthesia, aspiration is performed with mechanical aspirators or syringe suctioning for small areas. There is an assortment of electric-powered aspirators available for purchase. Most machines have a vacuum system that generates 1 atmosphere of negative pressure. Control dials are used to decrease the pressure in sensitive areas.

FIGURE 7.2   Twenty-two gauge, 3.5-inch spinal needle.

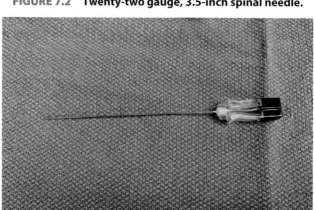

FIGURE 7.3   Sixty-milliliter Toomey syringe.

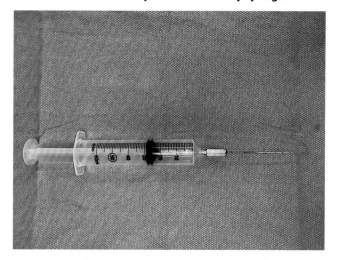

Syringes are the simplest way to accomplish aspiration. These create negative pressure from manually withdrawing the plunger on a large-volume syringe. Typically, a 60-mL Toomey syringe is used (Figure 7.3). A lock is placed on the withdrawn plunger to maintain the vacuum during aspiration.

Liposuction cannulas are made in various sizes, tip shapes, diameters, and hole configurations (Figure 7.4). Depending on the treatment site, typical sizes range from 10 to 25 cm in length and from 2 to 4 mm in diameter. The tips can be blunt, bullet, spatula, or "V" shaped. Less aggressive treatment starts with smaller diameter cannulas with blunt tips and a single port. As you increase the diameter of the cannula, number of ports, or change the tip shape, treatment is more aggressive.

There are powered cannulas available to assist the surgeon in the back and forth motion of aspiration. One benefit is that these devices enable smaller diameter cannulas (i.e., 2 mm) to be used for the entire procedure.

FIGURE 7.4   Examples of different cannulas and handles used in tumescent liposuction.

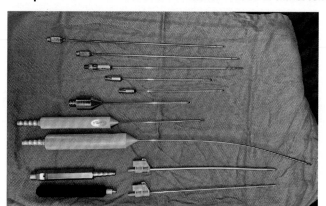

Procedural Approach

Careful marking with the patient in standing position using a permanent ink is helpful to delineate treatment areas and sections of peripheral feathering (Figure 7.5). This is important to do in order to set clear patient expectations of treatment areas and to mark any asymmetries and the exact desired areas of adipose tissue prior to swelling from the tumescent anesthesia occurs.

In order to access the subcutaneous adipose tissue, incisions through the skin are made with a 15 blade, 11 blade, or punch biopsy tool. They should be sized to the cannula. For example, if using a 2 mm cannula, a 2 mm punch tool can be used. Entry points can be anesthetized with the same tumescent solution used for the fat compartment, but some use injection of 0.5 to 1 mL of 1% lidocaine with 1:100,000 epinephrine. Some undermining can be helpful to facilitate cannula entry. The number of incisions depends on the area treated and the reach of the cannula. They should be oriented to allow the cannula to travel along the long axis of the site and to enable overlapping treatment in a triangular criss-cross pattern. After surgery, some surgeons suture the entry points, but often these wounds are left open to heal by second intention and facilitate drainage.

Once the entry sites have been made, anesthetic solution is infused into the fat compartment. One hand is placed on the target area to feel tissue tumescence. The end point is achieved when the maximum volume of anesthesia has been infused and/or the tissue is noted to be appropriately tumesced with blanching and a peau d'orange pebbled appearance of the skin is visible. To maximize patient comfort, the infusion is started slowly (i.e., 1 mL/min) and is increased as tolerated. The entire area to be treated is anesthetized in a pattern that minimizes needle repositioning. Anesthesia should be infused a few centimeters beyond the edge of the treated area.

After infiltration is complete, wait at least 10 minutes before aspiration, or start with the first area anesthetized. This allows for full onset of the vasoconstrictive effect of epinephrine. Aspiration of fat is patterned similar to the anesthesia, often in an overlapping fanned pattern. To ensure even results, make crossing tunnels at different depths in the fat. This often requires multiple passes over the treatment area from each access point with progressively larger cannulas.

FIGURE 7.5   Marking prior to liposuction of the flank/lower back. Circles indicates areas of adipose tissue, with fullest areas marked with "x" and straight lines to indicate areas of feathering during treatment.

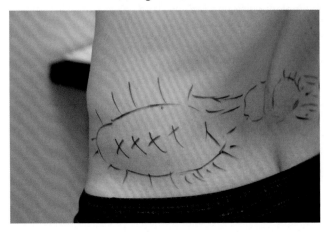

When handling the cannula, the near dominant hand is used to move it back and forth and the far "safe" hand is positioned overlying the treatment area to gauge position and depth. Grasping the fat with the far hand can help move the cannula into different areas. The cannula is continuously repositioned at slightly different angles in both radial and axial planes such that small tunnels are made throughout the treatment area. The cannula is feathered into adjacent tissues to ensure sufficient blending. The end point is reached once the goal volume of aspirate is obtained. Gently pinching the skin between the thumb and the second finger can be used to measure adequacy of fat removal. These authors recommend carefully standing the patient once to twice during the treatment session to assess symmetry with the aid of the original placed markings.

Postprocedural Care and Recovery

After the procedure is complete, the wounds are dressed with a sterile compression dressing. This is composed of an absorbent pad, netting, and a compression wrap or garment. The patient can expect active drainage during the first day, decreasing over the next several days. They will need to clean the entry points with antimicrobial soap and replace the dressings as they become saturated, likely several times per day the first 48 hours after treatment. Compression can be used for several days and is beneficial for up to 2 weeks.

The most commonly reported side effects of liposuction include swelling, bruising, itching, and numbness in the treated area. These usually subside over 1 to 2 weeks. Some patients will have persistent focal areas of numbness as well as palpable bumpiness or nodularity in the fat that can be massaged and treated with warm compresses. There are no reports of death among patients receiving liposuction from dermatologists using tumescent local anesthesia. The overall serious adverse event rate (per case) ranges from 0% to 0.16%.[2,3,7,17-20] Reported events include infection, venous thromboembolism, hematoma/seroma formation, and allergic reactions to antibiotics or garments. A meta-analysis of 24 liposuction studies showed that tumescent anesthesia alone had the lowest serious adverse event rate when compared to other methods that incorporated systemic anesthesia.[21]

Laser-Assisted Liposuction

Laser-assisted liposuction (LAL) augments manual aspiration by using selective photothermolysis to target fat and promote collagen contraction.[22] This can be performed during liposuction or before it as a separate procedure. Lasers used include the 980 nm diode, 1064 nm neodymium-doped yttrium aluminum garnet (Nd:YAG), 1064/1320 nm Nd:YAG, and 1440 nm. There are a variety of devices available commercially. Many use a combination of wavelengths to both target vasculature within the adipose tissue and stimulate collagen formation and skin tightening. Laser cannulas are small and minimally invasive. These "microcannulas" are ~1 mm in diameter and contain a smaller laser fiber within the cannula.

A recent meta-analysis comparing LAL to traditional liposuction found LAL to have better fat reduction, skin tightening, and patient satisfaction.[23] However, many of the included studies had a high risk of bias. Complication rate and severity from LAL do not differ significantly from traditional liposuction.[19]

▶ CRYOLIPOLYSIS

Background and Clinical Development

Although tumescent liposuction remains a popular choice for the removal of unwanted fat, it is an invasive surgical procedure. In recent years, there have been significant advancements in technology for noninvasive body contouring. This includes cryolipolysis, radiofrequency, and ultrasound devices. These devices target the physical properties inherent to fat. They carry the promise of decreasing the risk of side effects and shortening recovery time.

Cryolipolysis is the newest and most popular addition to the armamentarium of noninvasive fat-loss treatments. The advent of cryolipolysis stems from the observation of cold-induced panniculitis.[24-26] Also known as "popsicle panniculitis", this was first reported in a child who presented with an isolated indurated plaque on the cheek followed by transient atrophy of subcutaneous tissues after eating a popsicle. This led to the discovery that adipocytes are more sensitive to cold injury than surrounding tissue. In 2007, Anderson and colleagues introduced the first device aimed at fat-reduction through cold-induced apoptosis.[27] Known as cryolipolysis, this technique involves applying a cold applicator at a set temperature and time to a targeted area resulting in selective adipocyte injury. This triggers an inflammatory response and apoptosis-mediated loss of adipocytes.[27]

Cryolipolysis (CoolSculpting™; Zeltiq, Pleasanton, CA) is US Food and Drug Administration (FDA) cleared for treatment of the abdomen, flanks, thighs, upper arms, and submental region in individuals with a BMI of 30 or less. Other areas that have been treated include the lower back and inframammary folds. Candidates for cryolipolysis are those who need small to moderate reductions in fat. Clinical studies performed to date report 10% to 30% reduction in fat volume over 2 to 6 months of follow-up.[28-37] The most common method to quantify fat loss is using ultrasound or calipers. While the greatest change in fat volume is after the first treatment, a second treatment may result in approximately one-half the loss seen in the first treatment.[34,36] Some may benefit from more than two treatment sessions, contingent upon response and tolerability. Treatments should be spaced at least 6 weeks apart.

Procedural Approach

The CoolSculpting™ System is composed of an applicator that is applied to the target surface and is held in place with vacuum suction. Applicators come in different sizes depending on the treatment area (Table 7.6). A lubricant gel is applied before placing the applicator on the skin. A disposable trap is used to prevent gel from getting suctioned into the vacuum. Once the applicator is in place, the vacuum suction is turned on and the treatment session starts. The device sustains a preset cooling temperature for the duration of the treatment period. Support straps are attached from the vacuum head to a support pillow to secure the applicator in place and increase patient comfort. Treatment temperature and duration vary depending on the anatomic site and applicator used.

The machine has a "Cool Intensity Factor" (CIF) which is a measure of the rate of heat removal from body tissue. Clinical studies report using a CIF of 34 or 42, corresponding to a fat temperature of −5°C and −10°C, respectively. The treatment duration is between 30 and 60 minutes. The newest applicators, CoolAdvantage Plus and the CoolAdvantage Petite, report a treatment profile of −11°C for 45 and 35 minutes, respectively.[38]

Postprocedural Care and Recovery

Once the treatment is completed and the applicator is removed, the tissue is firm and cold to touch. A "butter stick" deformity of elevated, edematous tissue is expected and resolves within 6 minutes[30] (Figure 7.6). Immediate posttreatment changes to the skin include erythema, edema, and purpura. Two to five minutes of posttreatment massage may enhance fat loss.[35] Study authors posited that massage may enhance reperfusion injury to adipocytes.

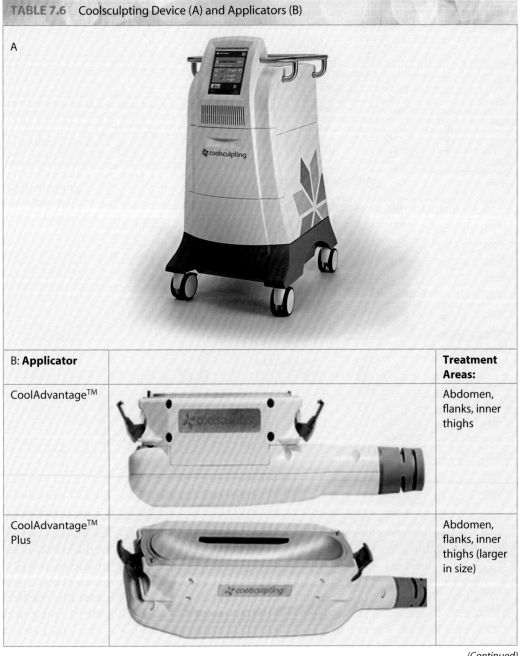

TABLE 7.6   Coolsculpting Device (A) and Applicators (B)

B: **Applicator**		**Treatment Areas:**
CoolAdvantage™		Abdomen, flanks, inner thighs
CoolAdvantage™ Plus		Abdomen, flanks, inner thighs (larger in size)

(Continued)

TABLE 7.6	Coolsculpting Device (A) and Applicators (B) (Continued)	
CoolMini™		Submental region
CoolSmooth PRO™		Non-pinchable fat (e.g., outer thighs)
CoolAdvantage Petite™		Upper arms

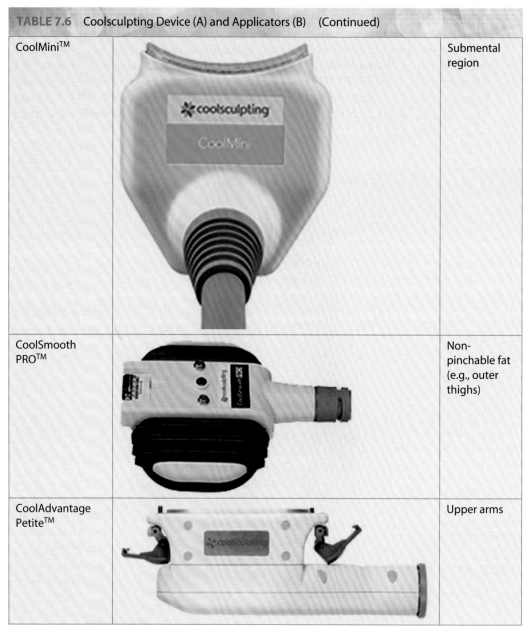

Following treatment, most patients experience edema, erythema, and purpura, which resolve within 1 to 2 weeks. Of sixty patients treated in the original pilot study, only three had mild swelling 1 week after treatment. Half of the patients reported numbness and 20% reported tingling at that time. These symptoms resolved in all patients by the 12-week follow-up visit. One study performed histologic analysis to further examine this reported side effect. Pre- and posttreatment biopsies did not reveal any quantitative or qualitative changes to peripheral nerves.[29]

FIGURE 7.6   A, "Butter stick" deformity of elevated, edematous tissue immediately after cryolipolysis, followed by resolution at 2 (B), 4 (C), and 6 (D) minutes.

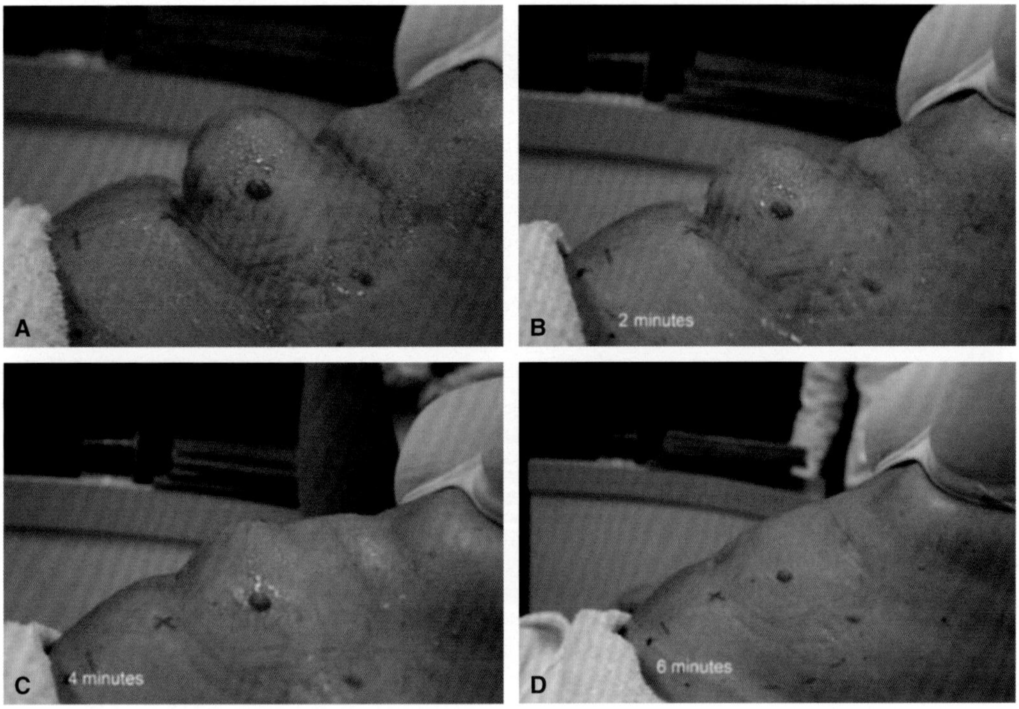

(Borrowed with permission from Dierickx CC, Mazer JM, Sand M, et al. Safety, tolerance, and patient satisfaction with noninvasive cryolipolysis. *Dermatol Surg.* 2013;39(8):1209-1216.)

Other less common adverse effects included temporary sensitivity, itching, and tenderness. One patient developed transient hyperpigmentation that resolved after 1 month.[39] There has been a single report of marginal mandibular nerve (MMN) injury after treatment of the submental region, resulting in asymmetric smile.[40] The symptoms completely resolved by 8 weeks after treatment. Multiple studies have examined the effect of treatment on lipid and transaminase levels. There was not an impact on cholesterol, triglycerides, or liver function tests.[31,33]

Another rare side effect described is paradoxical adipose hyperplasia (PAH). The initial report estimated an incidence of 0.0051%.[41] However, this may reflect underreporting as other authors have experienced significantly higher incidence rates (0.47%-0.78%).[41-46] Despite initial response, these patients present 2 to 3 months after treatment with a nontender fat mass in the treated area. This presents a management challenge as it is exacerbated by further cryolipolysis treatments and does not subside with time. Patients often need corrective liposuction if they desire improvement. The incidence appears higher in men and those of Hispanic descent, and the pathogenesis is not known. Hypotheses include activation of preexisting adipocytes by stem cells or a tissue hypoxia–induced rebound hyperplasia. Karcher et al. recommends against treating the lower abdomen of men and when treating the area in women, using two small applicators instead of one large applicator.[42] There is no published data to support these recommendations. Large, multicenter studies are needed to establish the incidence of this difficult to manage side effect and to develop strategies to minimize its occurrence.

Potential Risks, Benefits, and Limitations

Cryolipolysis provides a safe and noninvasive alternative for fat reduction without significant downtime. All reported side effects were temporary, with the exception of PAH. No long-term serious or systemic adverse events have been reported.

One potential pitfall during treatment is device interference. This occurs when the vacuum cup sensors detect an unexpected change in temperature, causing the device to discontinue the treatment cycle. Possible triggers include patient movement, electrical noise, or condensation.[39] If the treatment session stops prematurely and the vacuum suction is disabled, a new disposable gel trap must be used to reinitiate suction, significantly increasing expendable costs. To minimize the possibility of interference, the patient should remain motionless and not speak during the treatment cycle. The strap to secure the vacuum applicator provides further stability. Patient comfort should be ensured prior to treatment initiation.

Overall, the device is easy to operate and requires minimal physician face-time during treatment. In contrast to other injectable or surgical treatments, this offers the provider with the advantage of performing other duties while simultaneously utilizing this therapy. It is important to consider that the area of treatment is limited to the size of the applicator and injectable alternatives may sometimes offer more control and customization of both dosing and the treatment area.

▶ OTHER DEVICES

Radiofrequency

Radiofrequency is a rapidly alternating current that delivers heat to tissue based on the amount of current applied and the resistance of the target. The treatment is delivered through one or more electrodes held approximately 1 cm from the skin. The heating of dermal and subcutaneous tissue can lead to denatured collagen and new collagen formation. This can result in a tightening effect, but does not directly cause fat loss.[47,48] One such device, Thermacool TC (Thermage, Hayward, CA) is cleared for the noninvasive treatment of facial and nonfacial rhytids.[49]

Radiofrequency devices have also been used to treat thighs and buttocks. Due to the low water content of fat compared to surrounding tissue, it acts as an insulator. As the energy travels through fatty tissue, fibrous septae carry more current due to their lower impedence. Tightening in these areas is of variable efficacy.[49]

Ultrasound

Ultrasound treatment for skin tightening (Ulthera, Inc., Mesa, AZ) utilizes microfocused ultrasound with visualization. This technology penetrates to a depth of up to 5 mm to induce new collagen formation within the dermis and superficial musculoaponeurotic system.[50] Like radiofrequency, this type of ultrasound treatment does not result in fat loss.

However, high-intensity focused ultrasound devices are used to treat unwanted adipose tissue on the flank and abdomen. These devices selectively heat subcutaneous fat causing coagulative necrosis.[51,52] An alternative method of nonthermal focused ultrasound (UltraShape; Syneron Medical Ltd, Yokneam, Israel) utilizes mechanical energy to cause cavitation and fat cell lysis. This allows more selective destruction than tissue heating, which carries the risk of damaging adjacent structures including blood vessels, lymphatic vessels, connective tissue, nerves, and muscle.[53] Clinical data for this modality are limited to non-head and neck sites.

❱ DEOXYCHOLIC ACID

Background

Submental fullness is a common complaint among cosmetic patients. A youthful and aesthetically pleasing neck has a well-defined mandibular border, a cervicomental angle of 105° to 120°, and visible landmarks including the anterior border of the sternocleidomastoid, thyroid cartilage, and subhyoid depression.[54] Submental fat accumulation obscures the mandibular line and contributes to an overweight and aged appearance. This can be a stubborn area of fat deposition, often unresponsive to diet and exercise. Genetic predisposition to accumulation of submental adipose tissue, as well as normal aging, can create discordance between submental fullness and overall body mass index. Reduction can significantly improve patient satisfaction in appearance.[55] Treatment of submental fullness with deoxycholic acid (DCA) targets excess adipose tissue in the preplatysmal compartment. If fat accumulation is subplatysmal, a surgical approach including lipectomy with or without submentoplasty is often required.[55-57]

Endogenous DCA is a bile acid important in solubilization, breakdown, and absorption of dietary fats in the gastrointestinal tract. The molecule ATX-101 (Kybella™ [United States], Allergan, Inc.) is an injectable form of synthetic DCA approved by the FDA in 2015 for the treatment of moderate to severe fullness of the submental fat compartment. Off-label treatment has been extended to the lateral neck and jowls. When injected into subcutaneous fat, synthetic DCA causes adipocyte lysis by disrupting the cell membrane. Tissue macrophages and fibroblasts are then activated to clear cellular debris and stimulate fibrosis[54] (Figure 7.7). Given the destruction of adipocytes following treatment, the results are long-lasting. In Phase III clinical trials, reduction in submental fullness was demonstrated across all outcome measures including patient-reported assessments, caliper measurements, and magnetic resonance imaging.[58-62]

Patient Selection and Preoperative Counseling

Patients with moderate or greater submental fullness due to preplatysmal fat accumulation are appropriate candidates for DCA. This can be assessed by having the patient flex the platysmal muscle while palpating the preplatysmal fat pad in the submental region.

DCA injections should be avoided in patients with submental fullness due to laxity rather than fat deposition. Patients with significant skin laxity may be more amenable to nonsurgical tightening devices or surgical intervention. Patients with a history of submental/anterior cervical surgery or a history of facial nerve paralysis or dysphagia are not optimal candidates for DCA injection. Clinicians should also avoid injecting into actively inflamed or indurated tissue.

Prior to treatment, patients should be examined for the presence of prominent platysmal bands. These may be accentuated following reduction of preplatysmal fat and can be addressed with neuromodulators or surgical intervention (i.e., platysmaplasty).[63]

When examining a patient for DCA injection, the submental region is carefully inspected to rule out other causes of submental fullness such as thyromegaly, salivary gland enlargement, or lymphadenopathy. The patient is examined in both the upright and supine positions to fully assess cervical fullness. Prior to treatment, swallowing is assessed to rule out dysphagia, and smile symmetry is noted. Asymmetry may indicate MMN dysfunction.[64]

Reasonable expectations are discussed prior to treatment. A range of one to six treatments may be required to achieve satisfactory results, and most patients need at least two treatments. The number of treatment sessions is based on the severity of fullness

FIGURE 7.7   Mechanism of action of deoxycholic acid.

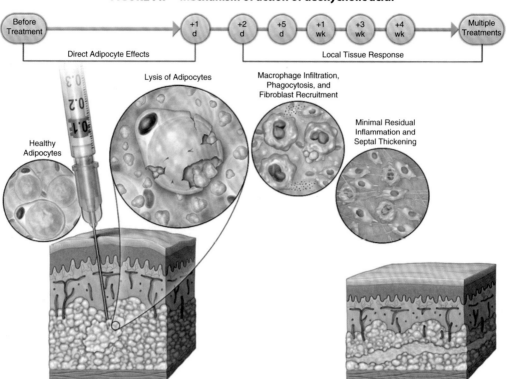

(Borrowed with permission from Dayan SH, Humphrey S, Jones DH, et al. Overview of ATX-101 (deoxycholic acid injection): a nonsurgical approach for reduction of submental fat. *Dermatol Surg.* 2016;42:S263-S270.)

prior to the onset of treatment. Submental fullness can be quantitatively assessed using the Clinician-Reported Submental Fat Rating Scale[61] (Figure 7.8). Most patients will see a noticeable difference with two to four treatments.[54]

Treatment sessions are spaced 1 month or greater apart, with 6 weeks being optimal in the authors' experience. Common adverse effects, discussed further below, are reviewed with the patient. DCA treatments can cost one to two thousand dollars per treatment, and if multiple treatments are required, it may be cost prohibitive for some patients.

Procedural Approach

Knowledge of relevant anatomy is essential for proper treatment. The MMN is susceptible to injury following DCA injection. This nerve innervates muscles that depress the lower lip, including the depressor anguli oris, depressor labii inferioris, orbicularis oris, and mentalis. The MMN exits from beneath the masseter muscle at the antegonial notch, curving slightly beneath the mandibular border before coursing upwards to innervate lower facial muscles (Figure 7.9). The nerve passes over the mandible with the facial artery and vein at the antegonial notch, which can be palpated at the anterior border of the clenched masseter muscle along the mid-mandible. As one ages, the MMN can drop beneath the mandibular border, making it more susceptible to injury. Direct injection of active drug should be avoided within the path of this nerve. Damage will result in temporary inability to depress the lower lip on the ipsilateral side of damage and smile asymmetry.[65]

FIGURE 7.8   The validated Clinican-Reported Submental Fat Rating Scale.

Scale	0	1	2	3	4
Submental convexity	Absent	Mild	Moderate	Severe	Extreme
Description	No localized submental fat evident	Minimal localized submental fat	Prominent localized submental fat	Marked localized submental fat	Extreme submental convexity
Representative photographs	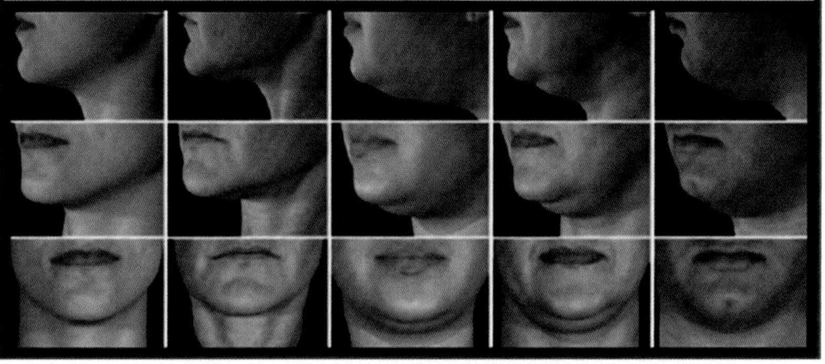				

(Reproduced from McDiarmid J, Ruiz JB, Lee D, et al. Results from a pooled analysis of two European, randomized, placebo-controlled, phase 3 studies of ATX-101 for the pharmacologic reduction of excess submental fat. *Aesthet Plast Surg.* 2014;38:849-860. Copyright © 2014 The Author(s). This article is published with open access at Springerlink.com.)

Preparation and Positioning

1. The patient is positioned comfortably in a semi-upright position, with the head reclined slightly and resting against a headrest.
2. The skin is cleansed thoroughly with an antiseptic solution.
3. The anatomic boundaries of the preplatysmal fat are marked with a surgical pen (Figure 7.10):
   - Superior boundary: inferior mandibular border and submental crease.
     - A line 1 to 1.5 cm below the mandibular border outlines a zone to avoid where the MMN may course beneath the mandible as it crosses at the antegonial notch.
   - Inferior boundary: hyoid bone.
   - Lateral boundary: inferior continuation of the labiomandibular fold.

The optimal concentration per treatment area is 2 mg/cm^2. A higher concentration of 4 mg/cm^2 has greater risk of adverse events without greater efficacy. Kybella™ is provided in 10 mg/mL vials. It is injected in 0.2 mL aliquots at 1 cm intervals, resulting in a concentration of 2 mg/cm^2. A temporary tattoo grid is superimposed onto the treatment area for precise injection spacing (Figure 7.11). To calculate the volume of DCA needed in milliliters, divide the number of tattoo grid points within the drawn treatment boundaries by five. For example, if there are 20 injection points, 4 mL of DCA is needed. Suggested delivery is via 1 mL syringes with a half-inch 30-gauge needle.[64] Measures to reduce pain are outlined in the *Rehabilitation and Recovery* section.

FIGURE 7.9 **Anatomy of the anterior neck with important anatomical landmarks. Marginal mandibular nerve is shown in yellow. Facial artery and vein are shown in red and blue, respectively.**

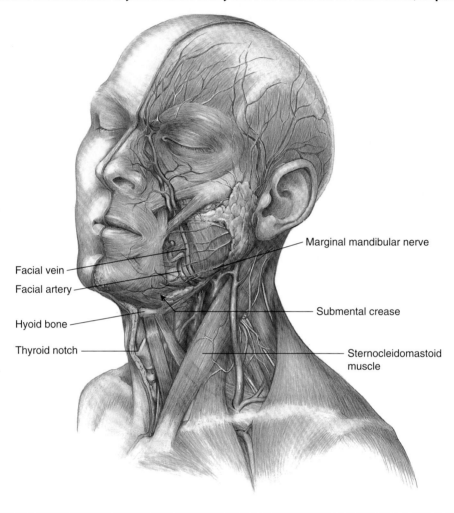

Facial vein

Facial artery

Hyoid bone

Thyroid notch

Marginal mandibular nerve

Submental crease

Sternocleidomastoid muscle

(Reprinted with permission from the Anatomical Charts Company.)

Injection Technique

1. Prep the patient as above with anatomical markings and the provided temporary tattoo grid for injection spacing (Figure 7.11).
2. Begin at most lateral point on the most inferior row. Pinch the preplatysmal fat between two fingers, insert needle perpendicular to skin into mid-subcutaneous fat. Avoid pinching skin or injecting too superficially, which can lead to skin necrosis. Inject first 0.2 mL aliquot into the first injection site.
3. Continue injecting 0.2 mL aliquots in each injection point, moving horizontally along the bottom row.
4. Once the bottom row is completed, move upward row by row until each injection point has been completed. Injections should end at a lateral edge of the most superior row.
5. The maximum recommended injection volume is 10 mL per treatment session.[54,66]
6. Repeat treatment sessions at a minimum of 28-day intervals. Histopathological inflammation is resolved by this time point.[54]

7. See Video 7.1.

FIGURE 7.10   **Anatomic boundaries of the preplatysmal fat, marked prior to injection with deoxycholic acid. Borders include the submental crease superiorly, caudal continuation of the labiomandibular folds laterally, and the hyoid bone inferiorly. Treatment should not be delivered in the gap between the inferior mandibular border and the submental crease, as risk of injury to the marginal mandibular nerve is greater in this region.**

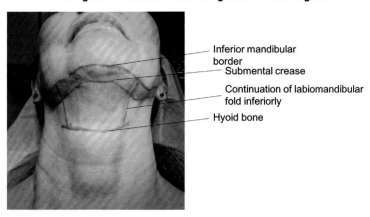

Inferior mandibular border
Submental crease
Continuation of labiomandibular fold inferiorly
Hyoid bone

Postprocedural Care and Recovery

Common treatment reactions following injection of DCA include pain, swelling, bruising, erythema, numbness, and induration.[59,60] Adverse reactions occurring in 2% or greater of patients receiving DCA and a greater incidence than placebo are shown in Table 7.7.[67] Mild edema and induration can persist for up to 4 weeks. Patients should contact the office if they experience smile asymmetry or difficulty in swallowing.

Pain can range from mild to severe in intensity. Measures to reduce pain include cold compresses, topical and injectable anesthetic, oral analgesics, oral antihistamines, and application of a chinstrap posttreatment. In one study of 83 patients, the use of both topical and injectable anesthetics decreased peak pain by 17% when compared to cold compresses alone. The addition of oral ibuprofen and oral loratadine prior to treatment, in addition to topical and injectable anesthetic, further decreased peak pain by 40%.[64] Measures to reduce pain are outlined in Table 7.8.[66]

FIGURE 7.11   **Temporary tattoo grid markings within the treatment area for deoxycholic acid injection shown prior to, during, and immediately following injection.**

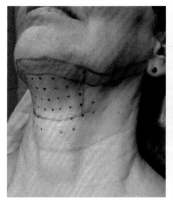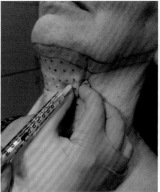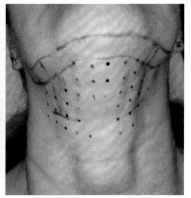

TABLE 7.7   Adverse Reactions in Pooled Trials 1 and 2[67,a]

Adverse Reaction	Kybella® (N = 513) n (%)	Placebo (N = 506) N (%)
Injection site reactions	492 (96%)	411 (81%)
Edema/swelling	448 (87)	218 (43)
Hematoma/bruising	368 (72)	353 (70)
Pain	356 (70)	160 (32)
Numbness	341 (66)	29 (6)
Erythema	136 (27)	91 (18)
Induration	120 (23)	13 (3)
Paresthesia	70 (14)	20 (4)
Nodule	68 (13)	14 (3)
Pruritus	64 (12)	30 (6)
Skin tightness	24 (5)	6 (1)
Site warmth	22 (4)	8 (2)
Nerve injury[b]	20 (4)	1 (<1)
Headache	41 (8)	20 (4)
Oropharyngeal pain	15 (3)	7 (1)
Hypertension	13 (3)	7 (1)
Nausea	12 (2)	3 (1)
Dysphagia	10 (2)	1 (<1)

[a]Adverse reactions that occurred in ≥2% Kybella®-treated subjects and at a greater incidence than placebo.
[b]Marginal mandibular nerve paresis.

Bruising occurs in the majority of patients. Oral agents that increase bleeding risk should be stopped 7 to 10 days before injection.[68] We do not recommend discontinuation of medically necessary blood thinners for patients who have had cardiovascular or clotting events. The vasoconstrictive effect of injected anesthetic with epinephrine may reduce the risk of significant purpura formation. Bothersome bruising can be managed in the posttreatment period with a pulsed-dye laser.

TABLE 7.8   Measures to Reduce Posttreatment Pain Following Deoxycholic Acid Injection[66]

Treatment	Comments
Cold compresses	• Applied 10-15 min pretreatment and posttreatment
Topical anesthetic	• 4% lidocaine cream applied under occlusion 45 min prior
Injectable anesthetic	• 1% lidocaine with epinephrine (1:100,000) within the area of treatment 15-30 min prior • Direct injection into the subcutaneous fat or infiltration with cannula
Oral antihistamine	• Loratadine 10 mg orally once daily for 7 d pretreatment and posttreatment
Oral analgesic	• Ibuprofen 600 mg, 1 h prior, continued 3 times daily for 3 d posttreatment • Acetaminophen 650 mg orally 1 h before treatment
Chinstrap	• Applied 15 min posttreatment and worn for at least 24 h

TABLE 7.9   Overview of Phase III Clinical Trials for ATX-101[57]

Study	Authors	Number of Subjects	Concentration of ATX-101, mg/cm^2	Percentage With One or Greater Improvement on a 5-Point Scale	P
European Phase III	Ascher et al.[58]	119	1	59.2	<.001
		121	2	65.3	<.001
European Phase III	Rzany et al.[62]	121	1	58.2	<.001
		122	2	68.3	<.001
US/Canadian Phase III (REFINE-1)	Jones et al.[60]	256	2	70.0	<.001
US/Canadian Phase III (REFINE-2)	Humphrey et al.[59]	258	2	66.5	<.001

Clinical Results

The safety and efficacy of ATX-101 have been studied in over 15 clinical trials, including four randomized, double-blind, placebo-controlled Phase III studies in Europe, the United States, and Canada.[58-62,69-71] Patients in the phase III studies needed to have "moderate to severe fullness" (Figure 7.2) to be considered for inclusion. Overall, 52% of subjects achieved a 1 or greater grade improvement in submental fullness after the second treatment with DCA. After the fourth treatment, this number increased to 72% of subjects. In two of the phase III trials, REFINE-1 and 2, MRI showed a significant reduction in submental fat (46.3% and 40.2%; $P < .001$ for both).[59,60] This corresponded to a reduction in submental fat thickness from baseline by a mean of 21.9 and 17.8 mm ($P < .001$). An overview of the Phase III clinical trials is presented in Table 7.9. Representative results are shown in Figure 7.12.

Phase IIIb studies for ATX-101 are ongoing in which partial and complete responders at 12 weeks posttreatment are being followed to monitor for sustained response. The majority of patients have been shown to maintain a partial (87.5%-95.4%) or complete response (87.4%-90.4%) at one and two-year follow-up intervals.[72] Considering DCA results in adipocyte cell death, it is reasonable to propose that fat reduction following treatment will be sustained.

Potential Risks, Benefits, and Limitations

The most common side effect of DCA is posttreatment pain, which can be moderate to severe in intensity. This is usually limited to a day or less in duration and can be reduced by measures outlined in Table 7.8.[64,68]

MMN paralysis is a known risk factor with DCA injection and occurred in 4% (11/258) of patients treated with ATX-101 in the REFINE phase III trials.[59,60] All incidences were described as mild to moderate in severity. Recovery time varied widely, ranging from 7 to 60 days. One severe case of MMN paralysis occurred and resolved at 85 days post treatment. One patient developed skin ulceration, likely due to dermal rather than mid-subcutaneous injection, and 2% (6/258) developed temporary dysphagia due to postinjection swelling and pain.

FIGURE 7.12   Treatment results from Phase III randomized clinical trials.

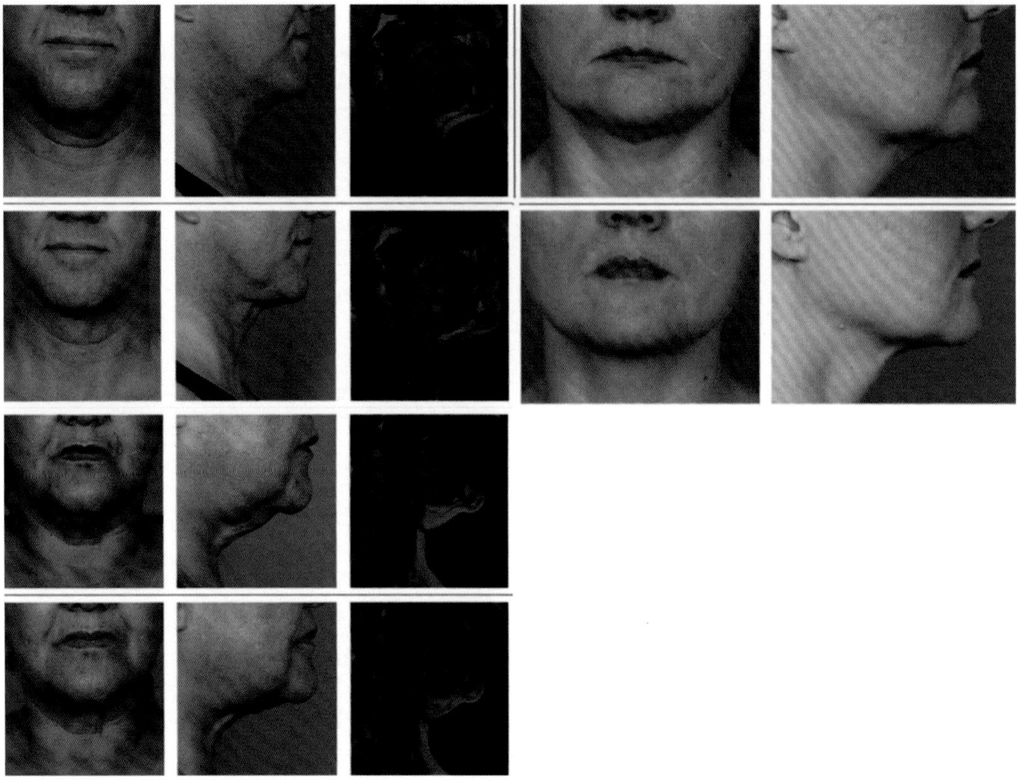

(Adapted from Humphrey S, Sykes J, Kantor J, et al. ATX-101 for reduction of submental fat: a phase III randomized controlled trial. *J Am Acad Dermatol.* 2016;75(4):788-797.e7. Copyright © 2016 American Academy of Dermatology, Inc. With permission.)

Despite submental fat reduction, increased skin laxity has not routinely been observed. Paradoxically, most patients (93%) in the REFINE-1 trial reported no change or improvement in submental skin laxity, possibly due to fibrosis and new collagen formation.

One potential side effect in men is alopecia in the area of treatment. In one study, this occurred in 8 of 39 men and resolved in all patients by the 6-week follow-up visit.[39]

No systemic adverse effects have been reported following subcutaneous injection of DCA, despite transient increases in plasma levels of endogenous DCA 12 to 24 hours after injection. In two Phase I clinical trials, there were no meaningful differences in heart rate, plasma concentration of lipids, proinflammatory cytokines, liver transaminases, or creatinine levels.[69,70] A separate Phase 1 study demonstrated no changes in QT intervals or other electrocardiogram parameters following subcutaneous administration of ATX-101.

▶ SUMMARY

The addition of noninvasive techniques to the armamentarium of fat loss treatments has greatly increased the number of procedures of this type performed by medical providers. As the technology continues to improve, they will only increase in popularity. When compared to liposuction and DCA injection, cryolipolysis has less downtime and potential adverse effects, but requires the practitioner to purchase and maintain the device. Thus, if size of the treatment area is amenable to the vacuum cup applicator, cryolipolysis is a good starting point. However, for larger areas of fat accumulation, liposuction is still the preferred modality, as cryolipolysis of multiple or large areas may be very time-consuming and expensive. Using the tumescent technique, this can be performed safely in the outpatient setting, without the need for systemic anesthesia. For small areas of submental fat or asymmetrical adipose hyperplasia, DCA injections offer a more tailored, targeted treatment approach. It can also be used to remove small areas of fat asymmetry or persistent accumulation following submental liposuction or cryolipolysis. All available options should be reviewed with the patient so he or she can make an informed decision based on risk tolerance and treatment goals.

REFERENCES

1. Klein JA. The tumescent technique for liposuction surgery. *Am J Cosmet Surg.* 1987;4:263-267.
2. Bernstein G, Hanke CW. Safety of liposuction: a review of 9478 cases performed by dermatologists. *J Dermatol Surg Oncol.* 1988;14(10):1112-1114.
3. Hanke CW, Bernstein G, Bullock S. Safety of tumescent liposuction in 15,336 patients. National survey results. *Dermatol Surg.* 1995;21(5):459-462.
4. Klein JA. Tumescent technique for regional anesthesia permits lidocaine doses of 35 mg/kg for liposuction. *J Dermatol Surg Oncol.* 1990;16(3):248-263.
5. Ostad A, Kageyama N, Moy RL. Tumescent anesthesia with a lidocaine dose of 55 mg/kg is safe for liposuction. *Dermatol Surg.* 1996;22(11):921-927.
6. Burk RW III, Guzman-Stein G, Vasconez LO. Lidocaine and epinephrine levels in tumescent technique liposuction. *Plast Reconstr Surg.* 1996;97(7):1379-1384.
7. Habbema L. Efficacy of tumescent local anesthesia with variable lidocaine concentration in 3430 consecutive cases of liposuction. *J Am Acad Dermatol.* 2010;62(6):988-994.
8. Lillis PJ. Liposuction surgery under local anesthesia: limited blood loss and minimal lidocaine absorption. *J Dermatol Surg Oncol.* 1988;14(10):1145-1148.
9. Rubin JP, Bierman C, Rosow CE, et al. The tumescent technique: the effect of high tissue pressure and dilute epinephrine on absorption of lidocaine. *Plast Reconstr Surg.* 1999;103(3):990-996; discussion 7-1002.
10. *Tumsecent Local Anesthesia: Recommendations from the American Academy of Dermatology*; 2017. Available at https://www.aad.org/practicecenter/quality/clinical-guidelines/office-based-surgery/tumescent-local-anesthesia.
11. *Xylocaine (Lidocaine)* [package insert]. Schaumburg, IL: APP Pharmaceuticals; 2010.
12. Moore DC, Bridenbaugh LD, Thompson GE, Balfour RI, Horton WG. Factors determining dosages of amide-type local anesthetic drugs. *Anesthesiology.* 1977;47(3):263-268.
13. Gordh T. Xylocaine – a new local anesthetic. *Aneaesthesia.* 1949;4:4-9.
14. Augustin M, Maier K, Sommer B, Sattler G, Herberger K. Double-blind, randomized, intraindividual comparison study of the efficacy of prilocaine and lidocaine in tumescent local anesthesia. *Dermatology.* 2010;221(3):248-252.
15. Breuninger H, Wehner-Caroli J. Slow infusion tumescent anesthesia. *Dermatol Surg.* 1998;24(7):759-763.
16. Lindenblatt N, Belusa L, Tiefenbach B, Schareck W, Olbrisch RR. Prilocaine plasma levels and methemoglobinemia in patients undergoing tumescent liposuction involving less than 2,000 ml. *Aesthet Plast Surg.* 2004;28(6):435-440.
17. Boeni R. Safety of tumescent liposuction under local anesthesia in a series of 4,380 patients. *Dermatology.* 2011;222(3):278-281.
18. Housman TS, Lawrence N, Mellen BG, et al. The safety of liposuction: results of a national survey. *Dermatol Surg.* 2002;28(11):971-978.
19. Chia CT, Albert MG, Del Vecchio S, Theodorou SJ. 1000 consecutive cases of laser-assisted liposuction utilizing the 1440 nm wavelength Nd:YAG laser: assessing the safety and efficacy. *Aesthet Plast Surg.* 2018;42(1):9-12.
20. Hanke W, Cox SE, Kuznets N, Coleman WP III. Tumescent liposuction report performance measurement initiative: national survey results. *Dermatol Surg.* 2004;30(7):967-977; discussion 78.
21. Halk AB, Habbema L, Genders RE, Hanke CW. Safety studies in the field of liposuction: a systematic review. *Dermatol Surg.* 2019;45(2):171-182.
22. Al Dujaili Z, Karcher C, Henry M, Sadick N. Fat reduction: pathophysiology and treatment strategies. *J Am Acad Dermatol.* 2018;79(2):183-195.
23. Pereira-Netto D, Montano-Pedroso JC, Aidar A, Marson WL, Ferreira LM. Laser-assisted liposuction (LAL) versus traditional liposuction: systematic review. *Aesthet Plast Surg.* 2018;42(2):376-383.
24. Duncan WC, Freeman RG, Heaton CL. Cold panniculitis. *Arch Dermatol.* 1966;94(6):722-724.
25. Epstein EH Jr, Oren ME. Popsicle panniculitis. *N Engl J Med.* 1970;282(17):966-967.
26. Rotman H. Cold panniculitis in children. Adiponecrosis E frigore of Haxthausen. *Arch Dermatol.* 1966;94(6):720-721.

27. Manstein D, Laubach H, Watanabe K, Farinelli W, Zurakowski D, Anderson RR. Selective cryolysis: a novel method of non-invasive fat removal. *Lasers Surg Med*. 2008;40(9):595-604.

28. Boey GE, Wasilenchuk JL. Enhanced clinical outcome with manual massage following cryolipolysis treatment: a 4-month study of safety and efficacy. *Lasers Surg Med*. 2014;46(1):20-26.

29. Coleman SR, Sachdeva K, Egbert BM, Preciado J, Allison J. Clinical efficacy of noninvasive cryolipolysis and its effects on peripheral nerves. *Aesthet Plast Surg*. 2009;33(4):482-488.

30. Dierickx CC, Mazer JM, Sand M, Koenig S, Arigon V. Safety, tolerance, and patient satisfaction with noninvasive cryolipolysis. *Dermatol Surg*. 2013;39(8):1209-1216.

31. Ferraro GA, De Francesco F, Cataldo C, Rossano F, Nicoletti G, D'Andrea F. Synergistic effects of cryolipolysis and shock waves for noninvasive body contouring. *Aesthet Plast Surg*. 2012;36(3):666-679.

32. Garibyan L, Sipprell WH III, Jalian HR, Sakamoto FH, Avram M, Anderson RR. Three-dimensional volumetric quantification of fat loss following cryolipolysis. *Lasers Surg Med*. 2014;46(2):75-80.

33. Lee KR. Clinical efficacy of fat reduction on the thigh of Korean women through cryolipolysis. *J Obes Weight Loss*. 2013;3:1-5.

34. Pinto HR, Garcia-Cruz E, Melamed GE. A study to evaluate the action of lipocryolysis. *Cryo Lett*. 2012;33(3):177-181.

35. Sasaki GH, Abelev N, Tevez-Ortiz A. Noninvasive selective cryolipolysis and reperfusion recovery for localized natural fat reduction and contouring. *Aesthet Surg J*. 2014;34(3):420-431.

36. Shek SY, Chan NP, Chan HH. Non-invasive cryolipolysis for body contouring in Chinese – a first commercial experience. *Lasers Surg Med*. 2012;44(2):125-130.

37. Ingargiola MJ, Motakef S, Chung MT, Vasconez HC, Sasaki GH. Cryolipolysis for fat reduction and body contouring: safety and efficacy of current treatment paradigms. *Plast Reconstr Surg*. 2015;135(6):1581-1590.

38. Zeltiq Aesthetics I. FDA 510(k); 2017 Available at https://www.accessdata.fda.gov/cdrh_docs/pdf17/k171069.pdf.

39. Kilmer SL, Burns AJ, Zelickson BD. Safety and efficacy of cryolipolysis for non-invasive reduction of submental fat. *Lasers Surg Med*. 2016;48(1):3-13.

40. Lee NY, Ibrahim O, Arndt KA, Dover JS. Marginal mandibular injury after treatment with cryolipolysis. *Dermatol Surg*. 2018;44(10):1353-1355.

41. Jalian HR, Avram MM, Garibyan L, Mihm MC, Anderson RR. Paradoxical adipose hyperplasia after cryolipolysis. *JAMA Dermatol*. 2014;150(3):317-319.

42. Karcher C, Katz B, Sadick N. Paradoxical hyperplasia post cryolipolysis and management. *Dermatol Surg*. 2017;43(3):467-470.

43. Kelly E, Rodriguez-Feliz J, Kelly ME. Paradoxical adipose hyperplasia after cryolipolysis: a report on incidence and common factors identified in 510 patients. *Plast Reconstr Surg*. 2016;137(3):639e-640e.

44. Singh SM, Geddes ER, Boutrous SG, Galiano RD, Friedman PM. Paradoxical adipose hyperplasia secondary to cryolipolysis: an underreported entity? *Lasers Surg Med*. 2015;47(6):476-478.

45. Stefani WA. Adipose hypertrophy following cryolipolysis. *Aesthet Surg J*. 2015;35(7):NP218-NP220.

46. Stroumza N, Gauthier N, Senet P, Moguelet P, Nail Barthelemy R, Atlan M. Paradoxical adipose hypertrophy (PAH) after cryolipolysis. *Aesthet Surg J*. 2018;38(4):411-417.

47. Arnoczky SP, Aksan A. Thermal modification of connective tissues: basic science considerations and clinical implications. *J Am Acad Orthop Surg*. 2000;8(5):305-313.

48. Goldberg DJ, Fazeli A, Berlin AL. Clinical, laboratory, and MRI analysis of cellulite treatment with a unipolar radiofrequency device. *Dermatol Surg*. 2008;34(2):204-209;discussion 9.

49. Sukal SA, Geronemus RG. Thermage: the nonablative radiofrequency for rejuvenation. *Clin Dermatol*. 2008;26(6):602-607.

50. Oni G, Hoxworth R, Teotia S, Brown S, Kenkel JM. Evaluation of a microfocused ultrasound system for improving skin laxity and tightening in the lower face. *Aesthet Surg J*. 2014;34(7):1099-1110.

51. Fatemi A, Kane MA. High-intensity focused ultrasound effectively reduces waist circumference by ablating adipose tissue from the abdomen and flanks: a retrospective case series. *Aesthet Plast Surg*. 2010;34(5):577-582.

52. Robinson DM, Kaminer MS, Baumann L, et al. High-intensity focused ultrasound for the reduction of subcutaneous adipose tissue using multiple treatment techniques. *Dermatol Surg*. 2014;40(6):641-651.

53. Coleman WP III, Coleman W, Weiss RA, Kenkel JM, Ad-El DD, Amir R. A multicenter controlled study to evaluate multiple treatments with nonthermal focused ultrasound for noninvasive fat reduction. *Dermatol Surg*. 2017;43(1):50-57.

54. Dayan SH, Humphrey S, Jones DH, et al. Overview of ATX-101 (deoxycholic acid injection): a nonsurgical approach for reduction of submental fat. *Dermatol Surg*. 2016;42(suppl 1):S263-S270.

55. Jordan JR, Yellin S. Direct cervicoplasty. *Facial Plast Surg*. 2014;30(4):451-461.

56. Vanaman M, Fabi SG, Cox SE. Neck rejuvenation using a combination approach: our experience and a review of the literature. *Dermatol Surg*. 2016;42(suppl 2):S94-S100.

57. Hurst E, Dietert J. *Nonsurgical treatment of submental fullness*. In: *Advances in Cosmetic Surgery*. Philadelphia, PA: Elsevier; 2018:1-15.

58. Ascher B, Hoffmann K, Walker P, Lippert S, Wollina U, Havlickova B. Efficacy, patient-reported outcomes and safety profile of ATX-101 (deoxycholic acid), an injectable drug for the reduction of unwanted submental fat: results from a phase III, randomized, placebo-controlled study. *J Eur Acad Dermatol Venereol*. 2014;28(12):1707-1715.

59. Humphrey S, Sykes J, Kantor J, et al. ATX-101 for reduction of submental fat: a phase III randomized controlled trial. *J Am Acad Dermatol*. 2016;75(4):788-797 e7.

60. Jones DH, Carruthers J, Joseph JH, et al. REFINE-1, a multicenter, randomized, double-blind, placebo-controlled, phase 3 trial with ATX-101, an injectable drug for submental fat reduction. *Dermatol Surg*. 2016;42(1):38-49.

61. McDiarmid J, Ruiz JB, Lee D, Lippert S, Hartisch C, Havlickova B. Results from a pooled analysis of two European, randomized, placebo-controlled, phase 3 studies of ATX-101 for the pharmacologic reduction of excess submental fat. *Aesthet Plast Surg*. 2014;38(5):849-860.

62. Rzany B, Griffiths T, Walker P, Lippert S, McDiarmid J, Havlickova B. Reduction of unwanted submental fat with ATX-101 (deoxycholic acid), an adipocytolytic injectable treatment: results from a phase III, randomized, placebo-controlled study. *Br J Dermatol*. 2014;170(2):445-453.

63. Koehler J. Complications of neck liposuction and submentoplasty. *Oral Maxillofac Surg Clin North Am*. 2009;21(1):43-52;vi.

64. Jones DH, Kenkel JM, Fagien S, et al. Proper technique for administration of ATX-101 (deoxycholic acid injection): insights from an injection practicum and roundtable discussion. *Dermatol Surg*. 2016;42(suppl 1):S275-S281.

65. Kenkel JM, Jones DH, Fagien S, et al. Anatomy of the cervicomental region: insights from an anatomy laboratory and roundtable discussion. *Dermatol Surg*. 2016;42(suppl 1):S282-S287.

66. Dover JS, Kenkel JM, Carruthers A, et al. Management of patient experience with ATX-101 (deoxycholic acid injection) for reduction of submental fat. *Dermatol Surg*. 2016;42(suppl 1):S288-S299.

67. *Kybella (Deoxycholic Acid)* [package insert]. Irvine, CA: Allergan; 2018.

68. Fagien S, McChesney P, Subramanian M, Jones DH. Prevention and management of injection-related adverse effects in facial aesthetics: considerations for ATX-101 (deoxycholic acid injection) treatment. *Dermatol Surg*. 2016;42(suppl 1): S300-S304.

69. Walker P, Fellmann J, Lizzul PF. A phase I safety and pharmacokinetic study of ATX-101: injectable, synthetic deoxycholic acid for submental contouring. *J Drugs Dermatol*. 2015;14(3):279-287.

70. Walker P, Lee D. A phase 1 pharmacokinetic study of ATX-101: serum lipids and adipokines following synthetic deoxycholic acid injections. *J Cosmet Dermatol*. 2015;14(1):33-39.

71. Glogau RG, Glaser DA, Callender VD, et al. A double-blind, placebo-controlled, phase 3b study of ATX-101 for reduction of mild or extreme submental fat. *Dermatol Surg*. 2019;45:1531-1541.

72. Dunican KC, Patel DK. Deoxycholic acid (ATX-101) for reduction of submental fat. *Ann Pharmacother*. 2016;50(10):855-861.

CHAPTER

8

Vascular Treatments of the Lower Extremity

Dillon Clarey, MD, and Ashley Wysong, MD, MS

Chapter Highlights

- Chronic venous disease secondary to valve reflux is a common and increasing problem.
- Numerous risk factors are present, including increasing age, family history, multiparity, and body mass.
- The disease has a significant impact on the quality of life for those affected in addition to increased economic burden to society.
- A thorough history (aching/tiredness, pain, tenderness, edema) and physical exam (varicose veins, reticular veins, telangiectasias, edema) are critical prior to choosing management modalities.
- Sclerotherapy is the mainstay of treatment for asymptomatic telangiectasias.
- Endovenous ablation has predominantly replaced high ligation and vein stripping in the management of saphenous vein varices.
- Ambulatory phlebectomy (mini-vein stripping) has been broadly replaced by minimally invasive techniques but is still used in select patients and on areas overlying bony prominences.

Broadly speaking, chronic venous disease (CVD) refers to the inability of blood to be returned from the lower extremities to the heart.[1,2] In a properly functioning vein, blood is propelled from the legs to the heart by calf contractions (muscular pump) and prevented from refluxing by bicuspid venous valves.[3] This combination enables a unidirectional flow.[4] Venous flow is influenced by both intrinsic (venous contractions, arterial inflow, thoracic/abdominal pressure, valve integrity, vein wall recoil) and extrinsic (gravity, atmospheric pressure, centrifugal force, compression) factors.[4]

The inability of a vein to return blood most commonly arises due to malfunctioning venous valves.[5] This is most often secondary to primary valve incompetence.[5] Incompetence can also result secondarily from trauma, deep venous thrombosis (DVT), lack of a muscular pump, or a congenital anomaly (May-Thurner, Ehlers-Danlos, Von Hippel-Lindau).[5] Risk factors for CVD include increasing age (decreased calf muscle mass leads to decreased muscle contraction, weakened vein walls, progressive inflammatory degradation of valves),[1] family history (risk as high as 90% if both parents are affected),[6] and multiparity (due to effects of hormones causing smooth muscle relaxation and increased abdominal pressure during pregnancy).[6-10] Refluxed blood travels from the deep venous system through the perforating venous system and ultimately into the superficial venous system.[5]

Nearly 60% to 70% (females > males) of the population has been estimated to have some degree of CVD, with the incidence of varicose veins at roughly 2% per year.[11] The incidence is typically higher in areas that are more industrialized, such as the Western countries.[2] Worldwide, CVD of the lower extremities costs billions of dollars a year.[12] In addition to the monetary impact, the psychological impact of CVD on the quality of life is significant, particularly in the case of venous ulceration.[12]

▶ LOWER EXTREMITY ANATOMY

The vein walls of the lower extremity are much thinner than arteries. They contain intimal, medial, and adventitial layers.[13] Each of these layers plays important roles in vein function. The primary role of the intimal layer is to serve an antithrombogenic function; it does this through a number of mechanisms (prostaglandin I2 production, tissue-type plasminogen activator [t-PA] production, others).[3] This antithrombogenic activity can be disturbed with damage to the intimal layer, leading to increased thrombogenicity.[3] Smooth muscle, collagen, and elastin compose the medial layer.[3,14] The adventitial layer, primarily composed of collagen, forms the outer layer and functions to provide veins with a degree of stiffness that enables the calf muscle pump to propel blood.[3] The lower extremity venous system is divided into three different compartments: deep, superficial (saphenous), and perforating (Figure 8.1).[15,16]

Deep Venous Compartment

The veins of the deep venous system lie beneath a muscular fascia and run with their associated arteries (Figure 8.1).[3] Due to this location, they function to drain the muscles of the lower extremity.[3] The deep compartment relies on calf muscle contraction and relaxation for propulsion of blood back toward the heart.[3] Functioning bicuspid valves of the deep and perforating system prevent reflux.[3]

FIGURE 8.1   **Diagrammatic representation of the three different compartments comprising the lower extremity.**

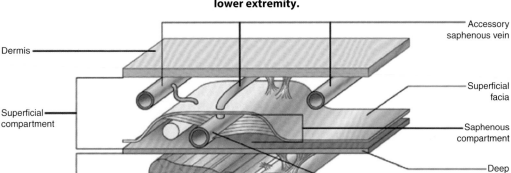

(Reprinted from Bergan J, Pascarella L. Chapter 4: Venous anatomy, physiology, and pathophysiology. In: *The Vein Book. Elsevier*; 2007:39-45. Copyright © 2007 Elsevier. With permission.)

FIGURE 8.2   Lower extremity deep venous system.

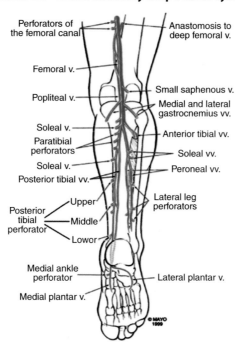

Perforators of
the femoral canal

Anastomosis to
deep femoral v.

Femoral v.

Popliteal v.

Small saphenous v.

Medial and lateral
gastrocnemius vv.

Soleal v.

Paratibial
perforators

Anterior tibial vv.

Soleal v.

Soleal vv.

Posterior tibial vv.

Peroneal vv.

Upper

Posterior
tibial
perforator

Middle

Lateral leg
perforators

Lower

Medial ankle
perforator

Lateral plantar v.

Medial plantar v.

© MAYO
1999

(Reprinted from Mozes G, Gloviczhi P. Chapter 2: Venous embryology and anatomy. In: *The Vein Book. Elsevier*, 2007:15-25. Copyright © 2007 Elsevier. With permission.)

Starting in the foot, the digital and metatarsal veins drain to form the deep plantar venous arch.[17] The deep plantar venous arch runs proximally over the foot to form the medial and lateral plantar veins (Figure 8.2).[17] At the ankle, the medial and lateral plantar veins drain into the posterior tibial vein. The anterior tibial vein is formed from the dorsal pedal vein.[3] The posterior tibial vein is responsible for draining blood from the posterior leg and medial and plantar foot, while the anterior tibial vein is responsible for the anterior lower leg and dorsal foot.[3] The peroneal vein drains blood from the lateral foot.[18] The posterior tibial vein receives drainage from the peroneal vein near the posteromedial fibula.[18] The anterior and posterior tibial vein join at the lower aspect of the posterior knee to form the tibioperoneal trunk and popliteal vein.[3] The popliteal vein ascends through the popliteal fossa and becomes the femoral vein upon entrance into the adductor hiatus.[3] The femoral vein joins the deep femoral vein to form the common femoral vein.[3] The saphenofemoral junction (SFJ), located 4 cm inferolateral to the pubic tubercle, is formed from the drainage of the great saphenous vein (GSV) into the common femoral vein.[18] The common femoral vein becomes the external iliac vein at the inguinal ligament.[18]

Superficial Venous Compartment

The location of the superficial venous system above the deep fascia allows these veins to drain the cutaneous circulation.[19] CVD is most prevalent in the superficial veins of the lower extremities secondary to their decreased muscular support compared to deeper veins.[3] The main vessels of this compartment include the truncal veins (e.g., GSV and small saphenous vein) as well as the named tributaries, or branches, off the saphenous system (e.g., anterior and posterior accessory of the GSV).[3,20] Reticular veins are a group

FIGURE 8.3   **Diagrammatic representation of the deep, perforating, and superficial venous systems.**

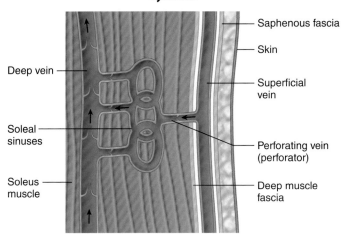

of veins that are located between the dermis and saphenous fascia and function to drain the skin and soft tissue (Figure 8.3).[3,20] The perforating venous system allows for communication of reticular veins to both the deep venous system and saphenous tributaries.[3,20]

The GSV lies in the saphenous compartment, an area in the superficial compartment bordered superficially and deep by saphenous fascia and muscular fascia, respectively (Figure 8.1).[3,20] The saphenous compartment also contains nerves and arteries associated with the saphenous vein but does not contain the reticular veins (more superficial).[3,21] The GSV originates on the dorsomedial foot from the dorsal pedal venous arch.[3,20-22] From there, the vein traverses superiorly anterior to the medial malleolus.[3] At the intersection of the middle and distal calf, the vein crosses and courses over to the posteromedial knee.[3] It then continues to ascend medially up the thigh to a point 3 to 4 cm inferolateral to the pubic tubercle. Here, it penetrates the deep fascia to join the common femoral vein at the SFJ.[3] At the SFJ, the superficial circumflex iliac vein (drains groin), superficial epigastric vein (drains abdominal wall) (Figure 8.4), and external pudendal vein (drains pelvis) are present.

As the saphenous vein courses up the mid-distal thigh, it may pierce the saphenous fascia to become more superficial.[22] A lack of fascial support has been proposed as a possible explanation for the more frequent presentation of varicose veins in these areas.[3,20] The GSV has also been shown to have duplication in the thigh (8%) and in the calf (25%).[3,21] These duplicated vessels lie within the saphenous compartment and later rejoin.[22] Of note, the saphenous nerve is present anterior to the GSV in the calf and must be monitored for in cases where GSV incompetence management ranges into the calf.[3]

The small saphenous vein arises from the dorsal pedal arch (Figure 8.5).[3,23] It ascends posterolateral to the lateral malleolus and has a variable termination into the popliteal vein.[3] Sixty percent of short saphenous veins (SSVs) join the popliteal vein within 8 cm of the knee, 20% join the GSV, and 20% join another deep vein (deep femoral, femoral, internal iliac).[3] The SSV can also continue superiorly as the vein of Giacomini and drain into the GSV via the posterior thigh circumflex vein.[3,24] The sural nerve, responsible for cutaneous sensation to the lateral foot and posterolateral leg, is located lateral to the SSV and Achilles tendon in the saphenous compartment. It pierces the muscular fascia prior to termination.[3]

FIGURE 8.4   Identification of laser positioned distal to the superficial epigastric vein.

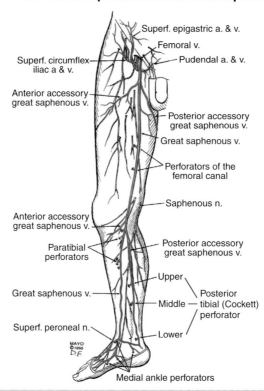

Superf. epigastric a. & v.
Femoral v.
Superf. circumflex iliac a & v.
Pudendal a. & v.
Anterior accessory great saphenous v.
Posterior accessory great saphenous v.
Great saphenous v.
Perforators of the femoral canal
Saphenous n.
Anterior accessory great saphenous v.
Posterior accessory great saphenous v.
Paratibial perforators
Upper
Great saphenous v.
Posterior tibial (Cockett) perforator
Middle
Superf. peroneal n.
Lower
Medial ankle perforators

(Reprinted from Caggiati A, Bergan JJ, Gloviczki P, et al. Nomenclature of the veins of the lower limbs: an international interdisciplinary consensus statement. *J Vasc Surg.* 2002;36(2):416-422. Copyright © 2002 The Society for Vascular Surgery and The American Association for Vascular Surgery. With permission.)

FIGURE 8.5   Lower extremity superficial venous system.

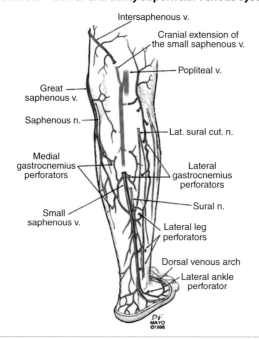

Intersaphenous v.
Cranial extension of the small saphenous v.
Popliteal v.
Great saphenous v.
Saphenous n.
Lat. sural cut. n.
Medial gastrocnemius perforators
Lateral gastrocnemius perforators
Sural n.
Small saphenous v.
Lateral leg perforators
Dorsal venous arch
Lateral ankle perforator

(Reprinted from Mozes G, Gloviczhi P. Chapter 2: Venous embryology and anatomy. In: *The Vein Book.* Elsevier; 2007:15-25. Copyright © 2007 Elsevier. With permission.)

Perforating Venous Compartment

The veins of the perforating venous system (average of 64 from the ankle to the groin) course through the muscular fascia and function to connect the superficial and deep venous compartments (Figure 8.3).[3] This allows blood to flow unidirectionally from superficial to deep.[21] There are four clinically significant groups of perforators based on location: foot, medial and lateral calf, and thigh.[3] These veins prevent reverse flow by closing their valves during the calf muscle pump, a time when there is increased deep venous pressure.[3] Conversely, the valves open up with relaxation of calf muscles to allow blood to flow superficially to deep along pressure gradients.[3] The only perforating system that does not direct blood in a superficial to deep direction is that found in the foot.[3]

▶ WORKUP FOR CHRONIC VENOUS DISEASE

A thorough history should be obtained upon initial evaluation.[1] This should include a description and duration of symptoms, precipitating and alleviating factors, number of pregnancies, pelvic symptoms (worse with menses, intercourse, standing), history of venous thromboembolism (VTE), family history of varicose veins, ulcers, VTE, coagulopathy,[25] peripheral vascular disease,[26] coronary artery disease,[26] and prior treatments.[1] CVD has a wide array of presentations.[27,28] The most common presenting symptom is aching/tired legs, although feelings of pain (throbbing, burning, pulling, stretching), swelling (most specific symptom), tenderness over a vein, and restless legs are also experienced.[3] Symptoms are worse with prolonged sitting or standing and improve with exercise, leg elevation, nonsteroidal anti-inflammatory drugs (NSAIDs), and compression therapy.[29,30]

Following a thorough history, a focused physical exam should then be performed.[1] On examination, it is imperative to check arterial pulses.[31] Confirmation of adequate arterial flow is required prior to usage of any compression therapy.[31] Examination findings include varicose veins (3-8 mm, Figure 8.6A), reticular veins (2-4 mm, blue, Figure 8.6B), telangiectasias (0.2-1 mm, red, "spider veins," Figure 8.6C), edema, ulceration (Figure 8.7), and skin color changes (Figure 8.8).[1] Noting the specific locations of varicosities and/or ulcerations can be beneficial in identifying the underlying pattern of insufficiency (Table 8.1). Importantly, abdominal, suprapubic, vulvar, inner thigh, or gluteal varicose veins are concerning for potential ilio-femoral obstruction/thrombosis and may necessitate further workup and imaging.[37] Engorgement of pelvic (Figure 8.9) and intrabdominal veins in these areas may present with pain of the low back, pelvis, vulva, and upper thigh areas. This syndrome, known as pelvic congestion syndrome, is characterized by chronic pelvic pain lasting for more than 6 months.[36] A history of multiple pregnancies and a family history of lower extremity varicose veins are common.[32]

Following completion of a history and physical examination, the algorithm in Figure 8.10 can be used to help guide work-up decisions. Any symptomatic patient should receive a bilateral duplex ultrasound performed by a registered vascular technologist. Gray scale ultrasound is used in identification of vein size and vein anatomy (mapping, congenital anomalies, ruling out of obstruction). Color doppler ultrasound is used for identification of flow direction and frequency shifts, and color flow with compression is helpful in ruling out DVT or other obstruction. Pulsed wave doppler can identify abnormal reflux: >0.5 seconds in the superficial system,[33] >1 second in the deep system,[33] and >0.35 seconds in perforators.[34] Other imaging modalities include conventional venography, computed tomography, and magnetic resonance venography/arteriography (MRV/MRA). If a patient is not symptomatic, however, and worrisome findings are noted on examination (lower extremity swelling, extensive varicosities, skin changes), a complete venous mapping and duplex ultrasound is performed. If symptoms and signs are not present, sclerotherapy can be utilized for reticular veins and telangiectasias.

FIGURE 8.6   **(A) Varicose veins, (B) reticular veins, and (C) telangiectasias.**

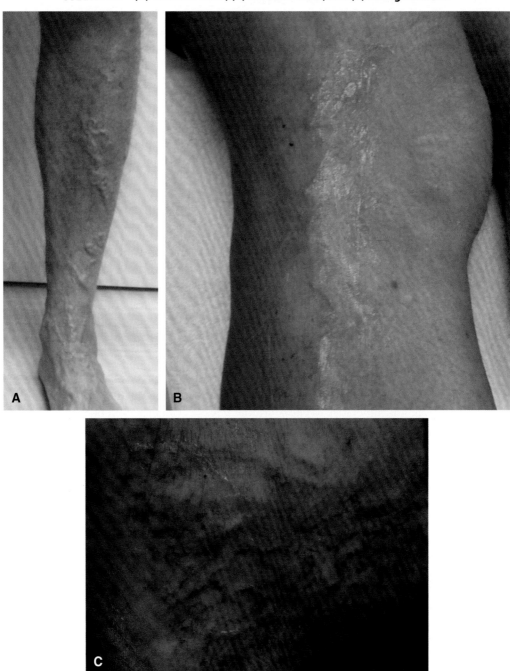

The Clinical-Etiology-Anatomy-Pathophysiology (CEAP) classification (Table 8.2) is a system that standardizes analysis of CVD and management alternatives.[35] It is not used as a measure of venous disease clinical severity or as a measure of response to therapy.[35] The clinical signs (C) of CEAP are used to categorize the observable signs of CVD. Those with C0-C3 or C4 disease are typically asymptomatic.[35]

FIGURE 8.7   Skin changes with ulceration over the medial malleolus in the distribution of the great saphenous vein.

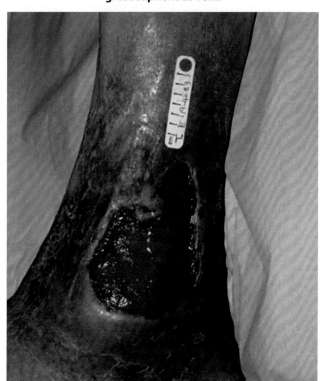

▶ TREATMENT OF CHRONIC VENOUS DISEASE

Medical Management

As with many diseases, management of CVD is initially conservative, starting with external compression stockings, elevation of the legs, and exercise therapy, sometimes referred to as the "EEE."[1] In addition, obese or overweight patients are encouraged to also focus on weight loss strategies. These are all efforts to decrease the pooling of blood in the legs, which will help mitigate the symptoms of CVD.[1] Additional systemic medications can be utilized, including NSAIDs (decrease pain/inflammation), rutosides (diminish aching/swelling),[36] horse chestnut seed extract (increases venous tone, decreases filtration, alters prostaglandins/histamine),[37] and pentoxifylline (improves blood flow).[38] For symptoms related to stasis dermatitis, topical management can be added (emollients, corticosteroids).[39]

Despite these efforts, conservative medical management will be unlikely to cure the underlying valvular dysfunction and venous insufficiency present in a large truncal vein. With technological advances, definitive management of CVD has progressed from ligation and vein stripping to more minimally invasive and endovenous approaches (Table 8.3).[40] The overall approach to minimally invasive vein treatments can be seen in Figure 8.10. The most commonly used procedures, endovenous thermal ablation (EVTA), sclerotherapy (visual and ultrasound guided), and ambulatory phlebectomy, will be discussed below.[40]

FIGURE 8.8   **Skin changes representing acute and chronic venous stasis dermatitis.**

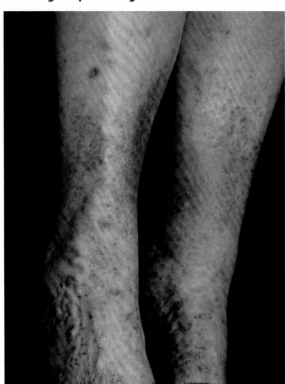

(Courtesy of Dr. Ryan M Trowbridge, MD.)

Endovenous Ablation: Thermal and Nonthermal

Endovenous ablation, a relatively new way of managing CVD, has replaced high ligation and stripping (HL and S) as the management gold standard for saphenous vein varices.[40] Endovenous ablation affords numerous benefits over HL and S, including its minimally invasive technique, ability to be performed on an outpatient basis, equivalent management success, decreased side effects (pain, wound infection, hematoma formation), decreased

TABLE 8.1   Clinical Patterns Aid in Identification of the Underlying Incompetent Vein

Skin Location	Affected Vein
Medial thigh/calf	Great saphenous vein (GSV)
Medial ankle	GSV
Lateral ankle	Short saphenous vein (SSV)
Posterior calf	SSV
Medial/proximal thigh	Pelvic (perineal, vulvar)
Labia	External pudendal, pelvic
Abdominal/suprapubic	Iliofemoral

FIGURE 8.9   **Retrograde flow in the ovarian veins with resulting engorgement of the deep pelvic veins (female equivalent of a varicocele) results in pelvic congestion syndrome.**[32]

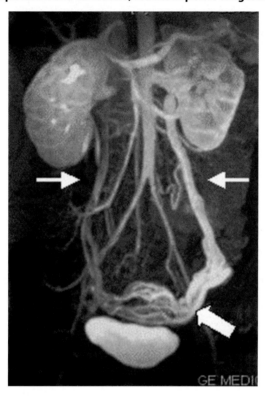

FIGURE 8.10   **Algorithm for chronic venous disease management.**

Evaluation Algorithm

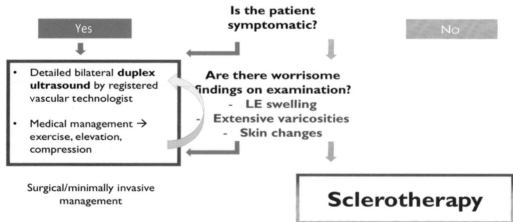

Is the patient symptomatic?

Yes

No

- Detailed bilateral **duplex ultrasound** by registered vascular technologist

- Medical management → exercise, elevation, compression

Are there worrisome findings on examination?
- LE swelling
- Extensive varicosities
- Skin changes

Surgical/minimally invasive management

Sclerotherapy

TABLE 8.2   Clinical-Etiology-Anatomy-Pathophysiology (CEAP)

Clinical Signs (C)		Etiology (E)		Anatomy (A)		Pathophysiology (P)	
C0	No signs of venous disease	Ec	Congenital	As	Superficial venous system	Pr	Venous reflux
C1	Telangiectatic/reticular spider veins only	Ep	Primary	Ap	Perforating veins	Po	Venous obstruction
C2	Simple varicose veins only	Es	Secondary	Ad	Deep venous system	Pr,o	Venous reflux and obstruction
C3	Edema of venous origin	En	Etiology not specified	An	Anatomy not specified	Pn	Reflux not specified
C4a	Hemosiderin pigmentation or eczema						
C4b	Lipodermatosclerosis						
C5	Healed venous ulcer						
C6	Active venous ulcer						

recurrence rates, and its ability to allow for a rapid return to activity.[40] It is often used in combination with sclerotherapy or phlebectomy, as addressing saphenous vein incompetence is imperative prior to management of lower extremity telangiectasias or reticular veins in order to decrease the recurrence risk.[41] Two main approaches to energy delivery comprise endovenous ablation: thermal (radiofrequency ablation (RFA) and endovenous laser therapy [EVLT]) and nonthermal (cyanoacrylate glue, VenaSeal, mechanochemical ablation [MOCA]).[42]

Thermal Ablation

EVLT and RFA comprise thermal endovenous ablation. The laser energy in EVLT is derived from a bare tip laser fiber (wavelengths 810-1470 nm). EVLT works by heating/boiling blood near the vein wall, which in turn causes steam bubble formation.[43] These steam bubbles, in combination with intraluminal red blood cell hemoglobin and vein wall water photothermal absorption, lead to vessel injury.[44] This leads to a loss of the antithrombogenic function of the tunica intima, fibrosis, occlusion through loss of tunica media collagen, and eventual vein ablation.[40] Vessel injury can be increased by decreasing the amount of space between the vessel wall and the laser fiber (tumescent anesthesia) and by increasing the quantity and length of heat contact.[44,45]

TABLE 8.3   Indications for Referral to a Vein Specialist

Venous ulceration (active or healed)
C4 disease (skin changes such as stasis dermatitis, lipodermatosclerosis, vasculopathy with negative workup, or livedoid vasculopathy)
C 2/3 disease with extensive varicose veins
Symptomatic V1 patients (even if only telangiectasias or reticular veins are present)
Failure of sclerotherapy

RFA utilizes radiofrequency energy from a bipolar radiofrequency catheter to damage the vein endothelium.[40] An electrode attached to the end of a catheter is placed into the affected vein. This electrode contacts the endothelium of the vein, radiofrequency energy is administered, and thrombosis of the vein occurs along with endothelial destruction.[46]

Both thermal endovenous ablation modalities have proven to be efficacious.[47] EVLT has been shown to have higher closure rates than RFA, especially at higher wavelengths (1320 nm), although the differences are minor.[48-57] Recurrence/recanalization of varicose veins after initial treatment is lower with EVLT than with RFA.[58] Few studies have noted a difference in minor complications, although postoperative pain is more likely to be associated with EVLT.[50,52,55,59-63] It has been hypothesized that this increase in pain is secondary to the increased maximum temperature and shorter time to maximum temperature seen with EVLT.[52-56,60,61,64,65] Ecchymoses are more common with EVLT than with RFA.[66] Serious side effects (DVT, pulmonary embolism [PE], endovenous heat-induced thrombosis) associated with EVTA are rare, although they are more commonly seen with the usage of HL and S.[52-56,59,64,67]

Endovenous Thermal Ablation Technique

To begin, a duplex ultrasound is operated to locate the diseased vein.[51,54,55,60-62,64,68] Using the Seldinger Technique, the vein is entered under ultrasound guidance with an 18-G needle and the endovenous location is confirmed with a pullback on the syringe showing blood and a normal saline flush (Figure 8.11). The syringe is removed allowing the guidewire to be placed through the 18-G needle. A small incision is made with an 11-blade in the skin at the site of the needle insertion to allow space for the catheter. The needle is removed and a catheter is infiltrated into and sent proximally in the diseased vein over the guidewire. The laser fiber or radiofrequency device is then placed in the vein. It is essential that the placement of the thermal device is confirmed to be distal to the superficial epigastric vein, typically 2 to 3 cm distal to the SFJ (Figure 8.12).[40] Once placement of the thermal device is confirmed, the catheter is withdrawn from the vein.

At this point, the provider or a trained ultrasound technician again utilizes the duplex ultrasound to ensure the laser fiber is in the desired location for management.[40] Tumescent anesthesia (lidocaine) is then administered into the perivenous space (saphenous compartment) to circumferentially surround the saphenous vein (Figure 8.13).[40] This serves a number of functions, notably to increase the space between the vein and the overlying skin and soft tissue (decreases cutaneous injury), increase the surface area of contact between the vein wall and laser fiber allowing for more effective ablation, and decrease pain.[40,69]

With the laser fiber now in the proper position and tumescent anesthesia obtained, the thermal energy is turned on.[40] As the energy is being delivered, the catheter is slowly withdrawn distally toward its starting position.[40] This enables for thermal damage to be delivered to the tunica intima throughout the course of the affected vein, effectively obliterating the entire vein.[40] The laser fiber is pulled out from the initial point of entry, the wound is properly closed, and compression is placed over the affected leg prior to leaving the clinic.[40] The procedure typically lasts 1 to 2 hours.

Nonthermal Ablation

Cyanoacrylate adhesive delivered via the VenaSeal Closure System and MOCA comprise the current nonthermal ablation options. Cyanoacrylate adhesive ("super glue") causes vein wall obliteration by promoting an inflammatory cascade secondary to polymerization upon injection.[68] MOCA applies a catheter with a rotating wire into the vein, effectively damaging the vein endothelium. This results in vain wall spasm.[46] The catheter is then slowly withdrawn, and while withdrawing, simultaneous injection of a sclerosant results in further endothelial damage and closure of the vein.[46]

FIGURE 8.11   Endovenous laser ablation (EVLA). (A) Vascular access into the saphenous vein is obtained under ultrasound guidance, and visualized with the needle in the vessel lumen (B). A typical surgical tray setup for EVLA (C).

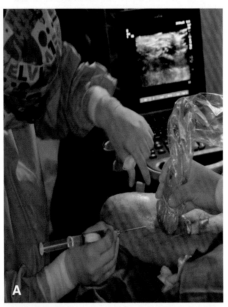

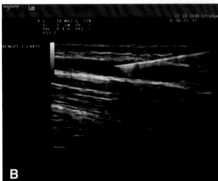

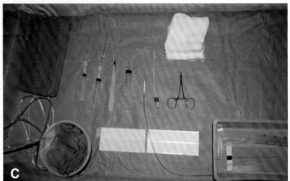

Nonthermal ablation provides treatment efficacy similar to thermal ablation, while also avoiding anesthesia and the morbidity associated with thermal energy, in terms of vein closure. This decreased morbidity has shown decreased rates of nerve injury.[69]

Sclerotherapy

Sclerotherapy (*sclero* = hard, *therapy* = treatment) is an outpatient procedure that involves the instillation of a sclerosing agent (liquid or foam) into a diseased vein.[70] This is done to damage the tunica intima with resulting fibrosis and to occlude the vessel via thrombosis.[12] Sclerotherapy is considered the standard of care for skin-level, superficial veins and for isolated small reticular veins and telangiectasias that do not have underlying truncal insufficiency.[71] Its uses are for cosmetically unacceptable and medically therapeutic reasons.[72] High-volume and high-potency ultrasound-guided

FIGURE 8.12   Thermal device distal to the superficial epigastric vein, typically 2 to 3 cm distal to the saphenofemoral junction.

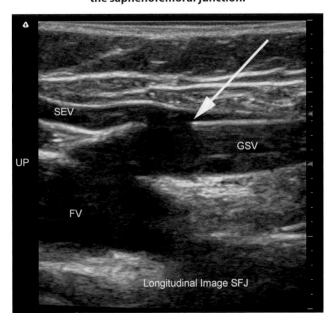

sclerotherapy (endovenous chemical ablation) can also be used with truncal vessels (GSV, SSV) when EVTA is contraindicated. Endovenous chemical ablation is used often in the management of tortuous, large incompetent branches not amenable to EVTA.[72]

FIGURE 8.13   Tumescent anesthesia surrounding laser fiber.

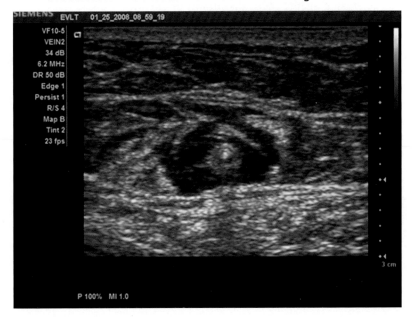

Sclerotherapy is guided by the principle of a minimal sclerosant concentration, which is the concentration of sclerosant needed to produce an effective sclerosis with the minimal amount of morbidity.[72] As the sclerosant is injected, it will diffuse away and become diluted by blood present in the vessel.[72] Thus, vessels with larger diameters will not see the sclerosant travel as far throughout the length of the vessel (Figure 8.14).[72] To counteract this, patients are ideally positioned with their legs elevated or supine, effectively decreasing the vessel size and allowing the sclerosant to diffuse throughout a greater length of the vessel (Figure 8.15).[73]

Three main categories of sclerosants are currently available: detergents, osmotics, and chemical irritants.[12] They are differentiated based on their mechanisms of action.[72]

Detergent Sclerosing Agents

Detergent sclerosing agents are fatty acids/alcohols that aggregate into lipid bilayers (micelles) upon injection, leading to denaturation of vein endothelial cell surface proteins via protein theft denaturation.[12] This disrupts the cell surface membrane of the endothelial lining, effectively lowering surface tension and causing the endothelial lining to shed.[12] Examples of detergent sclerosants include sodium tetradecyl sulfate (STS, trade name Sotradechol®) and polidocanol (trade name Asclera®).

Osmotic Sclerosing Agents

Osmotic sclerosing agents work by causing osmotic cellular dehydration, which results in cell death.[72,74] Injection of a higher concentration sclerosing agent causes fluid to shift from the cells, leading to denaturation of endothelial cell surface proteins, thrombosis, and fibrosis formation.[72] This category is associated with moderate discomfort and muscle cramps secondary to extravasation and necrosis.[72] Osmotic sclerosants also lose efficacy and concentration quickly due to rapid dilution in blood.[72,75] An advantage to the usage of hypertonic solutions is their lack of allergenicity. Due to the numerous disadvantages listed above, the usage of this class of sclerosing agents has decreased in recent years.[72]

Chemical Sclerosing Agents

Chemical sclerosing agents cause disruption of chemical bonds, leading to cell surface protein death and subsequent cellular death.[72] Examples include polyiodinated iodine

FIGURE 8.14   Volume of dilution versus distance from point of injection based on body position.

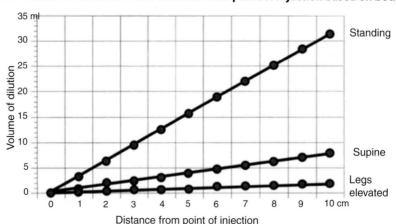

(From Goldman MP, Weiss RA. Sclerotherapy: Treatment of Varicose and Telangiectatic Leg Veins. New York, NY: Elsevier Health Science; 2016.)

FIGURE 8.15   Effects of body position on vein vessel size.

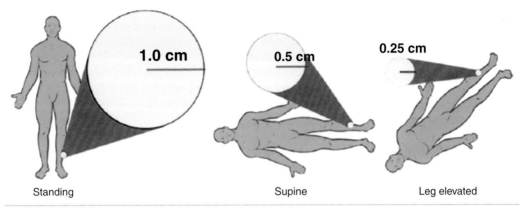

(From Goldman MP, Weiss RA. Sclerotherapy: Treatment of Varicose and Telangiectatic Leg Veins. New York, NY: Elsevier Health Science; 2016.)

(highest potency), ethanol, and glycerin.[72] Glycerin is available as a 72% solution and mixed with 1% lidocaine and epinephrine; these components are added to decrease pain with injection and to increase vasoconstriction, respectively.[72] Ethanol and polyiodinated iodine are rarely used.[72] A summary of sclerosing agents is provided in Table 8.4.

Sclerotherapy has proven more effective with recent advances, including duplex ultrasound usage, better visualization procedures, and the ability to utilize foam sclerosants.[71,72,76-78] Detergent sclerosing agents are the only type of sclerosing agents that have the ability to be injected as a foam.[12,72] Foam allows for a larger surface area that displaces more blood, allowing for increased contact of the sclerosant with the endothelium.[74] This allows the foam sclerosant to be much more efficacious (twice the potency and four times less toxicity) with less volume required than a liquid.[72] Foaming is performed by mixing liquid with gas.[74] The most utilized way is to use two syringes, one with room air and one with liquid detergent sclerosant (usually 1:4 ratio of solution to air).[72] Next, a three-way stopcock is connected to the two syringes (Tessari). The syringes are then plunged and released roughly 10 to 15 times to mix the two syringes until the ideal foam consistency is obtained.[72,79] As the foam contents are susceptible to degradation within 1 to 2 minutes, mixing them shortly before injection is necessary.[72,79] If necessary, vein lights and duplex ultrasound can be used to gain greater visualization of the vein as foam is more echogenic

TABLE 8.4	Summary of Sclerosing Agent Usage by Vessel Size			
Size of Vessel	**Sclerosant**	**Minimum Effective**	**Maximum Effective**	**Foamed?**
Reticular (1-3 mm)	Sodium tetradecyl sulfate (STS)	0.1%	0.25%	Yes
	Polidocanol	0.25%	0.5%	Yes
Telangiectasias (0.2-1 mm)	STS	0.1%	0.2%	No
	Polidocanol	0.2%	0.5%	No
	Glycerin	72%	72%	No
	Sclerodex	10% HS + 25% dextrose	10% HS + 25% dextrose	No

than liquid.[72] Foam has been shown to be associated with better closure rates.[72,80] Foam sclerotherapy is typically reserved for veins >1 mm and varicosities (Table 8.5).[72] It is typically withheld and/or used in smaller amounts or potencies in the management of small vessels (<1 mm) as there is an increased risk of hyperpigmentation and rupture.[72,81,82] Prior to its usage, it is important to inquire on a past medical history of a patent foramen ovale (PFO) or other right to left cardiac shunt and migraines with aura (higher risk of undiagnosed cardiac shunt) as patients with a PFO can develop air embolisms.[83,84] Those who experience migraines with aura should have an echocardiogram with a bubble study performed prior to foam sclerotherapy administration.[12]

Contraindications to sclerotherapy usage include patients with SFJ/SPJ reflux, those who are bedridden or otherwise immobile; have a history of superficial or deep venous thrombosis, trauma, local infection; are pregnant or lactating; have inability to ambulate, coagulopathies, and a previous allergic reaction to a sclerosing agent.[85,86]

Sclerotherapy Technique: Endovenous Chemical Ablation and Direct Visual Sclerotherapy

Prior to initiation of sclerotherapy, it is important to note that the highest-pressure vessels should be treated first (saphenous/truncal veins [GSV/SSV], large branches of saphenous/truncal veins, varicosities, reticular veins, venulectasias, and then telangiectasias).[72] If this is not done, it is expected that telangiectasias will continue to recur as reflux in deeper saphenous and reticular veins continues.[72]

Endovenous chemical ablation is a nonsterile procedure that utilizes high potency, foam sclerotherapy under ultrasound guidance to shut large, tortuous branches off the truncal veins that are not amenable to EVTA. After identifying under ultrasound guidance an enlarged, incompetent branch with documented reflux, a relatively straight segment, not overlying a bony prominence, is identified as the entry site. The area is cleansed with alcohol or chlorhexidine; the setup for this is shown in Figure 8.16A. A butterfly needle is then placed under ultrasound guidance and placement is confirmed with an air and saline flush. It is important to use ultrasound, to identify and mark perforator veins, and to ensure that the injection of the foam sclerotherapy (Figure 8.16B) is intravascular as the procedure utilizes high potency foam sclerosants, typically 5 to 10 mL of 0.5% to 1% polidocanol.

The remainder of reticular veins and telangiectasias ("spider veins") are treated by direct visual sclerotherapy. The first step is to cleanse the affected area with alcohol. Next, the patient is placed in the recumbent position. Direct cannulation with a 27/30 gauge needle on a 3 mL syringe should be used for reticular veins while telangiectasias require a larger syringe (5 mL). Due to the superficial nature of telangiectasias, the needle may be bent at 10° to 30° with the bevel up. Loop magnification with or without polarized light can be used to help identify the vessels for injection. The syringe is held between the index

TABLE 8.5   Summary of Options for Foam Sclerotherapy Based on Vessel Size

Vein Type	Size of Vessel	Instruments	Type of Sclerotherapy
Large branches off great saphenous vein/short saphenous vein	3-6 mm Blue	Ultrasound	Foam
Reticular veins	2-4 mm Blue	Vein light	Foam or liquid
Spider veins/telangiectasias	0.2-1 mm Red	Loops Polarized light	Liquid

FIGURE 8.16   (A) Setup for endovenous chemical ablation. (B) Foaming can be utilized in endovenous chemical ablation.

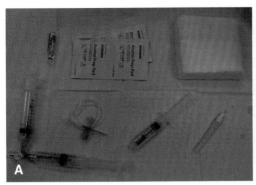
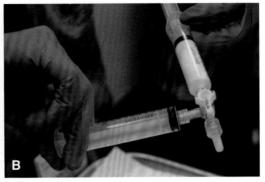

and middle fingers, and the thumb is placed on the plunger. The fourth and fifth fingers and opposite hand can rest on the lower extremity to decrease movement during injection. The sclerosant should be injected slowly with minimal pressure on the syringe. For each site, about 0.1 to 0.2 mL should be injected. Expect blanching in a radius of about 2 cm from the site of injection.[76] If at any time a bleb forms or there is extravasation or pain, the injection should be stopped immediately. In the treatment of telangiectasias, the concentration of sclerosant must be lowered: examples include 0.1% to 0.2% STS, 0.2% to 0.4% polidocanol, 72% glycerin, and Sclerodex® (10% hypertonic saline/25% dextrose).[76] With telangiectasias, a larger syringe (30G) will deliver less pressure at the needle tip.[87] Foam is typically not used.

Following any sclerotherapy procedure, the patient should walk for about 20 to 30 minutes. Compression stockings are worn to bring vessel walls in closer proximity, allowing for more thorough endothelial damage. This results in increased venous occlusion and a decreased risk of thrombophlebitis.[88] It also has the effect of decreasing telangiectatic matting, edema, bruising, and recanalization.[89] Compression stockings should be worn at all times for the next 24 to 48 hours and then during waking hours for the next 2 to 3 weeks.[90] Thigh-high compression stockings are used most often to allow for management of the entire affected area.[72] For telangiectasias only, 15 to 20 mm Hg of compression may be utilized, while 20 to 30 mm Hg is recommended for reticular veins.[91] During this time period, exercise is encouraged, but it is important to avoid heavy resistance movements or forceful muscular contractions as these will elevate abdominal and ultimately venous pressure.[91] If results are not initially satisfactory, do not retreat the same area for at least 4 to 8 weeks as immediately following treatment bruising, matting, and pigmentation changes are to be expected to clear over the upcoming 2 to 4 weeks. If the patient continues to have a poor response to treatment, reevaluation for reticular vessels, truncal varices, deeper reflux, and incompetent perforating veins should be performed, as one study reported 46% of women with spider veins alone had GSV or SSV reflux.[92] Two to four weeks post sclerotherapy, microthrombectomy may be performed to remove coagula present at the injection site and to reduce side effects (Figure 8.17).[93]

Side effects to monitor for include hyperpigmentation, temporary swelling, telangiectatic matting, pain, localized urticaria, and recurrence.[91] Hyperpigmentation present is secondary to hemosiderin deposition following blood extravasation at the site of injection.[91] Hyperpigmentation is most common with STS and lowest with glycerin.[94] Its incidence can be decreased by the removal of post-sclerotherapy coagula and it can be treated with a Q-switched laser (e.g., Nd:YAG).[95]

FIGURE 8.17   Removal of coagula 2-4 weeks post sclerotherapy. Small blade is used to scrape epidermis for coagula visualization (top). Coagula visualized below epidermis (bottom).

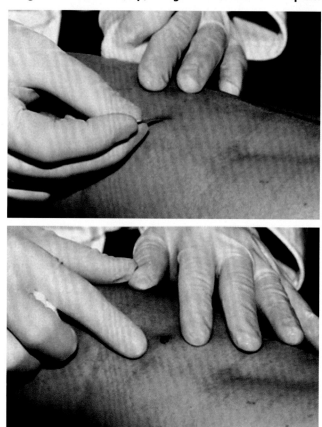

Complications of sclerotherapy are as follows: cutaneous necrosis (polidocanol is least toxic but necrosis can occur secondary to arteriolar occlusion); superficial thrombophlebitis; transient visual disturbances (seen with foam sclerotherapy in those with a history of migraines or PFOs); allergic reactions (highest with sodium morrhuate at 3% and lowest with STS at 0.3%); nerve damage (saphenous, sural); DVT; PE; embolic stroke; hematuria (seen with glycerin); and arterial injections[96] (pain, paresthesia, necrosis, compartment syndrome), seen most often in the posterior tibial artery over the posterior medial malleolus, external pudendal artery in the groin, and the peroneal artery in the knee.[97]

Ambulatory Phlebectomy

Ambulatory phlebectomy, or mini-vein stripping, has been largely replaced by the minimally invasive techniques above; however, it is still occasionally utilized in areas overlying bony prominences (not amenable to sclerotherapy) or in patients with allergy or contraindication for sclerotherapy.[40] It can be successfully combined with other CVD management options, including endovenous ablation and sclerotherapy, and in our therapeutic ladder (Figure 8.10), it is typically reserved for the final step.[98]

Ambulatory Phlebectomy Technique

The first step of the procedure is to inject local anesthesia at the sites of desired skin micro-incisions.[99] Tumescent anesthesia can also be utilized to increase vein compression and reduce blood loss.[98] Next, slit-like microincisions (1-3 mm) in the skin surface near the vein are made.[100] A number of devices, such as a number 11 blade or an 18-gauge cutting needle, can be used to make incisions in the skin surface.[98] Hooks are then utilized to grasp the vein and bring it through the skin incisions.[98] Hooks vary by size, shape, and sharpness; they include Muller and Oesch among many others.[98] Clamps are then inserted on both ends of the hook.[98,101] Clamps should have a fine tip that allows for close grip near the skin surface.[98] A scissors is used to split the vein between the clamps.[98] One end of the vein is then pulled out of the incision site with a clamp.[98] As the vein is extracted, clamps are continually placed on it as it may tear.[98] Ligation may be performed but is typically not done.[98,102] The sites of microincisions are then closed with sutures or may be covered with Steri-Strips™, dressed, and then wrapped with soft gauze.[98] Compression stockings (30-40 mm Hg) should be worn for a minimum of 2 weeks.[98] As the incisions in the skin are very small, minimal scarring is noted.[98] Complications and side effects associated with the procedure are very rare.[98,102]

▶ TREATMENT OF CHRONIC VENOUS ULCERS

Chronic venous ulcers (Figure 8.18) lead to significant pain and have a profound impact on an individual's quality of life.[1] Traditional treatments used in the management of chronic venous insufficiency are rarely curative.[1]

Standardized guidelines are available for venous ulcer management.[103] Venous ulcers should be dressed with nonadherent bandages.[103] Compression therapy (graduated, multilayered, high) has shown effectiveness in venous ulcer management.[103] Inelastic compression (short stretch) and Unna boot are more effective with regard to pump function than elastic compression (long stretch).[103] Pentoxifylline (400 mg three times daily for up to 6 months) is beneficial when used in combination with compression therapy.[103] Antibiotics are indicated with signs of classic infection.[103] Calf muscle exercises are recommended to help with the calf muscle pump.[103] There is currently no evidence for benefit of low-level laser therapy for venous ulcer improvement.[103] Other supportive measures, including hyperbaric oxygen, skin grafting, and vacuum-assisted closure, have

FIGURE 8.18   **Venous ulcer located over the medial malleolus in the distribution of the great saphenous vein. Guidewire placement (bottom).**

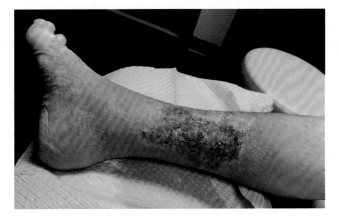

FIGURE 8.19   Before endovenous laser ablation (EVLA) (left) and EVLA 4-month follow-up (right).

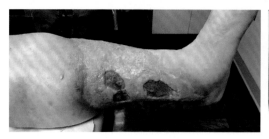 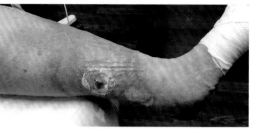

lower levels of evidence.[103] Surgical management and minimally invasive strategies (as described in Figure 8.10) can be very effective for patients with chronic venous leg ulcers and superficial venous disease (Figure 8.19).[99] If management is successful, preventing recurrence is the next important step. Evidence is strong for usage of below-knee compression hosiery.[103]

REFERENCES

1. Eberhardt RT, Raffetto JD. Chronic venous insufficiency. *Circulation*. 2014;130(4):333-346. Available at http://www.ncbi. nlm.nih.gov/pubmed/25047584.
2. Rabe E, Berboth G, Pannier F. Epidemiologie der chronischen Venenkrankheiten. *Wiener Medizinische Wochenschrift*. 2016;166(9-10):260-263. Available at http://link.springer.com/10.1007/s10354-016-0465-y.
3. Meissner MH. Lower extremity venous anatomy. *Semin Intervent Radiol*. 2005;22(3):147-156. Available at http://www. ncbi.nlm.nih.gov/pubmed/21326687.
4. Bazigou E, Makinen T. Flow control in our vessels: vascular valves make sure there is no way back. *Cell Mol Life Sci*. 2013;70(6):1055-1066. Available at http://www.ncbi.nlm.nih.gov/pubmed/22922986.
5. Goldman MP, Weiss RA, Bergan JJ. Diagnosis and treatment of varicose veins: a review. *J Am Acad Dermatol*. 1994;31(3 pt 1):393-413;quiz 414-416. Available at http://www.ncbi.nlm.nih.gov/pubmed/8077464.
6. Cornu-Thenard A, Boivin P, Baud JM, et al. Importance of the familial factor in varicose disease. Clinical study of 134 families. *J Dermatol Surg Oncol*. 1994;20(5):318-326. Available at http://www.ncbi.nlm.nih.gov/pubmed/8176043.
7. Komsuoğlu B, Göldeli O, Kulan K, et al. Prevalence and risk factors of varicose veins in an elderly population. *Gerontology*. 1994;40(1):25-31. Available at https://www.karger.com/Article/FullText/213571.
8. Hirai M, Naiki K, Nakayama R. Prevalence and risk factors of varicose veins in Japanese women. *Angiology*. 1990;41(3):228-232. Available at http://journals.sagepub.com/doi/10.1177/000331979004100308.
9. Fowkes F, Lee A, Evans C, et al. Lifestyle risk factors for lower limb venous reflux in the general population: Edinburgh Vein Study. *Int J Epidemiol*. 2001;30(4):846-852. Available at http://www.ncbi.nlm.nih.gov/pubmed/11511615.
10. Scott TE, LaMorte WW, Gorin DR, et al. Risk factors for chronic venous insufficiency: a dual case-control study. *J Vasc Surg*. 1995;22(5):622-628. Available at http://www.ncbi.nlm.nih.gov/pubmed/7494366.
11. Fowkes FGR, Evans CJ, Lee AJ. Prevalence and risk factors of chronic venous insufficiency. *Angiology*. 2001;52(1 suppl):S5-S15. Available at http://www.ncbi.nlm.nih.gov/pubmed/11510598.
12. Duffy DM. Sclerosants: a comparative review. *Dermatol Surg*. 2010;36(suppl 2):1010-1025. Available at http://www.ncbi. nlm.nih.gov/pubmed/20590708.
13. DFriedman, VMishra, JHsu. Treatment of Varicose Veins and Telangiectatic Lower-Extremity Vessels. In: Fitzpatrick's Dermatology. 9th ed. New York, NY: McGraw-Hill Medical; 2019. Available at https://accessmedicine.mhmedical.com/ content.aspx?bookid=2570&sectionid=210447008.
14. Nawroth PP, Handley DA, Esmon CT, et al. Interleukin 1 induces endothelial cell procoagulant while suppressing cell-surface anticoagulant activity. *Proc Natl Acad Sci U S A*. 1986;83(10):3460-3464. Available at http://www.ncbi.nlm.nih. gov/pubmed/3486418.
15. Kahn SR, M'lan CE, Lamping DL, et al. Relationship between clinical classification of chronic venous disease and patient-reported quality of life: results from an international cohort study. *J Vasc Surg*. 2004;39(4):823-828. Available at http://www.ncbi.nlm.nih.gov/pubmed/15071450.
16. van Korlaar I, Vossen C, Rosendaal F, et al. Quality of life in venous disease. *Thromb Haemost*. 2003;90(1):27-35. Available at http://www.ncbi.nlm.nih.gov/pubmed/12876622.
17. Ricci S, Moro L, Incalzi RA. The foot venous system: anatomy, physiology and relevance to clinical practice. *Dermatol Surg*. 2014;40(3):225-233. Available at http://www.ncbi.nlm.nih.gov/pubmed/24372905.

18. Lee DK, Ahn KS, Kang CH, et al. Ultrasonography of the lower extremity veins: anatomy and basic approach. *Ultrason (Seoul, Korea)*. 2017;36(2):120-130. Available at http://www.ncbi.nlm.nih.gov/pubmed/28260355.

19. Chwała M, Szczeklik W, Szczeklik M, et al. Varicose veins of lower extremities, hemodynamics and treatment methods. *Adv Clin Exp Med*. 2015;24(1):5-14. Available at http://www.advances.umed.wroc.pl/en/article/2015/24/1/5/.

20. Somjen GM. Anatomy of the superficial venous system. *Dermatol Surg*. 1995;21(1):35-45. Available at http://www.ncbi.nlm.nih.gov/pubmed/7600017.

21. Thomson H. The surgical anatomy of the superficial and perforating veins of the lower limb. *Ann R Coll Surg Engl*. 1979;61(3):198-205. Available at http://www.ncbi.nlm.nih.gov/pubmed/485047.

22. Caggiati A, Bergan JJ, Gloviczki P, et al. Nomenclature of the veins of the lower limbs: an international interdisciplinary consensus statement. *J Vasc Surg*. 2002;36(2):416-422. Available at http://www.ncbi.nlm.nih.gov/pubmed/12170230.

23. Notowitz LB. Normal venous anatomy and physiology of the lower extremity. *J Vasc Nurs*. 1993;11(2):39-42. Available at http://www.ncbi.nlm.nih.gov/pubmed/8274376.

24. Abramson DI. Diseases of the veins: pathology, diagnosis and treatment. *J Am Med Assoc*. 1988;260(24):3680. Available at http://jama.jamanetwork.com/article.aspx?doi=10.1001/jama.1988.03410240150061.

25. Blomgren L, Johansson G, Siegbahn A, et al. Parameter der Koagulation und Fibrinolyse bei Patienten mit chronischer venöser Insuffizienz. *Vasa*. 2001;30(3):184-187. Available at http://www.ncbi.nlm.nih.gov/pubmed/11582948.

26. Matic M, Matic A, Djuran V, et al. Frequency of peripheral arterial disease in patients with chronic venous insufficiency. *Iran Red Crescent Med J*. 2016;18(1):e20781. Available at http://www.ncbi.nlm.nih.gov/pubmed/26889387.

27. Burnand K. The physiology and hemodynamics of chronic venous insufficiency of the lower limb. *Handb Venous Disord Guidel Am Venous Forum*. 2001;2nd:49-57.

28. Mozes G, Carmichael SWGP. *Development and anatomy of the venous system.*In: *Handbook of Venous Disorders: Guidelines of the American Venous Forum*. 2nd ed. London, England: Arnold; 2011:11-24.

29. Jawien A. The influence of environmental factors in chronic venous insufficiency. *Angiology*. 2003;54(1 suppl):S19-S31. Available at http://journals.sagepub.com/doi/10.1177/0003319703054001S04.

30. Lacroix P, Aboyans V, Preux PM, et al. Epidemiology of venous insufficiency in an occupational population. *Int Angiol*. 2003;22(2):172-176. Available at http://www.ncbi.nlm.nih.gov/pubmed/12865883.

31. Shabani Varaki E, Gargiulo GD, Penkala S, et al. Peripheral vascular disease assessment in the lower limb: a review of current and emerging non-invasive diagnostic methods. *Biomed Eng Online*. 2018;17(1):61. Available at http://www.ncbi.nlm.nih.gov/pubmed/29751811.

32. Durham JD, Machan L. Pelvic congestion syndrome. *Semin Intervent Radiol*. 2013;30(4):372-380. Available at http://www.ncbi.nlm.nih.gov/pubmed/24436564.

33. Konoeda H, Yamaki T, Hamahata A, et al. Quantification of superficial venous reflux by duplex ultrasound-role of reflux velocity in the assessment the clinical stage of chronic venous insufficiency. *Ann Vasc Dis*. 2014;7(4):376-382. Available at http://www.ncbi.nlm.nih.gov/pubmed/25593622.

34. Labropoulos N, Tiongson J, Pryor L, et al. Definition of venous reflux in lower-extremity veins. *J Vasc Surg*. 2003;38(4):793-798. Available at http://www.ncbi.nlm.nih.gov/pubmed/14560232.

35. Moneta G. *Classification of Lower Extremity Chronic Venous Disorders – UpToDate*. UpToDate. 2019. Available at https://www.uptodate.com/contents/classification-of-lower-extremity-chronic-venous-disorders.

36. Martinez-Zapata MJ, Vernooij RW, Uriona Tuma SM, et al. Phlebotonics for venous insufficiency. *Cochrane Database Syst Rev*. 2016;4:CD003229. Available at http://www.ncbi.nlm.nih.gov/pubmed/27048768.

37. Pittler MH, Ernst E. Horse chestnut seed extract for chronic venous insufficiency. *Cochrane Database Syst Rev*. 2012;11:CD003230. Available at http://www.ncbi.nlm.nih.gov/pubmed/23152216.

38. Jull A, Waters J, Arroll B. Pentoxifylline for treatment of venous leg ulcers: a systematic review. *Lancet*. 2002;359(9317):1550-1554. Available at http://www.ncbi.nlm.nih.gov/pubmed/12047963.

39. Sundaresan S, Migden MR, Silapunt S. Stasis dermatitis: pathophysiology, evaluation, and management. *Am J Clin Dermatol*. 2017;18(3):383-390. Available at http://link.springer.com/10.1007/s40257-016-0250-0.

40. Ahadiat O, Higgins S, Ly A, et al. Review of endovenous thermal ablation of the great saphenous vein. *Dermatol Surg*. 2018;44(5):679-688. Available at http://insights.ovid.com/crossref?an=00042728-900000000-98787.

41. Schuller-Petrovic S. Endovenöse ablation der Stammvenenvarikose. *Wiener Medizinische Wochenschrift*. 2016;166(9-10):297-301. Available at http://www.ncbi.nlm.nih.gov/pubmed/27295103.

42. Brasic N, Lopresti D, McSwain H. Endovenous laser ablation and sclerotherapy for treatment of varicose veins. *Semin Cutan Med Surg*. 2008;27(4):264-275. Available at http://www.ncbi.nlm.nih.gov/pubmed/19150298.

43. Parente EJ, Rosenblatt M. Endovenous laser treatment to promote venous occlusion. *Lasers Surg Med*. 2003;33(2):115-118. Available at http://www.ncbi.nlm.nih.gov/pubmed/12913883.

44. van Ruijven PWM, Poluektova AA, van Gemert MJC, et al. Optical-thermal mathematical model for endovenous laser ablation of varicose veins. *Lasers Med Sci*. 2014;29(2):431-439. Available at http://link.springer.com/10.1007/s10103-013-1451-x.

45. Proebstle TM, Sandhofer M, Kargl A, et al. Thermal damage of the inner vein wall during endovenous laser treatment: key role of energy absorption by intravascular blood. *Dermatol Surg*. 2002;28(7):596-600. Available at http://www.ncbi.nlm.nih.gov/pubmed/12135514.

46. Kiguchi MM, Dillavou ED. Thermal and nonthermal endovenous ablation options for treatment of superficial venous insufficiency. *Surg Clin North Am*. 2018;98(2):385-400. Available at https://www.sciencedirect.com/science/article/pii/S003961091730230X?via%3Dihub.

47. Vuylsteke MF, Martinelli T, Van Dorpe J, et al. Endovenous laser ablation: the role of intraluminal blood. *Eur J Vasc Endovasc Surg*. 2011;42(1):120-126. Available at http://www.ncbi.nlm.nih.gov/pubmed/21524926.

48. Puggioni A, Kalra M, Carmo M, et al. Endovenous laser therapy and radiofrequency ablation of the great saphenous vein: analysis of early efficacy and complications. *J Vasc Surg*. 2005;42(3):488-493. Available at http://www.ncbi.nlm.nih.gov/pubmed/16171593.

49. Luebke T, Brunkwall J. Systematic review and meta-analysis of endovenous radiofrequency obliteration, endovenous laser therapy, and foam sclerotherapy for primary varicosis. *J Cardiovasc Surg (Torino)*. 2008;49(2):213-233. Available at http://www.ncbi.nlm.nih.gov/pubmed/18431342.

50. van den Bos R, Arends L, Kockaert M, et al. Endovenous therapies of lower extremity varicosities: a meta-analysis. *J Vasc Surg*. 2009;49(1):230-239. Available at http://www.ncbi.nlm.nih.gov/pubmed/18692348.

51. Ravi R, Trayler EA, Barrett DA, et al. Endovenous thermal ablation of superficial venous insufficiency of the lower extremity: single-center experience with 3000 limbs treated in a 7-year period. *J Endovasc Ther*. 2009;16(4):500-505. Available at http://jet.sagepub.com/lookup/doi/10.1583/09-2750.1.

52. Goode SD, Chowdhury A, Crockett M, et al. Laser and radiofrequency ablation study (lara study): a randomised study comparing radiofrequency ablation and endovenous laser ablation (810nm). *Eur J Vasc Endovasc Surg*. 2010;40(2):246-253. Available at http://www.ncbi.nlm.nih.gov/pubmed/20537570.

53. Krnic A, Sucic Z. Bipolar radiofrequency induced thermotherapy and 1064 nm Nd:Yag laser in endovenous occlusion of insufficient veins: short term follow up results. *Vasa*. 2011;40(3):235-240. Available at https://econtent.hogrefe.com/doi/10.1024/0301-1526/a000098.

54. Nordon IM, Hinchliffe RJ, Brar R, et al. A prospective double-blind randomized controlled trial of radiofrequency versus laser treatment of the great saphenous vein in patients with varicose veins. *Ann Surg*. 2011;254(6):876-881. Available at http://content.wkhealth.com/linkback/openurl?sid=WKPTLP:landingpage&an=00000658-201112000-00008.

55. Mese B, Bozoglan O, Eroglu E, et al. A comparison of 1,470-nm endovenous laser ablation and radiofrequency ablation in the treatment of great saphenous veins 10 mm or more in size. *Ann Vasc Surg*. 2015;29(7):1368-1372. Available at http://www.ncbi.nlm.nih.gov/pubmed/26122425.

56. Sydnor M, Mavropoulos J, Slobodnik N, et al. A randomized prospective long-term (>1 year) clinical trial comparing the efficacy and safety of radiofrequency ablation to 980 nm laser ablation of the great saphenous vein. *Phlebology*. 2017;32(6):415-424. Available at http://journals.sagepub.com/doi/10.1177/0268355516658592.

57. Balint R, Farics A, Parti K, et al. Which endovenous ablation method does offer a better long-term technical success in the treatment of the incompetent great saphenous vein? Review. *Vascular*. 2016;24(6):649-657. Available at http://journals.sagepub.com/doi/10.1177/1708538116648035.

58. Weiss RA, Weiss MA, Eimpunth S, et al. Comparative outcomes of different endovenous thermal ablation systems on great and small saphenous vein insufficiency: long-term results. *Lasers Surg Med*. 2015;47(2):156-160. Available at http://doi.wiley.com/10.1002/lsm.22335.

59. Gale SS, Lee JN, Walsh ME, et al. A randomized, controlled trial of endovenous thermal ablation using the 810-nm wavelength laser and the ClosurePLUS radiofrequency ablation methods for superficial venous insufficiency of the great saphenous vein. *J Vasc Surg*. 2010;52(3):645-650. Available at https://linkinghub.elsevier.com/retrieve/pii/S0741521410010566.

60. Tesmann JP, Thierbach H, Dietrich A, et al. Radiofrequency induced thermotherapy (RFITT) of varicose veins compared to endovenous laser treatment (EVLT): a non-randomized prospective study concentrating on occlusion rates, side-effects and clinical outcome. *Eur J Dermatol*. 2011;21(6):945-951. Available at http://www.ncbi.nlm.nih.gov/pubmed/21914582.

61. Rasmussen L, Lawaetz M, Serup J, et al. Randomized clinical trial comparing endovenous laser ablation, radiofrequency ablation, foam sclerotherapy, and surgical stripping for great saphenous varicose veins with 3-year follow-up. *J Vasc Surg Venous Lymphat Disord*. 2013;1(4):349-356. Available at https://linkinghub.elsevier.com/retrieve/pii/S2213333X13000966.

62. Bozoglan O, Mese B, Eroglu E, et al. Comparison of endovenous laser and radiofrequency ablation in treating varices in the same patient. *J Lasers Med Sci*. 2017;8(1):13-16. Available at http://www.ncbi.nlm.nih.gov/pubmed/28912938.

63. Woźniak W, Mlosek RK, Ciostek P. Complications and failure of endovenous laser ablation and radiofrequency ablation procedures in patients with lower extremity varicose veins in a 5-year follow-up. *Vasc Endovascular Surg*. 2016;50(7):475-483. Available at http://journals.sagepub.com/doi/10.1177/1538574416671247.

64. Almeida JI, Kaufman J, Göckeritz O, et al. Radiofrequency endovenous ClosureFAST versus laser ablation for the treatment of great saphenous reflux: a multicenter, single-blinded, randomized study (recovery study). *J Vasc Interv Radiol*. 2009;20(6):752-759. Available at http://www.ncbi.nlm.nih.gov/pubmed/19395275.

65. Shepherd AC, Gohel MS, Brown LC, et al. Randomized clinical trial of VNUS® ClosureFAST™ radiofrequency ablation versus laser for varicose veins. *Br J Surg*. 2010;97(6):810-818. Available at http://www.ncbi.nlm.nih.gov/pubmed/20473992.

66. Malskat WSJ, Stokbroekx MAL, van der Geld CWM, et al. Temperature profiles of 980- and 1,470-nm endovenous laser ablation, endovenous radiofrequency ablation and endovenous steam ablation. *Lasers Med Sci*. 2014;29(2):423-429. Available at http://link.springer.com/10.1007/s10103-013-1449-4.

67. Dermody M, O'Donnell TF, Balk EM. Complications of endovenous ablation in randomized controlled trials. *J Vasc Surg Venous Lymphat Disord*. 2013;1(4):427-436.e1. Available at http://www.ncbi.nlm.nih.gov/pubmed/26992769.

68. Moul DK, Housman L, Romine S, et al. Endovenous laser ablation of the great and short saphenous veins with a 1320-nm neodymium:yttrium-aluminum-garnet laser: retrospective case series of 1171 procedures. *J Am Acad Dermatol.* 2014;70(2):326-331. Available at https://linkinghub.elsevier.com/retrieve/pii/S0190962213010578.

69. Manfrini S, Gasbarro V, Danielsson G, et al. Endovenous management of saphenous vein reflux. Endovenous reflux management study group. *J Vasc Surg.* 2000;32(2):330-342. Available at http://www.ncbi.nlm.nih.gov/pubmed/10917994.

70. Chiesa R, Marone EM, Limoni C, et al. Chronic venous insufficiency in Italy: the 24-cities cohort study. *Eur J Vasc Endovasc Surg.* 2005;30(4):422-429. Available at http://www.ncbi.nlm.nih.gov/pubmed/16009576.

71. Goldman MP, Weiss RA, Duffy NSS DM. Guidelines of care for sclerotherapy treatment of varicose and telangiectatic leg veins. American Academy of Dermatology. *J Am Acad Dermatol.* 1996;34(3):523-528. Available at http://www.ncbi.nlm.nih.gov/pubmed/8609276.

72. Weiss MA, Hsu JTS, Neuhaus I, et al. Consensus for sclerotherapy. *Dermatol Surg.* 2014;40(12):1309-1318. Available at http://www.ncbi.nlm.nih.gov/pubmed/25418805.

73. Pollack AA, Taylor BE, Myers TT, et al. The effect of exercise and body position on the venous pressure at the ankle in patients having venous valvular defects. *J Clin Invest.* 1949;28(3):559-563. Available at http://europepmc.org/backend/ptpmcrender.fcgi?accid=PMC439636&blobtype=pdf.P

74. Goldman MP, Guex J-J, Ramelet A-A, Ricci S. *Sclerotherapy Treatment of Varicose and Telangiectatic Leg Veins.* 5th ed. Edinburgh, TX: Elsevier; 2011. 416.

75. Dietzek CL. Sclerotherapy: introduction to solutions and techniques. *Perspect Vasc Surg Endovasc Ther.* 2007;19(3):317-324. Available at http://www.ncbi.nlm.nih.gov/pubmed/17966153.

76. Sadick NS. Choosing the appropriate sclerosing concentration for vessel diameter. *Dermatol Surg.* 2010;36(suppl 2):976-981. Available at http://insights.ovid.com/crossref?an=00042728-201006002-00003.

77. Erkin A, Kosemehmetoglu K, Diler MS, et al. Evaluation of the minimum effective concentration of foam sclerosant in an ex-vivo study. *Eur J Vasc Endovasc Surg.* 2012;44(6):593-597. Available at https://linkinghub.elsevier.com/retrieve/pii/S1078588412006600.

78. Palm MD. Commentary: choosing the appropriate sclerosing concentration for vessel diameter. *Dermatol Surg.* 2010;36(suppl 2):982. Available at http://insights.ovid.com/crossref?an=00042728-201006002-00004.

79. Tessari L, Cavezzi A, Frullini A. Preliminary experience with a new sclerosing foam in the treatment of varicose veins. *Dermatol Surg.* 2001;27(1):58-60. Available at http://www.ncbi.nlm.nih.gov/pubmed/11231246.

80. Bergan J. Sclerotherapy: a truly minimally invasive technique. *Perspect Vasc Surg Endovasc Ther.* 2008;20(1):70-72. Available at http://www.ncbi.nlm.nih.gov/pubmed/18403470.

81. Kahle B, Leng K. Efficacy of sclerotherapy in varicose veins – prospective, blinded, placebo-controlled study. *Dermatol Surg.* 2004;30(5):723-728;discussion 728. Available at http://doi.wiley.com/10.1111/j.1524-4725.2004.30207.x.

82. Rathbun S, Norris A, Morrison N, et al. Performance of endovenous foam sclerotherapy in the USA. *Phlebol J Venous Dis.* 2012;27(2):59-66. Available at http://www.ncbi.nlm.nih.gov/pubmed/21893552.

83. StÜCker M, Kobus S, Altmeyer P, et al. Review of published information on foam sclerotherapy. *Dermatol Surg.* 2010;36(suppl 2):983-992. Available at http://www.ncbi.nlm.nih.gov/pubmed/20590705.

84. Hamel-Desnos C, Allaert FA. Liquid versus foam sclerotherapy. *Phlebol J Venous Dis.* 2009;24(6):240-246. Available at http://journals.sagepub.com/doi/10.1258/phleb.2009.009047.

85. Gillet J-L, Guedes JM, Guex J-J, et al. Side-effects and complications of foam sclerotherapy of the great and small saphenous veins: a controlled multicentre prospective study including 1,025 patients. *Phlebology.* 2009;24(3):131-138. Available at http://journals.sagepub.com/doi/10.1258/phleb.2008.008063.

86. Sarvananthan T, Shepherd AC, Willenberg T, et al. Neurological complications of sclerotherapy for varicose veins. *J Vasc Surg.* 2012;55(1):243-251. Available at https://linkinghub.elsevier.com/retrieve/pii/S0741521411013358.

87. Mann MW. Sclerotherapy: it is back and better. *Clin Plast Surg.* 2011;38(3):475-487. Available at https://www.plasticsurgery.theclinics.com/article/S0094-1298(11)00007-1/fulltext.

88. Cavezzi A, Tessari L. Foam sclerotherapy techniques: different gases and methods of preparation, catheter versus direct injection. *Phlebology.* 2009;24(6):247-251. Available at http://journals.sagepub.com/doi/10.1258/phleb.2009.009061.

89. Goldman MP. Compression in the treatment of leg telangiectasia: theoretical considerations. *J Dermatol Surg Oncol.* 1989;15(2):184-188. Available at http://www.ncbi.nlm.nih.gov/pubmed/2644328.

90. Weiss RA, Sadick NS, Goldman MP, et al. Post-sclerotherapy compression: controlled comparative study of duration of compression and its effects on clinical outcome. *Dermatol Surg.* 1999;25(2):105-108. Available at http://www.ncbi.nlm.nih.gov/pubmed/10037513.

91. Bergan JJ. *The Vein Book.* Elsevier Academic Press; 2007:617.

92. Engelhorn CA, Engelhorn Al V, Cassou MF, et al. Patterns of saphenous venous reflux in women presenting with lower extremity telangiectasias. *Dermatol Surg.* 2007;33(3):282-288. Available at http://www.ncbi.nlm.nih.gov/pubmed/17338684.

93. Scultetus AH, Villavicencio JL, Kao T-C, et al. Microthrombectomy reduces postsclerotherapy pigmentation: multicenter randomized trial. *J Vasc Surg.* 2003;38(5):896-903. Available at http://www.ncbi.nlm.nih.gov/pubmed/14603191.

94. Ramadan W, El-Hoshy K, Shabaan D, et. al. Clinical comparison of sodium tetradecyl sulfate 0.25% versus polidocanol 0.75% in sclerotherapy of lower extremity telangiectasia. *Gulf J Dermatol Venereol.* 2011;18:33-40.

95. Ianosi G, Ianosi S, Calbureanu-Popescu MX, et al. Comparative study in leg telangiectasias treatment with Nd:YAG laser and sclerotherapy. *Exp Ther Med.* 2019;17(2):1106-1112. Available at http://www.ncbi.nlm.nih.gov/pubmed/30679981.

96. Hafner F, Froehlich H, Gary T, et al. Intra-arterial injection, a rare but serious complication of sclerotherapy. *Phlebol J Venous Dis*. 2013;28(2):64-73. Available at http://www.ncbi.nlm.nih.gov/pubmed/22422795.

97. Munavalli GS, Weiss RA. Complications of sclerotherapy. *Semin Cutan Med Surg*. 2007;26(1):22-28. Available at http://scmsjournal.com/article/buy_now/?id=378.

98. Kabnick LS, Ombrellino M. Ambulatory phlebectomy. *Semin Intervent Radiol*. 2005;22(3):218-224. Available at http://www.ncbi.nlm.nih.gov/pubmed/21326696.

99. Wysong A, Taylor BR, Graves M, et al. Successful treatment of chronic venous ulcers with a 1,320-nm endovenous laser combined with other minimally invasive venous procedures. *Dermatol Surg*. 2016;42(8):961-966. Available at http://content.wkhealth.com/linkback/openurl?sid=WKPTLP:landingpage&an=00042728-201608000-00006.

100. Smith SR, Goldman MP. Tumescent anesthesia in ambulatory phlebectomy. *Dermatol Surg*. 1998;24(4):453-456. Available at http://www.ncbi.nlm.nih.gov/pubmed/9568202.

101. Dortu J, Raymond-Martimbeau P. *Ambulatory Phlebectomy*. Houstan, TX: PMR Edition; 1993.

102. Ramelet AA. Müller phlebectomy. A new phlebectomy hook. *J Dermatol Surg Oncol*. 1991;17(10):814-816. Available at http://www.ncbi.nlm.nih.gov/pubmed/1918588.

103. Rai R. Standard guidelines for management of venous leg ulcer. *Indian Dermatol Online J*. 2014;5(3):408-411. Available at http://www.ncbi.nlm.nih.gov/pubmed/25165686.

Cosmeceuticals

Michelle Henry, MD

Chapter Highlights

- Cosmeceuticals are topically applied, over-the-counter skincare products containing key active ingredients.
- Sunscreens are topical preparations that reflect or absorb ultraviolet radiation and can be physical, chemical, or combination products.
- To be labeled as "broad-spectrum", sunscreens must block both ultraviolet A and ultraviolet B radiation.
- Retinoids are vitamin A derivatives used in topical preparations for their antiaging effects.
- Various skin-lightning agents, including hydroquinone, retinoids, and ascorbic acid, are available in over-the-counter cosmeceuticals.
- Individuals with sensitive skin must be familiar with and avoid common antigens in skincare products; these individuals may benefit from patch testing.

Increasingly, patients are looking for cost-effective noninvasive methods to prevent and reverse the signs of skin aging. Topically applied, over-the-counter skincare products containing key active ingredients, commonly referred to as cosmeceuticals, are the first line of defense against aging and are ubiquitously used for a variety of aesthetic indications. Compared to other noninvasive or minimally invasive strategies such as energy-based devices, fillers, and neurotoxins, the use of cosmeceuticals has the lion's share of the market due to their ease of use and the fact that they are accessible to consumers regardless of their socioeconomic status. According to the latest data, the global cosmeceuticals market was USD 45.47 billion in 2017 and is estimated to reach 72.99 billion by 2023 at a compound annual growth of 8.21% during the forecasted period. In fact, the global cosmeceuticals market is outpacing all other product segments in the personal care products and cosmetics industry.[1]

Albert Kligman coined the term "cosmeceutical" in 1984 to refer to substances that exerted both cosmetic and therapeutic benefits.[2] According to Kligman, a product should address three main questions to qualify as a cosmeceutical. First, does the active ingredient penetrate the stratum corneum and reach in sufficient concentrations to its intended target in the skin? Second, does it have a known specific biochemical mechanism of action in the target cell or tissue in human skin? Finally, are there published, peer-reviewed, double-blind, placebo-controlled, statistically significant, clinical trials to substantiate the efficacy claims? Since cosmeceuticals are an amalgamation of cosmetics and pharmaceuticals, with the exception of sunscreens, they remain an unrecognized category by the US Food and Drug Administration and stringent regulatory pathways do not exist to guide research and marketing. Only recently have there been efforts to address quality control, substantiate marketing claims, and establish industry standards, since cosmeceuticals intend to deliver results on a higher level than cosmetics that simply color and scent the skin.[3]

Applications of cosmeceuticals can range from improving skin radiance and texture, reducing acne, decreasing pigmentation, and by far the most sought-after indication, antiaging. Most cosmeceuticals are made from marine algae, fruits, herbs, botanicals, or cell culture extracts. This chapter will focus on cosmeceuticals used for skin protection, retinoids for antiaging, formulations for skin brightening, and products that are safe to use in sensitive skin.

▶ SUNSCREENS

Sunscreens are topical preparations containing filters that reflect or absorb radiation in the ultraviolet (UV) wavelength range. While sunlight is essential for vitamin D synthesis and can boost well-being, chronic or acute exposure to UV radiation (290-400 nm) can have detrimental effects on human skin such as sunburn, photoaging, and skin cancer. The UV radiation that reaches the earth's surface contains 5% ultraviolet B (UVB) (290-320 nm) and 95% ultraviolet A (UVA) (320-400 nm). UVB radiation includes the most biologically active wavelengths that are responsible for sunburn, inflammation, and skin cancer, while UVA rays are those that significantly contribute to photoaging and play a major role in the development of sunspots, dyschromias, and fine lines.[4-6]

Topical photoprotection works primarily through either scattering and reflection of UV energy or absorption of UV energy. Many current sunscreens contain ingredients that work through both mechanisms in terms of UV protection. In the United States, where sunscreens are considered to be over-the-counter drugs that need to be FDA-approved, there are 17 different UV filters, while many other UV filters are available in Europe, Canada, and Australia.[7-9] They are classified as organic (formerly known as chemical sunscreens) and inorganic (formerly known as physical sunscreens). Since no single agent effectively provides adequate protection from both UVA and UVB radiation, nearly all commercially available sunscreen products contain agents from both groups. Two or more sunscreen active ingredients may be combined with each other in a single product when used in the concentrations approved by the FDA for each agent. Broad-spectrum sunscreens are generally combinations of sunscreen products that are able to absorb both UVB and UVA radiation.

Organic filters (Table 9.1) include a variety of aromatic compounds that protect the skin by absorbing UV energy and transforming it into a negligible amount of heat energy.[19] Specifically, the sunscreen chemical, after being excited to a higher energy state from its ground state via the absorption of UV radiation, returns to the ground state emitting energy in the form of longer wavelengths, typically as very weak red light or mild infrared radiation. The most common sunscreen organic agents, salicylates and cinnamates, both absorb UVB. Salicylates were the first UV chemical absorbers used in commercially available sunscreen preparations with a UV absorbance of about 300 nm. The salicylate

TABLE 9.1   Sunscreens

Sunscreen	Range of Protection
Organic	
Salicylates	
• Octisalate (octyl salicylate) • Homosalate • Trolamine salicylate	UVB
Cinnamates	
• Octinoxate • Cinoxate	UVB
Benzophenones	
• Oxybenzone • Sulisobenzone • Dioxybenzone	UVB, UVA2
Others	
• Octocrylene • Ensulizole • Avobenzone • Ecamsule • Drometrizole • Meradimate • Bemotrizinol • Bisoctrizole	• UVB • UVB • UVA1 • UVB, UVA2 • UVB, UVA2 • UVA2 • UVB, UVA2 • UVB, UVA2
Inorganic	
Titanium dioxide	UVB, UVA1, UVA2
Zinc oxide	UVB, UVA1, UVA2

group of sunscreen agents includes octyl salicylate and homomenthyl salicylate. Among cinnamates, octinoxate is the most widely used UVB filter worldwide. Cinnamates, chemically related to balsam of Peru, coca leaves, cinnamic aldehyde, and cinnamic oil, have a peak absorption wavelength of about 305 nm. The chemical structure of the cinnamates, as a group, makes the molecule insoluble in water, requiring more frequent reapplication of the preparation.

Benzophenone derivates and anthranilates are effective at absorbing UVA radiation. Although the primary protective range for benzophenone is in the UVA range, a secondary protective band is also noted in the UVB range. The most commonly used benzophenone agents are oxybenzone and dioxybenzone. Although these ingredients are much less allergenic than first-generation sunscreen, they still carry a risk of contact allergy. Other agents such as avobenzone can be combined with UVB filters such as homosalate and octisalate to yield a broad-spectrum coverage.

Inorganic filters (Table 9.1) are mineral compounds, the most common being zinc oxide and titanium dioxide. These are believed to reflect and scatter UV light over a wide range of wavelengths, effectively serving as a physical barrier to incident UV and visible light.[20] However, studies have shown that these compounds, and in particular micronized preparations, absorb rather than reflect UV radiation. Their popularity has grown in recent years due primarily to their low toxicity profile. Aside from being effective in protecting against both UVA and UVB, these agents are fairly photostable and have not been shown to induce phototoxic or photoallergic reactions. Early formulations of physical sunscreen agents were not widely accepted because the particulate matters had to be incorporated in high concentrations, resulting in an opaque film on the skin that was not cosmetically acceptable. Newer formulations provide "micronized" formulations that allow for adequate protection while having a translucent appearance that leads to improved cosmetic results. Considering zinc oxide and titanium dioxide, the former was shown to provide superior protection for UVA in the 340 to 380 nm range and tends to be less pasty on the skin.

When determining the efficacy of a sunscreen, the most important assay is the sun protection factor (SPF). The SPF refers to the ratio of the minimal dose of solar radiation that produces perceptible erythema (minimal erythema dose) on sunscreen-protected skin compared with unprotected skin. Thus, it measures a sunscreen's ability to prevent development of erythema and sunburn upon exposure to primarily UVB radiation. The SPF value is assessed under experimental conditions using a light source that simulates the solar radiation on the skin of light-skinned volunteers who have applied an amount of sunscreen corresponding to 2 mg/cm^2. Since SPF does not adequately measure protection from UVA, the FDA issued new regulations, effective in 2012, for labeling sunscreen products. Under these new regulations, only sunscreen products that can pass the FDA's test for protection against both UVA and UVB rays will be labeled as "broad spectrum."

Broad-spectrum sunscreen products that contain an SPF of 15 or higher may have the following statement on the label: "If used as directed with other sun-protection measures, decreases the risk of skin cancer and early skin aging caused by the sun." Those that fail the broad-spectrum test or have an SPF <15 must add the following to their label: "Skin cancer/skin aging alert: Spending time in the sun increases your risk of skin cancer and early skin aging. This product has been shown only to help prevent sunburn, not skin cancer or early skin aging." Moreover, the FDA no longer allows sunscreen products to be labeled "sweat proof" or "water proof." Sunscreens can be labeled as "water resistant" or "very water resistant" if they maintain their SPF after 40 or 80 minutes of swimming or sweating, respectively. Sunscreen products with SPF 15 are generally recommended for daily use, whereas cosmetics that contain sunscreen (e.g., facial moisturizers, foundations) may improve the photoprotection compliance.[21] Most cosmetic products are formulated to provide an SPF of 15 to 30 and may or may not be labeled as broad spectrum. Broad-spectrum sunscreen products with SPF 30 or higher are recommended for individuals performing outdoor work, sports, or recreational activities.

The benefits of sunscreens in protecting against the development of several conditions, from photoaging to skin cancer, have been documented in clinical studies. For example, both observational and randomized trials have demonstrated that sunscreens prevent the development of actinic keratoses and squamous cell carcinomas.[22-25] Sunscreens, by protecting the skin against external stimuli that lead to aging, can also shield it against skin changes such as pigmentation and wrinkling.[26] Broad-spectrum sunscreens with high SPF are generally used for the prevention of photodermatoses, which can be elicited by either UVB or UVA.

Despite its importance in protecting the skin and preventing skin disease, compliance still remains a challenge. Common reasons for noncompliance have included the stickiness of the product, which is greater with higher SPF, while cosmetic elegance, including texture, absorbability, absence of greasiness, and pleasant smell, was the most common positive feature of a sunscreen product cited by consumers.[27,28] Since sunscreen ingredients are oil-soluble, the most widely commercialized sunscreen products are oil-in-water emulsions, in which microscopic drops of oily materials are dispersed in a continuous water phase that also typically contains other polar ingredients like glycerin or glycols.[29] Lotions are thinner and less greasy than creams and are generally preferred for application over large body areas. Adopting simple application techniques that can be incorporated in an individual's daily routines can also assist with compliance. For example, the so-called "teaspoon rule" that involves applying approximately one teaspoon of sunscreen to the face and neck and each upper extremity and two teaspoons to the front, back torso, and each lower extremity can help adequate application of sunscreen.[30-32] The time of application is also important as sunscreens should be applied 15 to 30 minutes before sun exposure to allow the formation of a protective film on the skin and should be reapplied at least every 2 hours.[33]

◗ RETINOIDS FOR ANTIAGING

Retinoids have been used for decades in both therapeutic and cosmeceutical settings. The term retinoid refers to a class of substances comprising vitamin A (retinol) and its derivatives, both natural and synthetic. Precursors of retinol are retinyl esters and retinaldehyde that can be oxidized into retinoic acid which is the biologically active form of vitamin A.[34,35] Retinol may also be esterified with fatty acids to form retinyl esters. Since retinoids are lipophilic molecules, they can diffuse through plasma membranes or cross the cutaneous barrier when applied topically. Inside the cells, retinol and its active metabolites can bind to nuclear receptors (retinoic acid receptor [RAR] or retinoid X receptor [RXR]). Then, the ligand-receptor complexes bind to a RAR-response element DNA sequence, resulting in the modulation of the expression of genes involved in cellular differentiation and proliferation.[36-38] This leads to an increase of procollagen production, inhibition of inflammatory mediator release, reduction of collagen breakdown enzymes such as MMPs, and improvement of dermal vasculature. Retinol-dependent biological cascades can lead to increased epidermal cell renewal, expansion of cell layers, strengthening of the skin barrier, and collagen remodeling.

Therapeutic retinoids are typically RAR or RXR ligands that are prescribed to treat conditions such as acne, psoriasis, actinic keratosis, and some types of cancer.[39] Other retinol metabolites that can bind to retinoid receptors and affect gene expression such as tretinoin, alitretinoin, isotretinoin, adapalene, and tazarotene are considered therapeutic retinoids.[40]

On the other hand, precursors of retinoic acids, such as retinyl esters; retinol; retinaldehyde; 4-oxoretinol, 4-oxoretinal, and 4-oxoretinoic acids that do not bind nuclear retinoid receptors, are considered and used in topical cosmeceutical products.[38] These agents have been used to prevent and treat aging skin for decades with retinoic acid having the strongest activity, followed by retinaldehyde, retinol, and finally retinyl esters.

Retinoic acid is considered the gold standard in antiaging topical therapy. It is the most extensively investigated topical retinoid, and its safety profile is well established. In the United States, retinoic acid is available by prescription and exists in cream, gel, microsphere gel, and emollient base formulations under branded names and as generic drugs. The optimal concentration needed to have antiaging benefits has not been established, but commercial products to date are available in 0.025%, 0.05%, and 0.1% formulations. Prior to initiating treatment with topical retinoids, patients should be warned that local side effects such as skin irritation, redness, scaling, dryness, burning, stinging, and peeling can occur, that peak during the first 2 weeks and subside thereafter.[41] Tretinoin, tazarotene, and adapalene can be used for treatment of photoaging and all three substances have been validated in clinical studies. In a meta-analysis of 12 randomized trials, it was shown that application of tretinoin cream once daily in concentrations of 0.02% to 0.1% for 16 to 48 weeks was more effective than placebo in overall improvement of photodamage.[41] A more recent trial evaluating the long-term efficacy and safety of daily application of tretinoin 0.05% cream in 204 subjects with moderate to severe photoaging demonstrated significant improvement in all signs of photodamage compared to placebo.[42] Tazarotene, typically reserved for individuals without skin sensitivity, has also been shown to be safe and efficacious for the treatment of photoaging at a concentration range of 0.05% to 0.1%.[43] Adapalene is the mildest type of prescription strength retinoic acid that has been shown in the concentration range of 0.1% to 0.3% to improve the appearance of cutaneous photoaging and fine lines.[44] Retinoic acid improves several manifestations of photoaging, including textural changes, dyschromias, and fine wrinkles within the first few weeks of usage. Changes such as improvement of wrinkles are not seen until at least 2 to 4 months of continuous application.

Natural retinoids, such as retinol, retinaldehyde, and retinyl esters, are used in innumerable cosmeceutical preparations for the treatment of photoaged skin. However, because these compounds are not regulated as drugs, indication and contraindication data are not available.

Retinol, less irritating when compared to retinoic acid, has been shown in several small-scale clinical and histological studies to improve the signs of aging. Still, the evidence linking retinol application with collagen production is lacking. A study evaluating the effects of all-trans-retinol, all-trans-retinoic acid, and vehicle, when applied to human skin. This study showed that retinol 1.6% significantly increased epidermal thickening to level was comparable to retinoic acid 0.025% but without the erythema associated with retinoic acid.[45] In another study, topical application of 1% retinol in 53 individuals for a week led to increased collagen synthesis and reduction of MMP enzymes.[46] Retinol has also been successfully combined with other substances such as vitamin C, hydroquinone, and other molecules in formulations, effectively increasing its antiaging effects.[47,48] In general, cosmeceutical preparations seem to have retinol concentrations ranging from 0.1% to 1%, with those with the higher concentration being more efficacious, but this information is often missing. Moreover, as retinol is extremely unstable and easily degraded, exposure to light and air, as well as the vehicle used for retinol delivery, plays a crucial role in eliciting its efficacy.

Retinaldehyde is another retinoid included in cosmeceutical preparations due to its favorable tolerability profile and its efficacy for treatment of aged and photoaged skin. A concentration of 0.05% appears to be effective and well tolerated, allowing for prolonged use on sensitive areas such as the face. There are fewer studies evaluating the efficacy of retinaldehyde compared to other retinoids; nonetheless, the body of evidence supports its use as an antiaging agent. In a study evaluating the effect of 0.05% retinaldehyde in 32 subjects with mild to moderate photoaging, considerable reduction in the surface roughness and coarse wrinkling was observed at the 4-month follow-up.[49] In another study, significant increase in epidermal and dermal thickness, as well as in cutaneous elasticity, was observed after use of 0.05% retinaldehyde in 40 patients.[50]

Retinyl esters such as retinyl-acetate and retinyl-palmitate are considered the least effective topical retinoids. Although they are widely present in cosmeceutical products, there is little data to support their use as an antiaging agent. Moreover, their permeability through the stratum corneum is greatly reduced compared to other retinoids. In a double-blind, randomized, placebo-controlled trial with 80 patients using a topical formulation containing retinyl esters, there was no improvement noted at the 24- or 48-week follow-up. Moreover, there was no histological evidence indicating the role of retinyl ester in extracellular matrix remodeling.[51]

▶ SKIN BLEACHING AGENTS

Cosmeceutical agents that selectively target hyperplastic melanocytes and inhibit key regulatory steps in melanin synthesis have been developed to treat various skin-pigmentation conditions such as melasma, postinflammatory pigmentation, and sunspots. The gold standard and most effective agent for pigment-lightning is hydroquinone; however, due to its side effects and safety profile, its use has been restricted in cosmeceuticals.[52] As an alternative, a variety of vitamins and botanicals have been studied and evaluated as skin-lightning agents. A summary of agents and clinical studies for pigment reduction is presented in Table 9.2.

Retinoids. Retinoids, aside from having antiaging properties as mentioned above, can act through multiple mechanisms as skin-lightning agents. These include inhibition of tyrosinase, inhibition of epidermal melanin dispersion, interference of pigment transfer to keratinocytes, as well as acceleration of pigment loss by increasing the epidermal cellular turnover.[53] In a clinical study, where tretinoin was used in 38 patients with melasma over a 40-week period, a 68% improvement was observed, as well as side effects such as erythema and desquamation.[54] A patient at baseline and at 3 months post daily use of a retinoid-containing cosmeceutical is shown in Figure 9.1.

Arbutin. Arbutin, a compound found in dried leaves of different plant species (including blueberry, cranberry, pear trees), is one of the most popular skin-lightning and depigmenting agents worldwide. Arbutin is derived from hydroquinone and can inhibit tyrosinase activity and melanocyte maturation.[55] Although there is paucity of trials on the efficacy of arbutin on hyperpigmentation, a trial using synthetic topical (deoxyarbutin) showed an enhanced sustained improvement, general skin lightning, and a safety profile comparable to hydroquinone.[56]

Ascorbic Acid (Vitamin C). Vitamin C, a naturally occurring antioxidant, has been shown to have biological properties that reduce tyrosinase activity and melanin synthesis.[57] It interferes with pigment production by interacting with copper ions at the tyrosinase active site and reducing dopaquinone production. As topical vitamin C derived from fruits and vegetables is unstable, derivatives such as magnesium-ascorbyl-phosphate have been developed that are stable and maintain the skin-lightning activity.[58] Topically applied vitamin C formulations may protect against UVB radiation–induced phototoxicity and improve hyperpigmentation disorders, such as melasma and postinflammatory hyperpigmentation (PIH).[59] In terms of tolerability profile, vitamin C is generally nonirritating and thus useful in dark-skinned ethnic groups in whom PIH is a concern.

Alpha-Tocopherol (Vitamin E): Vitamin E is a major lipophilic antioxidant found in the plasma, membrane, and tissues. There are eight naturally occurring molecules possessing vitamin E activity, with alpha-tocopherol being the most abundant followed by gamma-tocopherol. Vitamin E has been shown to have skin-lightning properties, and there is a large body of experimental evidence proving its photoprotective effects.[60] It causes depigmentation by interfering with lipid peroxidation of melanocyte membranes, increasing intracellular glutathione content, and inhibition of tyrosinase.[61] Vitamin E together with vitamin C has been shown to have synergistic effects in skin lightning. In a double-blind study on the therapeutic effect of a combination preparation of vitamins E and C in comparison with single preparation of vitamin C in the treatment of chloasma or pigmented contact dermatitis, combination treatment resulted in significantly better clinical improvement than treatment with vitamin C alone in both diseases.[62] Allergic reactions or side effects are rare with vitamin E, and most products on the market contain alpha-tocopherol at a maximum concentration of 5%.

TABLE 9.2 Cosmeceuticals With Skin-Lightning Action

Active Ingredient	Patients	Placebo Controlled	Study End points	Route of Administration	Treatment	Results	Reference Number
5% Vitamin C vs 4% HQ	16	–	Melasma	Topical	16 wk	62.5% versus 93% improvement 6.2% versus 68.7% side effects	10
Niacinamide	18	+	Hyperpigmentation	Topical	4 wk	Significant decrease in hyperpigmentation	11
Kojic acid versus HQ	80	–	Mild/moderate dyschromia	Topical	12 wk	Equivalent efficacy	12
Grape seed extract	12	–	Chloasma	Oral	6 mo	Significant improvement	13
Orchid extract versus 3% vitamin C	48	–	Melasma, lentigo	Topical	8 wk	Equivalent efficacy	14
Coffeeberry extract	30	+	Hyperpigmentation	Topical	6 wk	Global improvement in skin lightning	15
Soy moisturizer	65	+	Moderate photodamage	Topical	12 wk	Significant improvement	15
Licorice extract	20	–	Melasma	Topical	4 wk	Significant improvement	16
2% NAG + 4% iacinamide	202	+	Hyperpigmentation	Topical	8 wk	Significant improvement	17
Natural ingredient product versus HQ	56	–	Hyperpigmentation	Topical	12 mo	Equivalent improvement with prescription	18

FIGURE 9.1   **Female, 58 y/o, before (A) and after (B) 3 months of daily application of a retinoid-containing cosmeceutical.**

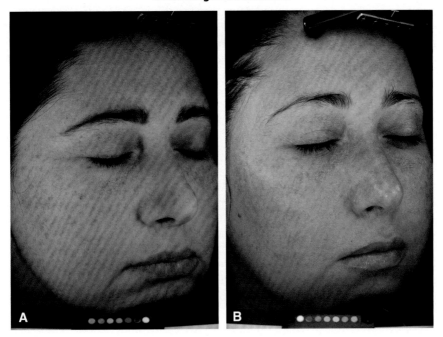

Niacinamide: Niacinamide, the active amine of vitamin B3, is commonly found in cosmeceuticals and has been shown to interfere with the interaction between keratinocytes and melanocytes, thereby inhibiting melanogenesis.[11] Aside from skin-lightning properties, niacinamide can reduce trans-epidermal water loss, improve barrier function, and can be used to treat photodamage. Clinical trials using 2% niacinamide have shown that it significantly reduces the total area of hyperpigmentation and increases skin lightness after 4 weeks of treatment. Although niacinamide has been shown to be less irritating than hydroquinone, as evidenced in a study comparing 4% niacinamide to 4% hydroquinone in the treatment of melasma, it requires a longer treatment duration to produce visible results, and the improvement in hyperpigmentation is not significantly better than with hydroquinone.[63] Cosmeceuticals with niacinamide can contain it up to a 5% concentration.

Kojic Acid: Kojic acid is a depigmenting agent derived from the *Acetobacter, Aspergillus,* and *Penicillium* species of fungi. It reduces pigment by inhibiting the production of free tyrosinase.[64] Aside from interfering with tyrosinase, kojic acid induces IL-6 production in melanocytes, a cytokine with antimelanogenic action.[65] Kojic acid is available in concentrations of 1% to 4%, but given its modest efficacy, it is often combined with arbutin, glycolic acid, licorice extract, mulberry extract, and vitamin C. Kojic acid can also be used together with hydroquinone and glycolic acid for the treatment of hyperpigmentation. Using these agents together may reduce irritant contact dermatitis, which is one of the common side effects of kojic acid.

Plant Extracts: Various plant extracts have been studied and shown promise for pigment-reduction. They typically have natural antioxidant properties, can inhibit tyrosinase, and lack side effects.[66] Such substances and their source include anthocyanins (found in red grapes, blueberries, strawberries, red cabbage), quercetin (found in onions, apple skins, berries, broccoli), catechins (found in green tea, cacao), isoflavones (found in soybeans), carotenoids (found in carrots, sweet peppers, oranges), lycopene (found in tomatoes), and oligomeric proanthocyanidins or procyanidins (found in grape seed extract).[14,15,67]

N-Acetyl Glucosamine: N-acetylglucosamine (NAG) is a monosaccharide that inhibits the conversion of protyrosinase to tyrosinase, thus decreasing pigmentation.[68] In a clinical study, 2% NAG was found to reduce facial hyperpigmentation after 8 weeks of application.[68] In another 10-week clinical study, use of a formulation containing the combination of niacinamide + NAG was shown to reduce the appearance of irregular pigmentation including hypermelanization, providing an effect beyond that achieved with SPF 15 sunscreen.[17]

▶ PRODUCTS FOR SENSITIVE SKIN

Sensitive skin is defined by the onset of symptoms such as erythema, pruritus, prickling, burning, or tingling sensations after exposure to various physical, chemical, psychological, or hormonal factors.[69,70] Sensitive skin is a frequent occurrence and epidemiological studies have shown that half the population worldwide is affected by sensitive skin. These studies show that the affected gender distribution is approximately 60% women and 40% men, and symptoms peak in the summer rather than in the winter.[71]

Individuals with sensitive skin demonstrate heightened reactivity of the cutaneous somatosensory system, which is not directly related to any immunological or allergic mechanism. Although research on sensitive skin was initially focused on the face where the skin is naturally more delicate, other locations have shown to present these symptoms, mainly the scalp and the hands.[72]

As the mechanisms driving skin reactivity are poorly understood, treatments remain a challenge and are not standardized. Factors that can aggravate the skin's sensitivity threshold include impaired skin barrier function, together with an increase in trans-epidermal water loss, as these increase exposure to irritants.[73] Thus, key to managing sensitive skin is strengthening the stratum corneum, hydration, and increasing the antioxidant capacity of the epidermis against external and internal triggers. Products such as cosmeceuticals can greatly benefit sensitive skin, as long as they are free from irritants and substances that can trigger flares.

To this end, ingredients that cause irritation and need to be avoided include alcohol, ketones, and xylene. Substances that are too acidic or alkaline also need to be avoided, and preference needs to be given to those with a pH of approximately 5.5. Common ingredients of cosmeceutical preparations are botanicals that can increase the risk of irritation as they can be highly allergenic. Some plants that have shown to have high allergenicity are tea tree oil, propolis, peppermint, lavender, lichens, and henna.[74,75] Other compounds that have the potential to cause phototoxic effects, thus leading to burning and erythema, include bergapten (aka 5-methoxypsoralen) and psoralens in fig leaves, and a naturally occurring furanocoumarin in bergamot oil that causes phototoxicity.[76-78] Severe adverse allergic reactions have been observed with German chamomile (*Matricaria recutita*), cayenne (*Capsicum annuum*), and echinacea (*Echinacea angustifolia*).[79,80] For individuals with sensitive skin, it is prudent to conduct a safety test prior to a cosmeceutical product such as the Repeat Insult Patch Test. This is a 1-month test that measures for irritant reactions in the first 10 days and allergic sensitization in the last 10 days.

Cosmeceutical agents that have been shown to be safe in conditions such as rosacea, eczema, and atopic dermatitis are also thought to be beneficial for individuals with sensitive skin. These include niacinamide, licorice extracts, feverfew, green tea, and aloe.[81]

Topical treatment with niacinamide has been shown to improve the stratum corneum barrier function and also improve red blotchiness in photoaged patients.[82] Hydroxypropyl chitosan and colloidal oatmeal are other common cosmeceutical agents that are protective to the skin barrier and have anti-inflammatory action.[83,84] Cosmeceuticals with antioxidant properties can also benefit sensitive skin as they reduce the amount of oxidative stress molecules in the skin and curb the strength of pro-inflammatory cascades. Such agents include vitamin C, tea extracts (green, red, white, black), coffeeberry extract and caffeine, aloe vera, turmeric, chamomile (bisabolol), and mushrooms.

▶ DISCUSSION

Laboratory and clinical data suggest that the use of cosmeceuticals is a very promising field, and their potential applications in various disease and aesthetic conditions are bountiful. Cosmeceutical products claiming to affect the structure and function of skin are beholden to higher standards of scientific substantiation than cosmetic products. These standards include at minimum being able to substantiate the three major questions proposed by Dr Albert Kligman: a clear understanding that the ingredient penetrates into skin, a defined mechanism of action, and that it has specific clinical effects with continued topical use. Since cosmeceutical products are expected to provide only subtle improvements in skin appearance, this creates a challenge for demonstrating efficacy compared to a vehicle control. Nonetheless, collectively the body of evidence points to their beneficial effects in protecting against photodamage, reversing the signs of aging, protecting sensitive skin, and lightning the skin. Importantly, apart from being stand-alone agents, cosmeceutical therapies can also be used adjuvant to chemical peels, lasers, and injectables, making antiaging regimens less painful and requiring less postprocedural healing time.[85] PIH can be decreased with some of the cosmeceuticals described, such as ascorbic acid.[86] Topical retinoids used prior to ablative laser treatments can aid re-epithelialization and reduce erythema.[87]

Regardless of all the caveats, the study of active ingredients used in cosmeceutical agents remains fruitful and compelling. Ongoing research can advance the general understanding of dermal signaling mechanisms and provide deeper insights into the mechanism of action of existing cosmetic procedures. Cosmeceutical studies can ameliorate the field by not only providing proof of clinical efficacy but by using gene, protein, and histologic evidence to ascertain their effectiveness. Consumers can have access to a better variety of noninvasive, cost, and time-effective options tailored to their specific skin needs and conditions, and clinicians can access comprehensive information to counsel and treat their patients accordingly.

REFERENCES

1. Global Cosmeceuticals Market 2017-2023: Cosmeceuticals Market is Outpacing all Other Product Segments in Personal Care. Globenewswire.com, Globe Newswire, 18 June 2018. Available at https://www.globenewswire.com/news-release/2018/06/11/1519409/0/en/Global-Cosmeceuticals-Market-2017-2023-Cosmeceuticals-Market-is-Outpacing-all-Other-Product-Segments-in-Personal-Care.html. Accessed August 17, 2020.
2. Kligman A. The future of cosmeceuticals: an interview with Albert Kligman, MD, PhD. Interview by Zoe Diana Draelos. *Dermatol Surg.* 2005;31(7 pt 2):890-891.
3. Amer M, Maged M. Cosmeceuticals versus pharmaceuticals. *Clin Dermatol.* 2009;27(5):428-430.
4. de Gruijl FR, Rebel H. Early events in UV carcinogenesis – DNA damage, target cells and mutant p53 foci. *Photochem Photobiol.* 2008;84(2):382-387.
5. Tewari A, Sarkany RP, Young AR. UVA1 induces cyclobutane pyrimidine dimers but not 6-4 photoproducts in human skin in vivo. *J Invest Dermatol.* 2012;132(2):394-400.
6. Yaar M, Gilchrest BA. Photoageing: mechanism, prevention and therapy. *Br J Dermatol.* 2007;157(5):874-887.
7. Fourtanier A, Moyal D, Seite S. UVA filters in sun-protection products: regulatory and biological aspects. *Photochem Photobiol Sci.* 2012;11(1):81-89.
8. Hexsel CL, Bangert SD, Hebert AA, Lim HW. Current sunscreen issues: 2007 Food and Drug Administration sunscreen labelling recommendations and combination sunscreen/insect repellent products. *J Am Acad Dermatol.* 2008;59(2):316-323.
9. Ou-Yang H, Stanfield JW, Cole C, Appa Y. An evaluation of ultraviolet A protection and photo-stability of sunscreens marketed in Australia and New Zealand. *Photodermatol Photoimmunol Photomed.* 2010;26(6):336-337.
10. Espinal-Perez LE, Moncada B, Castanedo-Cazares JP. A double-blind randomized trial of 5% ascorbic acid vs. 4% hydroquinone in melasma. *Int J Dermatol.* 2004;43(8):604-607.

11. Hakozaki T, Minwalla L, Zhuang J, et al. The effect of niacinamide on reducing cutaneous pigmentation and suppression of melanosome transfer. *Br J Dermatol*. 2002;147(1):20-31.

12. Draelos ZD, Yatskayer M, Bhushan P, Pillai S, Oresajo C. Evaluation of a kojic acid, emblica extract, and glycolic acid formulation compared with hydroquinone 4% for skin lightning. *Cutis*. 2010;86(3):153-158.

13. Yamakoshi J, Sano A, Tokutake S, et al. Oral intake of proanthocyanidin-rich extract from grape seeds improves chloasma. *Phytother Res*. 2004;18(11):895-899.

14. Tadokoro T, Bonté F, Archambault JC, et al. Whitening efficacy of plant extracts including orchid extracts on Japanese female skin with melasma and lentigo senilis. *J Dermatol*. 2010;37(6):522-530.

15. Wallo W, Nebus J, Leyden JJ. Efficacy of a soy moisturizer in photoaging: a double-blind, vehicle-controlled, 12-week study. *J Drugs Dermatol*. 2007;6(9):917-922.

16. Amer M, Metwalli M. Topical liquiritin improves melasma. *Int J Dermatol*. 2000;39(4):299-301.

17. Kimball AB, Kaczvinsky JR, Li J, et al. Reduction in the appearance of facial hyperpigmentation after use of moisturizers with a combination of topical niacinamide and N-acetyl glucosamine: results of a randomized, double-blind, vehicle-controlled trial. *Br J Dermatol*. 2010;162(2):435-441.

18. Thornfeldt C, Rizer RL, Trookman NS. Blockade of melanin synthesis, activation and distribution pathway by a nonprescription natural regimen is equally effective to a multiple prescription-based therapeutic regimen. *J Drugs Dermatol*. 2013;12(12):1449-1454.

19. Sambandan DR, Ratner D. Sunscreens: an overview and update. *J Am Acad Dermatol*. 2011;64(4):748-758.

20. Cole C, Shyr T, Ou-Yang H. Metal oxide sunscreens protect skin by absorption, not by reflection or scattering. *Photodermatol Photoimmunol Photomed*. 2016;32(1):5-10.

21. Draelos ZD. The multifunctional value of sunscreen-containing cosmetics. *Skin Ther Lett*. 2011;16(7):1-3.

22. Darlington S, Williams G, Neale R, Frost C, Green A. A randomized controlled trial to assess sunscreen application and beta carotene supplementation in the prevention of solar keratoses. *Arch Dermatol*. 2003;139(4):451-455.

23. Green A, Williams G, Neale R, et al. Daily sunscreen application and betacarotene supplementation in prevention of basal-cell and squamous-cell carcinomas of the skin: a randomised controlled trial. *Lancet*. 1999;354(9180):723-729.

24. Sanchez G, Nova J, Rodriguez-Hernandez AE, et al. Sun protection for preventing basal cell and squamous cell skin cancers. *Cochrane Database Syst Rev*. 2016;7:CD011161.

25. van der Pols JC, Williams GM, Pandeya N, Logan V, Green AC. Prolonged prevention of squamous cell carcinoma of the skin by regular sunscreen use. *Cancer Epidemiol Biomarkers Prev*. 2006;15(12):2546-2548.

26. Hughes MC, Williams GM, Baker P, Green AC. Sunscreen and prevention of skin aging: a randomized trial. *Ann Intern Med*. 2013;158(11):781-790.

27. Draelos ZD. Compliance and sunscreens. *Dermatol Clin*. 2006;24(1):101-104.

28. Xu S, Kwa M, Agarwal A, Rademaker A, Kundu RV. Sunscreen product performance and other determinants of consumer preferences. *JAMA Dermatol*. 2016;152(8):920-927.

29. Tanner PR. Sunscreen product formulation. *Dermatol Clin*. 2006;24(1):53-62.

30. Isedeh P, Osterwalder U, Lim HW. Teaspoon rule revisited: proper amount of sunscreen application. *Photodermatol Photoimmunol Photomed*. 2013;29(1):55-56.

31. Jeanmougin M, Bouloc A, Schmutz JL. A new sunscreen application technique to protect more efficiently from ultraviolet radiation. *Photodermatol Photoimmunol Photomed*. 2014;30(6):323-331.

32. Schneider J. The teaspoon rule of applying sunscreen. *Arch Dermatol*. 2002;138(6):838-839.

33. Beyer DM, Faurschou A, Haedersdal M, Wulf HC. Clothing reduces the sun protection factor of sunscreens. *Br J Dermatol*. 2010;162(2):415-419.

34. Castenmiller JJ, West CE. Bioavailability and bioconversion of carotenoids. *Annu Rev Nutr*. 1998;18:19-38.

35. Paik J, Vogel S, Piantedosi R, Sykes A, Blaner WS, Swisshelm K. 9-cis-retinoids: biosynthesis of 9-cis-retinoic acid. *Biochemistry*. 2000;39(27):8073-8084.

36. Fisher GJ, Datta SC, Talwar HS, et al. Molecular basis of sun-induced premature skin ageing and retinoid antagonism. *Nature*. 1996;379(6563):335-339.

37. Napoli JL. Biochemical pathways of retinoid transport, metabolism, and signal transduction. *Clin Immunol Immunopathol*. 1996;80(3 pt 2):S52-S62.

38. Sorg O, Antille C, Kaya G, Saurat JH. Retinoids in cosmeceuticals. *Dermatol Ther*. 2006;19(5):289-296.

39. Dawson MI. Synthetic retinoids and their nuclear receptors. *Curr Med Chem Anticancer Agents*. 2004;4(3):199-230.

40. Sorg O, Saurat JH. Topical retinoids in skin ageing: a focused update with reference to sun-induced epidermal vitamin A deficiency. *Dermatology*. 2014;228(4):314-325.

41. Samuel M, Brooke RC, Hollis S, Griffiths CE. Interventions for photodamaged skin. *Cochrane Database Syst Rev*. 2010;86(3):CD001782.

42. Kang S, Bergfeld W, Gottlieb AB, et al. Long-term efficacy and safety of tretinoin emollient cream 0.05% in the treatment of photodamaged facial skin: a two-year, randomized, placebo-controlled trial. *Am J Clin Dermatol*. 2005;6(4):245-253.

43. Kang S, Leyden JJ, Lowe NJ, et al. Tazarotene cream for the treatment of facial photodamage: a multicenter, investigator-masked, randomized, vehicle-controlled, parallel comparison of 0.01%, 0.025%, 0.05%, and 0.1% tazarotene creams with 0.05% tretinoin emollient cream applied once daily for 24 weeks. *Arch Dermatol*. 2001;137(12):1597-1604.

44. Kang S, Goldfarb MT, Weiss JS, et al. Assessment of adapalene gel for the treatment of actinic keratoses and lentigines: a randomized trial. *J Am Acad Dermatol*. 2003;49(1):83-90.

45. Kang S, Duell EA, Fisher GJ, et al. Application of retinol to human skin in vivo induces epidermal hyperplasia and cellular retinoid binding proteins characteristic of retinoic acid but without measurable retinoic acid levels or irritation. *J Invest Dermatol*. 1995;105(4):549-556.

46. Varani J, Warner RL, Gharaee-Kermani M, et al. Vitamin A antagonizes decreased cell growth and elevated collagen-degrading matrix metalloproteinases and stimulates collagen accumulation in naturally aged human skin. *J Invest Dermatol*. 2000;114(3):480-486.

47. Draelos ZD. Novel approach to the treatment of hyperpigmented photodamaged skin: 4% hydroquinone/0.3% retinol versus tretinoin 0.05% emollient cream. *Dermatol Surg*. 2005;31(7 pt 2):799-804.

48. Seite S, Bredoux C, Compan D, et al. Histological evaluation of a topically applied retinol-vitamin C combination. *Skin Pharmacol Physiol*. 2005;18(2):81-87.

49. Vienne MP, Ochando N, Borrel MT, Gall Y, Lauze C, Dupuy P. Retinaldehyde alleviates rosacea. *Dermatology*. 1999;199(suppl 1):53-56.

50. Diridollou S, Vienne MP, Alibert M, et al. Efficacy of topical 0.05% retinaldehyde in skin aging by ultrasound and rheo-logical techniques. *Dermatology*. 1999;199(suppl 1):37-41.

51. Green C, Orchard G, Cerio R, Hawk JL. A clinicopathological study of the effects of topical retinyl propionate cream in skin photoageing. *Clin Exp Dermatol*. 1998;23(4):162-167.

52. Nordlund J, Grimes P, Ortonne JP. The safety of hydroquinone. *J Cosmet Dermatol*. 2006;5(2):168-169.

53. Ortonne JP. Retinoid therapy of pigmentary disorders. *Dermatol Ther*. 2006;19(5):280-288.

54. Griffiths CE, Finkel LJ, Ditre CM, Hamilton TA, Ellis CN, Voorhees JJ. Topical tretinoin (retinoic acid) improves melasma. A vehicle-controlled, clinical trial. *Br J Dermatol*. 1993;129(4):415-421.

55. Maeda K, Fukuda M. Arbutin: mechanism of its depigmenting action in human melanocyte culture. *J Pharmacol Exp Ther*. 1996;276(2):765-769.

56. Boissy RE, Visscher M, DeLong MA. DeoxyArbutin: a novel reversible tyrosinase inhibitor with effective in vivo skin lightning potency. *Exp Dermatol*. 2005;14(8):601-608.

57. Choi YK, Rho YK, Yoo KH, et al. Effects of vitamin C vs. multivitamin on melanogenesis: comparative study in vitro and in vivo. *Int J Dermatol*. 2010;49(2):218-226.

58. Farris PK, Topical vitamin C: a useful agent for treating photoaging and other dermatologic conditions. *Dermatol Surg*. 2005;31(7 pt 2):814-817;discussion 818.

59. Kameyama K, Sakai C, Kondoh S, et al. Inhibitory effect of magnesium L-ascorbyl-2-phosphate (VC-PMG) on melano-genesis in vitro and in vivo. *J Am Acad Dermatol*. 1996;34(1):29-33.

60. Thiele JJ, Hsieh SN, Ekanayake-Mudiyanselage S. Vitamin E: critical review of its current use in cosmetic and clinical dermatology. *Dermatol Surg*. 2005;31(7 pt 2):805-813;discussion 813.

61. Badreshia-Bansal S, Draelos ZD. Insight into skin lightning cosmeceuticals for women of color. *J Drugs Dermatol*. 2007;6(1):32-39.

62. Hayakawa R, Ueda H, Nozaki T, et al. Effects of combination treatment with vitamins E and C on chloasma and pig-mented contact dermatitis. A double blind controlled clinical trial. *Acta Vitaminol Enzymol*. 1981;3(1):31-38.

63. Navarrete-Solis J, Castanedo-Cázares JP, Torres-Álvarez B, et al. A double-blind, randomized clinical trial of niacinamide 4% versus hydroquinone 4% in the treatment of melasma. *Dermatol Res Pract*. 2011;2011:379173.

64. Kim YJ, Uyama H. Tyrosinase inhibitors from natural and synthetic sources: structure, inhibition mechanism and per-spective for the future. *Cell Mol Life Sci*. 2005;62(15):1707-1723.

65. Choi H, Kim K, Han J, et al. Kojic acid-induced IL-6 production in human keratinocytes plays a role in its anti-melanogenic activity in skin. *J Dermatol Sci*. 2012;66(3):207-215.

66. Sarkar R, Arora P, Garg KV. Cosmeceuticals for hyperpigmentation: what is available? *J Cutan Aesthet Surg*. 2013;6(1):4-11.

67. No JK, Soung DY, Kim YJ, et al. Inhibition of tyrosinase by green tea components. *Life Sci*. 1999;65(21):241-246.

68. Bissett DL, Robinson LR, Raleigh PS, et al. Reduction in the appearance of facial hyperpigmentation by topical N-acetyl glucosamine. *J Cosmet Dermatol*. 2007;6(1):20-26.

69. Muizzuddin N, Marenus KD, Maes DH. Factors defining sensitive skin and its treatment. *Am J Contact Dermat*. 1998;9(3):170-175.

70. Saint-Martory C, Roguedas-Contios AM, Sibaud V, Degouy A, Schmitt AM, Misery L. Sensitive skin is not limited to the face. *Br J Dermatol*. 2008;158(1):130-133.

71. Willis CM, Shaw S, De Lacharrière O, et al. Sensitive skin: an epidemiological study. *Br J Dermatol*. 2001;145(2):258-263.

72. Misery L, Rahhali N, Ambonati M, et al. Evaluation of sensitive scalp severity and symptomatology by using a new score. *J Eur Acad Dermatol Venereol*. 2011;25(11):1295-1298.

73. Seidenari S, Francomano M, Mantovani L. Baseline biophysical parameters in subjects with sensitive skin. *Contact Dermatitis*. 1998;38(6):311-315.

74. Corazza M, Borghi A, Gallo R, et al. Topical botanically derived products: use, skin reactions, and usefulness of patch tests. A multicentre Italian study. *Contact Dermatitis*. 2014;70(2):90-97.

75. Jack AR, Norris PL, Storrs FJ. Allergic contact dermatitis to plant extracts in cosmetics. *Semin Cutan Med Surg*. 2013;32(3):140-146.

76. Pathak MA. Phytophotodermatitis. *Clin Dermatol*. 1986;4(2):102-121.

77. Bassioukas K, Stergiopoulou C, Hatzis J. Erythrodermic phytophotodermatitis after application of aqueous fig-leaf extract as an artificial suntan promoter and sunbathing. *Contact Dermatitis*. 2004;51(2):94-95.

78. Bollero D, Stella M, Rivolin A, Cassano P, Risso D, Vanzetti M, et al. Fig leaf tanning lotion and sun-related burns: case reports. *Burns.* 2001;27(7):777-779.
79. Kircik LH. Comparative study of the efficacy and tolerability of a unique topical scar product vs white petrolatum following shave biopsies. *J Drugs Dermatol.* 2013;12(1):86-90.
80. Mammone T, Muizzuddin N, Declercq L, et al. Modification of skin discoloration by a topical treatment containing an extract of Dianella ensifolia: a potent antioxidant. *J Cosmet Dermatol.* 2010;9(2):89-95.
81. Draelos ZD. Cosmeceuticals for rosacea. *Clin Dermatol.* 2017;35(2):213-217.
82. Christman JC, Fix DK, Lucus SC, et al. Two randomized, controlled, comparative studies of the stratum corneum integrity benefits of two cosmetic niacinamide/glycerin body moisturizers vs. conventional body moisturizers. *J Drugs Dermatol.* 2012;11(1):22-29.
83. Veraldi S, Raia DD, Schianchi R, De Micheli P, Barbareschi M. Treatment of symptoms of erythemato-telangiectatic rosacea with topical potassium azeloyl diglycinate and hydroxypropyl chitosan: results of a sponsor-free, multicenter, open study. *J Dermatolog Treat.* 2015;26(2):191-192.
84. Wu J. Treatment of rosacea with herbal ingredients. *J Drugs Dermatol.* 2006;5(1):29-32.
85. Wisniewski JD, Ellis DL, Lupo MP. Facial rejuvenation: combining cosmeceuticals with cosmetic procedures. *Cutis.* 2014;94(3):122-126.
86. Davis EC, Callender VD. Postinflammatory hyperpigmentation: a review of the epidemiology, clinical features, and treatment options in skin of color. *J Clin Aesthet Dermatol.* 2010;3(7):20-31.
87. Orringer JS, Kang S, Johnson TM, et al. Tretinoin treatment before carbon-dioxide laser resurfacing: a clinical and biochemical analysis. *J Am Acad Dermatol.* 2004;51(6):940-946.

Miscellaneous Aesthetic Procedures

**Lindsey M. Voller, BA, Rachit Gupta, BS,
Noora S. Hussain, BS, Charles E. Crutchfield III, MD,
Javed A. Shaik, PhD, MS, Maria K. Hordinsky, MD,
Neil S. Sadick, MD, and, Ronda S. Farah, MD**

Chapter Highlights

- Microdermabrasion utilizes mild mechanical abrasion to resurface the outer epidermis, promoting skin rejuvenation and enhancing cosmesis.
- Cellulite is a common complaint of the female aesthetic patient; treatments include topicals, injectables, subcision, and the use of various energy-based devices.
- Microneedling is an aesthetic technique that uses focal tissue injury to stimulate remodeling and neocollagenesis.
- Platelet-rich plasma has numerous uses in the aesthetic medicine, including for rejuvenation, treatment of alopecia, and improvement in the appearance of scars.

▶ MICRODERMABRASION

Introduction

Microdermabrasion (MDA) is a simple, nonsurgical exfoliation procedure that utilizes mild mechanical abrasion to resurface the outer epidermis.[1] The superficial injuries induced by MDA promote skin rejuvenation and improve cosmetic appearance as the tissue heals. Monteleone first described the clinical use of MDA in 1988 following its development in Italy in 1985.[2] MDA has since become a commonly performed minimally invasive procedure across a variety of clinical settings. The American Society for Aesthetic Plastic Surgery estimates that MDA is the third most widely utilized skin rejuvenation procedure after chemical peels and intense pulsed light (IPL).[3] MDA has been used to address an assortment of aesthetic concerns, including photodamage, wrinkles, uneven skin tone and texture, melasma, striae, pores, tattoo removal, and superficial acne scars.[1,4,5] MDA has also been shown to improve transdermal delivery of certain medications via increased permeability of the skin barrier.[6] This section provides an overview of microdermabrasion and its current utility in clinical practice.

Devices

MDA devices are classified as type I devices with the US Food and Drug Administration (FDA) exemption.[7] Traditional MDA consists of two main elements constituting a closed-loop system: an abrasive, exfoliating component and a vacuum pump or compressed air power source (Figure 10.1).[5] The abrasive component may contain inert crystals—typically aluminum oxide—that are projected onto the skin under negative pressure from a sterilizable or disposable handpiece. The propelled crystals subsequently transfer their kinetic energy to the stratum corneum, which causes corneocyte detachment and removal of surface debris.[1,5] Alternatively, crystal-free systems utilize diamond- or crystal-embedded handpieces or bristles as the abrasive stimulus (Table 10.1). Level of abrasiveness can vary based on handpiece coarseness. Vacuum suction simultaneously collects debris as the device moves along the skin.

In addition to stratum corneum removal, MDA causes melanosome redistribution within the epidermis and flattening of the dermal-epidermal junction.[1,8-10] Increased density of collagen has also been reported.[1,8,11] Rajan et al. demonstrated increased stratum corneum hydration with concurrent decrease in transepidermal water loss 1 week after MDA, suggesting improved skin barrier function associated with the procedure.[12] Improvement in lipid barrier function through enhanced ceramide production has also been documented.[13] The combined effects of MDA improve cosmesis as the skin undergoes remodeling.

Since the introduction of the first MDA system in 1985, devices have evolved considerably. Crystal-free systems are largely replacing traditional aerosolized crystal devices due to their decreased risk of ocular irritation and particle inhalation.[14] Certain devices also incorporate topical medication administration to enhance transdermal drug absorption. Some authors have administered low-molecular-weight compounds such as vitamin C and 5-fluorouracil in conjunction with MDA; however, additional studies are needed investigating this purpose.[6,15] Notably, at-home devices are becoming exceedingly popular among skincare consumers, and numerous options are now on the market. While

FIGURE 10.1   Schematic depicting a typical microdermabrasion device.

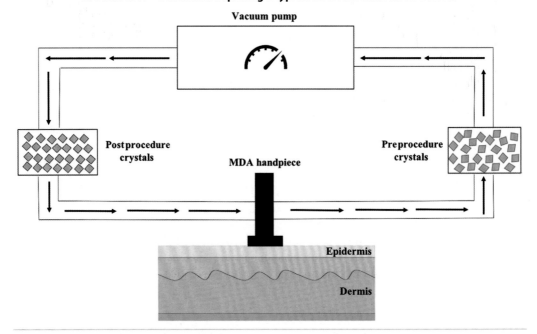

(Image courtesy of Ronda S. Farah, MD, University of Minnesota, Department of Dermatology, MN, USA.)

TABLE 10.1 Comparison of Crystal and Crystal-free Devices

	Crystal Devices	**Crystal-Free Devices**
Abrasive medium	Inert crystals (e.g., aluminum oxide or sodium chloride)	Diamond- or crystal-embedded handpiece
Mechanism	Crystals propelled onto skin, causing corneocyte detachment	Abrasive handpiece directly exfoliates and disrupts skin surface
Risks	Increased risk of particle inhalation, corneal abrasion	No risk of particle inhalation or corneal abrasion

these devices are often considered less aggressive than in-office systems, patients should consider completing a pretreatment visit with a board-certified dermatologist to ensure they are an appropriate candidate.

An additional crystal-free alternative is the newly developing technique of hydradermabrasion. Hydradermabrasion employs an abrading system consisting of an oxygen- and water-based solution, suction pressure cleansing, and MDA to exfoliate the outer epidermis.[16] Through hydradermabrasion, microcanals are widened in the epidermis and dermis while also providing cutaneous hydration. The effects of hydradermabrasion were investigated in a 2008 trial by Freedman et al.[17] Ten healthy female volunteers underwent six treatment sessions of hydradermabrasion with polyphenolic antioxidant serum at 7 to 10 day intervals, while 10 volunteers received antioxidant serum only. Skin biopsy demonstrated significantly increased epidermal and papillary dermal thickness compared to pretreatment in the hydradermabrasion + antioxidant serum group; changes were nonsignificant in the serum-only group.[17] Administration of topical polyphenolic antioxidants in this setting may enhance overall treatment effects of MDA, leading to greater clinical improvements in fine lines, skin texture, pore size, and hyperpigmentation.[18] As hydradermabrasion becomes increasingly widespread, it will likely become a routine alternative to traditional MDA. However, current literature on this technique is sparse and further investigation is warranted.

Reported Uses

Many patients are suitable candidates for MDA given its minimally invasive nature and overall excellent safety profile. Indeed, MDA can be performed safely on any Fitzpatrick skin type (I-VI), although authors have suggested proceeding more conservatively with patients of darker skin tones (types IV-VI) to decrease the risk of postinflammatory pigmentary changes.[5]

As procedure effectiveness depends largely on presenting skin concern, practitioners should select patients on the basis of projected responsiveness to treatment. However, few well-designed clinical trials exist that evaluate MDA and compare its efficacy to other minimally invasive procedures.[1] Among existing evidence, it appears that patients with superficial skin conditions—such as facial rhytides, fine lines, skin dullness, enlarged pores, and/or texture concerns—are likely to derive the most benefit from MDA treatment.[7,19,20] MDA may be useful in treating select cases of acne scarring but may require longer treatment and/or deeper ablation.[9,21] Mild to moderate improvements in striae distensae have also been reported.[1] Evidence is mixed on the utility of MDA for treatment of acne vulgaris, dyspigmentation disorders such as melasma, and erythematous disorders including rosacea and telangiectasias.[14,19,22,23] Patients interested in undergoing MDA should therefore receive appropriate counseling on treatment indications, alternatives, risks, and benefits; it is also critical to set realistic expectations prior to a patient's first treatment session. Furthermore, a thorough medical history and skin examination should be conducted to ensure there are no major contraindications to treatment.

An additional consideration when planning MDA with interested patients is treatment cost. As a cosmetic procedure, MDA is not typically covered by insurance companies and prices may differ based on provider, geographic region, and extent/duration of treatment. Ballpark treatment costs may be $100 or more and prices vary widely across the United States. Additionally, multiple sessions are recommended to achieve maximum results.[14] Estimated total cost must be discussed upfront with patients to ensure understanding of financial implications prior to initiating a treatment plan.

Technique

MDA is performed in outpatient clinical and nonclinical settings (e.g., clinics, salons, and medical spas) by various trained professionals—including dermatologists, plastic surgeons, nurses, and licensed aestheticians (Figure 10.2). Topical anesthetic is not required, and the procedure should be discontinued if the patient is experiencing excessive discomfort. A general operating procedure as adapted from Small et al. and Karimipour et al. is outlined in Table 10.2,[14,19] although standard technique may differ significantly based on the practitioner. Treatment technique will also vary based on device manufacturer recommendations. Note that surface ablation may be altered through adjustments to device head size, particle size, number of passes, speed of probe movement, abrasion depth, crystal flow rate, exposure time, and vacuum pressure.[6]

Postprocedure instructions may also vary based on treatment parameters. Similar to laser-based procedures, moisturizers, sunscreen, avoidance of irritants, and sun avoidance are typically recommended. More pronounced results may be achieved through multiple sessions over a longer period of time; weekly or biweekly treatments for 4 to 6 weeks are often recommended for visible improvement.[19] Following treatment plan completion, touch-up sessions may be provided on an individual basis to maintain and/or enhance results.

FIGURE 10.2   Photograph depicting a typical microdermabrasion procedure.

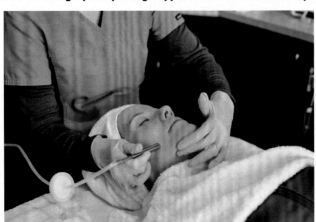

(Courtesy of Dr. Charles E Crutchfield III, Crutchfield Dermatology, Eagan, MN.)

TABLE 10.2	Description of Typical Microdermabrasion Preparations and Treatment Techniques
1-2 weeks prior to procedure	• Consider discontinuing irritating skin products (e.g., retinoids, glycolic acid) • Consider herpes and varicella prophylaxis in patients with history of herpes simplex virus (HSV) or varicella zoster virus (VZV) infection
Day of procedure	• Consent patient • Confirm patient has not been recently tanned • Inspect skin for active infection, severe pustular acne, cutaneous malignancy in the treatment area, and other dermatoses • Obtain baseline photographs • Consider performing test spot in nontreatment area (especially in higher Fitzpatrick skin types)
Procedure preparation	• Provide protective eyewear • Cleanse skin and degrease treatment area • Allow area to dry completely • Select device treatment settings. Recommended parameters depend on device being utilized; follow manufacturer guidelines accordingly
Procedure	• Confirm device treatment settings • Place device handpiece on skin • Consider application of tension and constant, even pressure • Perform passes per manufacturer recommendations; use of three passes in varying directions has been proposed[18] • Consider using decreased suction and pressure on areas with thinner skin
Patient monitoring	• Continuously monitor patient for signs of excessive discomfort, irritation, or development of immediate petechiae/purpura • Continue until treatment end point of mild erythema
Postprocedure	• Remove debris with moistened washcloth • Apply moisturizer and broad-spectrum sunscreen • Counsel patient to avoid skin irritants (e.g., retinoids, glycolic acid) for 1-2 wk • Sanitize or sterilize device per manufacturer recommendations

Treatment Pearls

At separate treatment visits, patients can be offered adjunct aesthetic procedures, including light-based devices, injectables, chemical peels, and skin tightening. This may enhance overall treatment effect. However, the authors do not recommend performing these procedures on the same day as MDA.

Risks and Contraindications

As a minimally invasive procedure, MDA is highly safe overall with a low risk of serious adverse events. Minor complications include tenderness at the treatment site, edema, and bruising. Patients should be counseled that mild redness can be expected shortly after the procedure, but it should resolve within 1 to 5 days.[14] For significant erythema, ice packs can be applied and topical steroids may be considered. Patients may also report mild transient discomfort and tingling. However, pain is not expected and should be reported immediately to the supervising physician. Lack of appropriate eye protection may lead to corneal irritation.[19] Similar to other dermatologic surgical procedures, excessive bruising may result if the patient has particularly thin skin or is taking an antiplatelet agent or anticoagulant at time of the procedure. Scarring and abrasions are rare but may occur if MDA is performed with overly aggressive treatment settings. As with any skin procedure, physicians should caution patients on the risks of hypo- and hyperpigmentation. Autoinoculation of viral infections (e.g., herpes simplex virus, warts, molluscum contagiosum) may occur; certain authors suggest pretreatment prophylaxis with acyclovir or valacyclovir among patients with a history of herpes simplex or varicella infection.[14] Devices should always be cleaned thoroughly or sterilized after use to avoid transmission of infectious disease. For staff members, there has been suggestion that inhalation of aluminum oxide crystals may be related to risk of fibrotic lung disease or Alzheimer dementia. Further research is needed to identify a direct relationship.[9,19]

Contraindications to MDA include, but are not limited to, pregnancy or breastfeeding, active infection, growing or bleeding lesions, history of keloidal or hypertrophic scarring, immunosuppression, skin atrophy, bleeding abnormality, dermatoses in the treatment area, cutaneous malignancy in the area, and severe pustular acne.[14] While dermabrasion was discussed in the 2017 isotretinoin consensus guidelines by Waldman et al. in *Dermatologic Surgery*, use of isotretinoin in conjunction with MDA was not explicitly addressed.[24]

Conclusion

This section highlighted the clinical utility of microdermabrasion, a minimally invasive procedure that utilizes mechanical abrasion to resurface the outer layer of the epidermis, promoting collagen formation and improving cosmesis as the skin heals. From its early introduction, MDA evolved quickly into a routine cosmetic procedure that can be incorporated into a variety of outpatient settings. Many patients are appropriate candidates for MDA given its low risk of adverse events, although clinical trials are limited due to FDA exemption status. Further research is needed to define the appropriate patient population that may benefit the most from treatment.

▶ TREATMENT OF CELLULITE

Introduction

Also known as gynoid lipodystrophy, adiposis edematosa, edematous fibrosclerotic paniculopathy, and nodular liposclerosis, cellulite is characterized by uneven dimpling or nodularity of the skin (Figure 10.3).[25-28] Cellulite is extremely common in women; it has been perpetuated in the literature that somewhere between 85% and 98% of women across all races experience some form of cellulite during their lifetime.[25,29,30] However, original publications examining the prevalence of cellulite are lacking. Cellulite occurs much less frequently in men with a prevalence of 1% to 2%, generally occurring only among men who have conditions presenting with relative androgen deficiency such as Klinefelter syndrome and congenital hypogonadism.[30-33] Despite the high prevalence of cellulite, data on epidemiology are sparse; it is, however, thought to be more common in Caucasian women compared to Asian women.[30] Cellulite typically tends to present in women between 20 to 30 years of age, but can be noticed by some women immediately after puberty, as early as 15 years old.[31]

Upon a search of PubMed, original articles studying the effect of cellulite on quality of life are limited. In a study performed by Hexsel et al. (published in *Cellulite: Pathophysiology and Treatment* by Goldman) evaluating 62 female patients with cellulite between the ages

FIGURE 10.3   This image illustrates a 34-year-old female with cellulite, displaying uneven dimpling and nodularity.

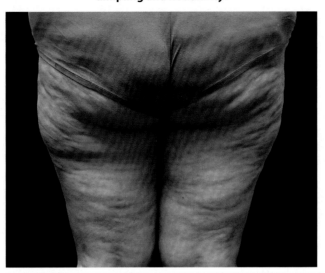

(Courtesy of Dr. Charles E Crutchfield III, Crutchfield Dermatology, Eagan, MN.)

of 18 and 45 years, 70% of all participants reported that cellulite "hampered their lives greatly."[34] Published in abstract form and also published in *Cellulite: Pathophysiology and Treatment* by Goldman, Hexsel et al. again evaluated 50 female volunteers and found that cellulite caused women to restrict their outdoor activities, types of clothes worn, resulted in feelings of poor self-esteem, and caused fear of spouses' attention and judgment.[35] However, full details of this study are not available. Additional studies needed to quantify cellulite's effect of quality on life are needed.

Although the term "cellulite" was first coined by the French in the mid-1800s, this condition was first studied in 1920 and thought to be an abnormality of water metabolism by French scientists Alquier and Paviot.[32,36] It would take another 50 years before the concept of cellulite made its way to households across the United States, due to an immensely popular book, titled *Cellulite: Those Lumps, Bump, and Bulges You Couldn't Lose Before*, about cellulite published by Nicole Ronsard, a New York salon owner.[37,38] Cellulite took hold of popular culture in the 1970s, sparking the development of an entire industry focused on treating this condition. The earliest treatments for cellulite focused on improving lymphatic flow and improving circulation to the affected areas, typically involving a combination of physical therapies, such as massage and topical anticellulite creams.[31] Treatments have gradually evolved to focus on the structural abnormalities seen in cellulite.[31]

In the 21st century, treatment of cellulite has become a large and still rapidly growing industry across the world. Several major categories of treatments have evolved over the last few decades: physical decompression, topical therapies, radiofrequency, acoustic wave therapy, microfocused ultrasound, cryolipolysis, injectables, and subcision. While many of these treatments are established for cellulite, others are used in off-label fashion and involve several major categories: a combination of physical and topical therapies, radiofrequency devices, subcision, and injectable treatments.[31] Treatments for patients can be quite costly. Peer-reviewed data on average cost of patients undergoing cellulite treatment are lacking. However, online websites hosting community reviews and costs for popular cosmetic procedures report that the average patient undergoing treatment for cellulite spends approximately $1,650 total, but can spend up to $5,000.[39]

Etiology

Goldman and Hexsel describe cellulite as a physiologic rather than pathologic state; it is thought that the purpose of cellulite is to ensure adequate stores of adipose tissue in post-pubertal women to guarantee sufficient calories for high energy–requirement states such as pregnancy and lactation.[40] The etiology of cellulite is poorly understood, but there are numerous known risk factors that cause a predisposition for development of cellulite. In addition to genetics, increasing age, female sex at birth, Caucasian race, estrogen, pregnancy, other hormonal changes, a diet excessively rich with carbohydrates, and sedentary lifestyle have all been associated with cellulite development (Table 10.3).[27,31,36]

The pathophysiology of cellulite development is controversial and has not been definitively elucidated, although there have been several major theories: anatomical differences between sexes, connective tissue laxity, and vascular and lymphatic dysfunction.[30] Originally described by Nürnberger and Müller, subcutaneous fat lobules protruding into the overlying layer of dermis termed "papillae adiposae" in women are larger in size and positioned more upright compared to fat lobules in men.[33,43] However, other studies have found an unclear correlation between the degree of fat lobule herniation and the appearance of cellulite.[33,45-47] Pierard et al. proposed that instead, vertical stretch of the hypodermis results in laxity of connective tissue, predisposing to papillae adiposae and the appearance of cellulite.[45] Meanwhile, other studies propose the role of lymphatic outflow abnormalities, chronic inflammation, and localized edema in the development of cellulite.[30,36,48,49] In reality, the development of cellulite is quite complex and likely involves a combination of the three pathways.

Clinical Evaluation and Physical Examination

As described by Goldman and Hexsel, cellulite is a physiologic state more common in women.[25,29,40] Cellulite typically presents asymptomatically in women; XXY syndrome, hypogonadism, and hormone therapy for prostate malignancy, however, may result in

TABLE 10.3	Proposed Risk Factors for Cellulite[31,36]
Genetics	• Variability in *ACE* and *HIF1A*[41] • Possible reduction in expression of the adiponectin gene[42]
Demographics	• Postpubertal patients[31,33] • Increased age[43] • Female sex at birth[32,33,40,43] • Increased in Caucasian women (compared to Asian or African-American women)[31,36]
Hormones	• Estrogen, possibly promoting lipogenesis[36] • Pregnancy and lactation[36] • Insulin promotes net production of adipose tissue[36] • Prolactin worsens cellulite appearance via localized edema[36]
Nutrition	• High-carbohydrate diet[30,36] • High-salt diet results in worsened appearance of cellulite due to increased fluid retention[36,44]
Social factors	• Low-activity lifestyles[36] • Alcohol use[36] • Increased body mass index (BMI)[36,43] • Tobacco use is associated with increased prevalence of cellulite[36]

ACE, angiotensin-converting enzyme; HIF1A, hypoxia-inducible factor 1-alpha.

cellulite in men.[30-33] During the physical examination, the area of skin suspected to have cellulite should be evaluated by the clinician in an effort to differentiate it from obesity or other cellulite-mimicking processes. While obesity and cellulite may appear similar, cellulite tends to occur more so in the skin of the abdomen, pelvic region, buttocks, and lower extremities.[27] Other abnormalities that can appear similar to cellulite and should be considered in the differential diagnosis include lipoedema, lymphedema, lipoatrophy, or infragluteal folds.[31,50] It is important for physicians to understand the differences between cellulite and skin findings associated with cellulite-mimicking processes, as treatments for cellulite can lead to worsening of other skin conditions.[31]

There are several methods for evaluating patients with cellulite. Examination of patients while standing can make underlying cellulite more evident.[26] A pinch test or muscle contraction can also be performed to make underlying cellulite more prominent.[26] High-definition photographs should be taken prior to starting any treatments, so as to document efficacy or lack of response to treatment.[31] It is important to ensure that lighting, background, and body positioning during photography are kept as consistent as possible; Nikolas et al. outlined a standardized method of photography for cellulite.[31,51,52] Diagnostic tools such as two-dimensional (2D) magnetic resonance imaging (MRI) and ultrasound imaging have also been utilized for evaluation of cellulite.[26]

Cellulite Grading

The severity of cellulite can be graded using several scales; two commonly used are the Nürnberger-Müller Scale and the Cellulite Survey Scale (CSS).[33,53,54] The Nürnberger-Müller Scale, one of the first scales devised for grading cellulite, describes the severity of cellulite based on what positions it can be visualized in and based on response to a pinch test or muscle contraction.[33,47] The CSS is a newer scale, incorporating other morphological features in addition to features assessed as part of the Nürnberger-Müller Scale. The CSS incorporates five factors into the overall score: number of depressions, depth of depressions, skin laxity, morphology of skin alterations, and the Nürnberger-Müller Scale.[54] Based on overall CSS scoring, different treatments can be considered on a per-patient basis. Most recently, new scales known as "Cellulite Dimples-At Rest" and "Cellulite Dimples-Dynamic" have been developed and validated by Hexsel et al.[55] The impact of cellulite on patients can also be measured in effect on quality of life; one way to assess this is the CelluQOL survey, created by Hexsel et al. in 2011.[35,56]

Interventions (Table 10.4)

Physical Decompression Therapy

One of the oldest methods of treating cellulite is simply with physical manipulation, including traditional massage. Recent device advances are combining positive pressure massage with negative pressure provided by vacuum-assisted technology.[26,47] With minimal side effects and contraindications, massage therapy is thought to help with outflow of lymphatic fluid and improve local blood flow, improving the appearance of cellulite.[26] The most commonly reported FDA-cleared massage device for cellulite on the market is Endermologie® (LPG Systems, Valence, France), a device that involves a combination of tissue massage, rolling, and manipulation.[57,58] The terminology Endermologie® originates from the words "ende" and "derm," meaning under and skin, respectively.[58] Endermologie®, a handheld device consisting of one vacuum compartment and two tissue

TABLE 10.4	Cellulite Treatments at a Glance[a]
Physical decompression	• Massage • Massage with vacuum suction and tissue manipulation (e.g., Endermologie®)
Topicals	• Methylxanthines • Retinoids • Herbal creams
Radiofrequency	• Monopolar (e.g., Thermage®, Exilis®, TruScuplt®) • Bipolar (e.g., Profound®, VelaShape®, VelaSmooth®) • Multipolar (e.g., Venus Freeze®, Venus Legacy®) • Unipolar (e.g., Accent®)
Acoustic wave	• For example, Cellactor®, Z-wave®
Microfocused ultrasound with visualization	• For example, UltraShape®, Ultherapy®
Cryolipolysis	• For example, CoolSculpt®
Injectables	• Collagenase • Fillers • Phosphatidylcholine
Carboxytherapy	
Subcision	• Manual • Vacuum-assisted (e.g., Cellfina®) • Laser (Cellulaze®)

[a]Disclaimer: While many of these treatments are specifically cleared by the FDA for treatment of cellulite, several of these treatments are not and instead used in an off-label fashion for cellulite treatment.

rollers, aims to mobilize deep tissue and subcutaneous fat by providing negative pressure and tissue manipulation.[57,58] The typical treatment regimen consists of ten 45-minute sessions twice a week, until an improvement in cellulite appearance is seen.[30,57,58] Despite being a popular treatment for cellulite, data on efficacy are limited. Some studies show mild improvement in cellulite,[57,58] while others show no statistically significant difference.[59] Collis et al. conducted a study on 52 women with cellulite, randomizing them to two treatment arms consisting of Endermologie® and topical aminophylline cream. Only 10 of 35 women treated with Endermologie® had improvement in cellulite appearance when assessed by study subjects. No statistical significance was found for either topical aminophylline cream or Endermologie®.[59] Evaluation for improvement by investigators did not reach this level of efficacy. Kutlubay et al. describe a statistically significant reduction in cellulite grade, as well as in mean body circumference. Gulec also demonstrated a mild statistically significant reduction in cellulite grade. Patient's weight loss and hydration status may also be impacting the results of these studies; Additional studies are needed to delineate efficacy of this therapy.

Topical Therapies

The earliest available and least invasive pharmacologic treatments for cellulite are cosmeceuticals. However, as these are topical products, their efficacy is limited by cutaneous penetration.[28] While cosmeceuticals are heavily marketed to consumers for treatment of cellulite, efficacy is limited and no topicals are known to cure cellulite.[57] While mechanism of action is not definitive, cosmeceuticals have been touted to increase circulation, promote lipolysis, stimulate production of collagen, and reduce inflammation.[31,60,61]

While there are numerous options for topicals, the most commonly used and best evaluated treatments are methylxanthines, such as caffeine and aminophylline, and retinoid compounds. Methylxanthines are grouped as beta-agonists and exert their effects by encouraging lipolysis and reducing lipogenesis. Methylxanthines are additionally thought to increase levels of cAMP through inhibition of phosphodiesterase.[31,62] Anecdotally, caffeine is thought to be the safest and most effective methylxanthine anecdotally, but literature search supporting the use of methylxanthines is limited.[60,63]

Topical retinoids are thought to decrease the appearance of cellulite primarily by increasing the formation of blood vessels and encouraging the synthesis of collagen and other connective tissue.[28,62] In a study by Kligman et al. evaluating the effect of 0.3% retinol cream on 19 patients, almost 70% of patients reported improvement in treated areas compared to the control group.[64] However, a study by Piérard-Franchimont concluded that despite improvements in elasticity and viscosity of skin, the overall dimpled appearance of cellulite showed little to no improvement.[65]

In addition to methylxanthines and retinoids, other cosmeceuticals have also been investigated for treatment of cellulite.[60] Hexsel and Soirefmann published a literature review in 2011 discussing other cosmeceutical options, including the following: *Ginkgo biloba*, pentoxifylline, *Centella asiatica*, *Ruscus aculeatus*, silicium, papaya *(Carica papaya)*, pineapple *(Ananas sativus)*, red grapes *(Vitis vinifera)*, *Cynara Scolymus*, ivy, *Melilotus officinalis*, vitamin E, and vitamin C.[60] As with methylxanthines and retinoids, little data exist currently to support their use for cellulite treatment.[60]

In general, topical treatments are tolerated very well by most patients. However, patients should be counseled about the mixed and often disappointing results of these treatments, as well as risks of allergic reactions such as contact dermatitis.[61,66] Additionally, long-term efficacy of these treatments is not well established as most publications examining these medications have been limited by sample size and duration of follow-up.[28]

Radiofrequency Device Therapies

The use of the medical devices for the management of cellulite has exploded over the last few decades. Radiofrequency (RF) has long been an FDA–cleared option for treatment of cellulite. RF devices have many other applications in aesthetic dermatology including but not limited to tightening of loose skin, body contouring, diminishment of scar appearance, and cellulite reduction.[67-69] RF devices generate thermal energy and deliver this in a targeted manner to the area of cellulite.[28] RF is thought to work by locally increasing temperature of body tissue, which stimulates production of new collagen while also degrading and remodeling existing collagen.[28] Several different categories of RF devices exist based on the number of electrodes used. The earliest generations of radiofrequency devices included unipolar, monopolar, bipolar, and tripolar options. More recent generations of RF devices are being released in multipolar, multigenerator, and temperature-controlled options (Figure 10.4).[28,70] RF devices can also be combined with other therapies, including vacuum, massage, ultrasound, targeted pressure energy, and more.[28,71,72]

Monopolar RF therapy is characterized by current administered between a single electrode and a grounding plate.[68,73] In general, monopolar devices penetrate more deeply than unipolar or bipolar devices, which may result in more pain experienced by patient.[68] Thermage® (Solta Medical, Hayward, CA) was the first monopolar RF device cleared by the FDA for cellulite (in 2002), but new devices cleared by the FDA for cellulite have since been released onto the market such as Exilis® (BTL Aesthetics, Prague, Czech Republic), TruSculpt® (Cutera, Brisbane, CA), and more.[68] Monopolar RF has supportive studies that demonstrate tolerability and improvement.[72]

FIGURE 10.4   **An illustration displaying probes and radiofrequency waves in monopolar, bipolar, and multipolar radiofrequency devices.**

Types of radiofrequency

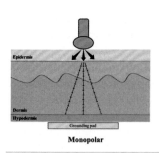
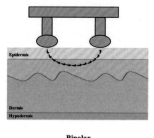
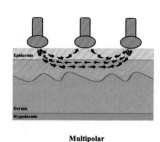

Monopolar   Bipolar   Multipolar

(Image courtesy of Ronda S. Farah, MD, University of Minnesota, Department of Dermatology, MN, USA.)

Bipolar radiofrequency involves current transmitted between two poles on a single handpiece probe, with the depth of penetration being determined by the distance between the two poles.[68,73] Bipolar therapy tends to be less deeply penetrating and therefore may be better tolerated by patients, but in some instances, less efficacious.[68] As reviewed by Beasley and Weiss in 2014, there are many bipolar RF devices on the market, each with their own variation of the bipolar RF technology.[68] For example, the Profound® RF device (Syneron/Candela, CA, USA) includes microneedling in addition to fractionated bipolar RF, while VelaShape® and VelaSmooth® (Syneron/Candela, CA, USA) incorporate infrared light in addition to bipolar RF.[74] All three of these devices have been cleared by the FDA for treatment of cellulite. Much of the literature focused on these devices is on body sculpting, rather than cellulite. VelaSmooth® and VelaShape® devices, combining bipolar RF with infrared light, suction, and massage, have been effective in clinical studies for the reduction of cellulite.[31,68,75-77] In a study evaluating the use of VelaSmooth® on thigh cellulite in 16 patients, more than half of patients had a 25% improvement in appearance of cellulite.[75] In a separate study evaluating 35 patients undergoing treatment with VelaSmooth®, Sadick et al. found that 70% of all patients experienced a reduction in thigh circumference and 100% of patients experienced some level of reduction in cellulite. However, improvement in both of these studies was assessed based on physician evaluations.[31,76] Furthermore, it is clear what degree of this improvement was related to radiofrequency as opposed to the other incorporated technologies discussed previously. Furthermore, these are industry-funded studies.

Multipolar radiofrequency devices employ the same concept as monopolar and bipolar radiofrequency devices, but use a minimum of three electrodes.[78,79] As described in a review of radiofrequency by Sadick et al., multipolar radiofrequency devices alternate which electrode serves as the positive pole, with all other electrodes serving as negative poles.[79] This alternation of positive poles between the multiple electrodes is thought to prevent unwanted tissue damage while delivering the same amount of targeted thermal energy to affected areas of skin.[78,79] As with other types of radiofrequency, multipolar radiofrequency can be combined with other technologies such as pulsed electromagnetic field (PEMF), suction, and vacuum.[79] Commonly used devices available on the market for cellulite treatment include the Venus Freeze® (not FDA-cleared for cellulite) and Venus Legacy® (FDA-cleared for cellulite) devices, developed by Venus Concept (Ontario, Canada) (Figure 10.5).[70] Studies evaluating the Venus Legacy® device, combining multipolar RF, PEMF, and suction, have demonstrated encouraging results; In 25 women undergoing 8 weeks of once weekly Venus Legacy treatments for abdominal cellulite by Wanitphakdeedecha et al., significant improvement in cellulite appearance was seen in as

FIGURE 10.5   A, Illustration of the Venus Legacy® device (Venus Concept, Ontario, Canada), a device using multipolar radiofrequency (RF) technology. B, A rendering of the Varipulse suction technology used in the Venus Legacy device. C, A portrayal of improvement in cellulite appearance in the buttocks after six treatments. D, A portrayal of improvement in cellulite appearance in the thighs after eight treatments.

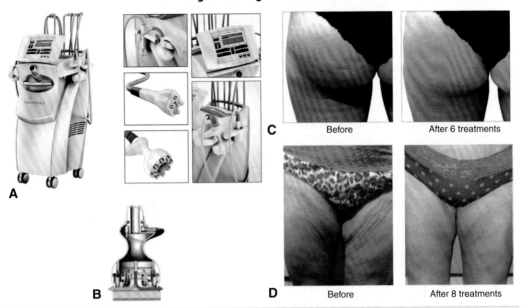

(Images (A) and (B) courtesy of Venus Concept.Images; (C) and (D) courtesy of Revive Wellness and Body Care by Angie, respectively, obtained through Venus Concept.)

little as 1 week after starting treatment and persisted for 12 weeks in many of the patients.[80] Side effects were minimal and 60% of patients were satisfied with the treatment.[80]

Unipolar devices have a single electrode and no grounding pad, with radiofrequency delivered in the form of electromagnetic radiation instead of current.[68,73] The most common FDA-approved device for cellulite treatment using unipolar RF technology is the Accent® device (Alma Lasers, Caesarea, Israel), which uses a combination of unipolar and bipolar RF.[73] A study by Goldberg et al. found 27 of 30 participants undergoing treatment with unipolar RF demonstrated clinical improvement in cellulite.[81] Another study conducted by Alexiades-Armenakas et al. evaluating efficacy of the same device on 10 subjects found visual improvement in cellulite in all participants, but without statistical significance.[73] Overall, results of unipolar RF therapy are encouraging, but literature review is limited due to lack of investigation.

Overall, RF devices are well tolerated.[68] They have well-established benefit, with participants in multiple studies experiencing visually significant skin tightening and improvement in cellulite.[53] RF devices are often used in combination with other therapies including massage and infrared energy, due to the differing but complementary mechanisms.[47] The nature and purpose of the procedure, associated risks, possible consequences, complications, and alternative methods of treatment should be thoroughly explained in detail to the patient. This includes but is not limited to heat sensation, erythema, swelling, pain, bruise, burn, scar, blistering, and skin discoloration.[73,81] The outcome could be any of the following: no improvement, slight improvement, and multiple treatments are required. Before and after photos should be standardized and obtained along with baseline and final weight as weight changes may impact final appearance. Clinicians should be aware of their device and its incorporated technologies. Clinicians need to be aware of anatomy, underlying structures, and screen for interactions with pacemakers/defibrillators, implants/plates, screws, magnets, or jewelry in the targeted area. Temperature is of utmost importance and should be precisely monitored due to the risk of burn with these devices. Generally, the procedure is repetitive and multiple treatments are required. Clinicians may also need to purchase gel or other disposable equipment for the operation of the devices. Overall, results are encouraging, and patients may see clinical improvements, but results are far from a cure. More well-designed studies evaluating RF devices are needed as much of the literature evaluating RF devices is of poor quality.[82]

Acoustic Wave Therapy

Acoustic waves, also known as extracorporeal shock waves, have recently been found to have numerous applications in aesthetic dermatology, including reduction of cellulite.[26] While the definitive mechanism is unclear, it is hypothesized to include a combination of the following: (1) disruption and weakening of the fibrous septae, (2) decreasing local lymphedema, (3) stimulation of lipolysis, (4) increasing local blood flow, and encouragement of new collagen and elastin formation.[26,28,83] There are two types of acoustic wave therapy that have been found to be effective for cellulite: focused and radial extracorporeal shock waves.[28]

Commonly used devices on the market cleared by the FDA for cellulite treatment are Cellactor® (Storz Medical AG, Switzerland) and Z-wave® (Zimmer Biomet, Warsaw, Indiana, USA).[28] A study by Hexsel et al. using the Cellactor® system on 25 patients found a statistically significant reduction in the Cellulite Severity Scale from 11.1 to 9.5 after 12 treatment sessions, indicating a reduction in the percentage of patients with severe cellulite.[84] Additionally, 89% of patients were satisfied with treatment results.[84] A meta-analysis conducted by Knobloch and Kraemer identified 11 clinical studies, five of which were randomized controlled trials, evaluating acoustic wave therapy which demonstrated evidence that both radial and focused acoustic wave therapy were efficacious in cellulite treatment.[85]

Similar to radiofrequency, this method of treatment is also noninvasive, minimally painful, with limited recovery time needed. All trials to date have involved approximately one to two sessions per week for a total of six to eight sessions for patients, with a mean follow-up of approximately 3 to 6 months.[85] Acoustic wave therapy can be used in combination with other therapies, including radiofrequency, cryolipolysis, and laser therapy. Reports of adverse events for patients are rare; physicians administering this treatment do report that the noise can be uncomfortable, so protective equipment is recommended.[83]

Microfocused Ultrasound With Visualization

Historically used for skin tightening of the face, chest, arms, thighs, and buttocks, microfocused ultrasound with visualization (MFU-V) is another noninvasive treatment modality for cellulite.[31,62,86,87] As discussed in a review by Khan et al., ultrasound waves are thought to result in localized adipose tissue destruction by a number of mechanisms including thermal injury, disruption of tissue microarchitecture, and cavitation.[62] The visualization component of this therapy allows the practitioner to confirm proper placement of the ultrasound transducer and thus deliver the ultrasound waves more effectively and accurately.[31] Efficacy of ultrasound therapy has not been well established, but a number of studies do demonstrate moderate improvement in cellulite appearance.[62,71,82]

Two commonly used MFU-V devices include Ultherapy® (Ulthera Inc, AZ, USA) and UltraShape® (Syneron/Candela, CA, USA), although neither are cleared by the FDA specifically for treatment of cellulite. Moreno-Moraga et al. evaluated 30 patients with three treatments of UltraShape® each at an interval of 1 month.[88] All 30 patients showed reduction in fat thickness, with a statistically significant reduction in average mean abdominal circumference of 3.95 cm.[88] No change in patient weight was noted, so improvement in fat thickness was attributed directly to UltraShape® therapy. Of note, this improvement was noted specifically in the nonobese group of patients, suggesting that this therapy may be better suited for thinner patients.[88] Davis et al. contribute their experience with cellulite treatment using MFU-V, noting that it provides significant benefit with tightening of skin and thus overall appearance of cellulite.[31] MFU-V therapy has a very patient-friendly side effect profile. In numerous studies, adverse events were rare and generally only included mild bruising, erythema, and pain self-resolving in 2 to 3 days.[88-90]

Cryolipolysis

Cryolipolysis, or freezing of localized subcutaneous adipose tissue, has been cleared by the FDA for fat reduction and cellulite treatment in recent years (e.g., CoolSculpting®, Zeltiq Aesthetics, CA, USA) and is thought to reduce the appearance of cellulite by creating localized cold-induced panniculitis.[91,92] As discussed in a review of cryolipolysis by Ingargiola et al., contraindications to cryolipolysis therapy include conditions exacerbated by exposure to low temperatures including but not limited to paroxysmal cold hemoglobinuria, cryoglobulinemia, and cold urticaria.[91] Evidence on effectiveness of cryolipolysis is sparse; some studies have shown modest benefit.[62] All 19 studies analyzed by Ingargiola et al. did find a reduction in localized adiposity in treated areas, but did not evaluate patients on the basis of reduction in cellulite appearance.[91] Cryolipolysis has also been demonstrated to have some benefit when used in combination with other treatments, including radiofrequency, acoustic wave, and microfocused ultrasound therapies.[31] One benefit for cryolipolysis is minimal side effects of pain and erythema, compared to other therapies for cellulite.[91] Because cryolipolysis procedures for treatment of cellulite are so new, treatment protocols have not been established and research is ongoing into analyzing long-term effectiveness.[26,91]

Injectable Therapies

Due to the wide prevalence of cellulite, there is a significant amount of research taking place into novel treatments. One such treatment modality is injectable therapies, such as injectable collagenase; produced by *Clostridium histolyticum*. Qwo was FDA-approved in 2020 and is the first collagenase *Clostridium histolyticum* to obtain this approval.[28,31] During this treatment, the collagenase, *Clostridium histolyticum* is given directly into areas of cellulite on the buttock or thighs.[93] The injectable collagenase is thought to improve the appearance of cellulite by disrupting the triple helix structures of collagen, especially in fibrous septae which adhere the dermal layer of skin to underlying fascia.[93] Side effects include bruising and injection site reactions including pain at the site of injection.[93]

Another possible emerging treatment for cellulite is injections of dermal fillers, typically including either calcium hydroxyapatite or poly-L-lactic acid.[28,31] However, the use of these fillers for cellulite is off-label and investigations demonstrating appropriate dilution, improvement, and long-term consequences and outcomes are needed.

Other injectable options requiring further investigation for cellulite treatment include phosphatidylcholine and carboxytherapy. Phosphatidylcholine is thought to improve cellulite appearance by causing apoptosis of adipose tissue and lipolysis possibly through the tumor necrosis factor (TNF)-α pathway.[94,95] Carboxytherapy in contrast involves the injection of carbon dioxide gas into the skin through use of a machine.[26] Intradermal carbon dioxide acts as a vasodilator, which improves cellulite appearance by increasing circulation of blood and lymph, improving elasticity of skin, and decreasing the amount of fatty deposits present.[26] A study from Eldsouky et al. indicates that both are similarly effective in treatment of cellulite, but larger studies with a longer period of follow-up are needed to better understand the role of these therapies.[96]

Subcision Therapy

Subcision is a minimally invasive procedure whereby a needle is inserted directly into the subcutaneous layer of adipose tissue, with the aim of disrupting fibrous septae. Maintaining proper depth of the subcision device is crucial for good results. Subcision deep to the target tissue may result in minimal improvement for the superficial dimpling of cellulite, while superficial subcision can lead to skin necrosis.[47] Previously, subcision has been categorized as manual, vacuum-assisted, and laser-assisted.[26,31,47]

Manual subcision has also been evaluated for the treatment of cellulite (Figure 10.6). During this procedure, the areas of cellulite are numbed with a topical anesthetic agent (vasoconstrictor with lidocaine), a needle (18 G) is inserted under the skin, and a fanning technique is used to release the fibrous cords of cellulite. In a study performed by Hexsel and Mazzuco, nearly 80% of patients were very satisfied with the procedure and another 20% of patients had a partial response to treatment.[97] Additionally, nearly 10% of patients experienced results persistently through 2 years of follow-up after undergoing only one treatment of subcision.[97] Although efficacious, the main drawbacks of this treatment are the side effects, including edema, discomfort, pain, and bruising.[97] Due to the risk of inconsistent results and significant side effects of pain and bruising, manual subcision has become less popular in recent years compared to vacuum-assisted and laser-assisted methods of subcision.[31,47]

Recently, a novel tissue stabilized–guided subcision (TS-GS) system (Cellfina System®; Merz North America, Inc., Raleigh, NC) was developed and FDA cleared for the improvement of cellulite in the buttocks and thigh areas of adult women.[26] The benefits of Cellfina®

FIGURE 10.6   Before and after images of a female patient having undergone manual subcision treatment for cellulite.

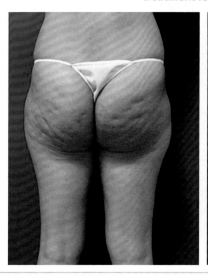
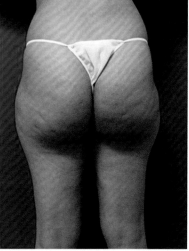

(Courtesy of Dr. Neil Sadick.)

over traditional manual subscision with a needle are its precise control of treatment depth and area of tissue (fibrous septae) and a unique vacuum-assisted design. Because this device is vacuum-assisted, this device has been marketed as accurate and reproducible with possibly longer-lasting effects than traditional manual subscision.[26] Cellfina® has been shown in multicenter clinical studies to improve cellulite with results lasting 3 years.[98] In the latest clinical study, 55 subjects were followed for an extended period of up to 3 years after receiving a single treatment using the TS-GS system. Another study completed by Geronemus et al. demonstrated significant improvement rated by study participants and physician raters in cellulite appearance, as well as statistically significant improvement in quality of life after only one session of TS-GS.[99] The results of this trial supported an FDA clearance of the device for the long-term reduction in the appearance of cellulite following TS-GS.[31,98]

Subscision technology has also evolved to include laser devices. Cellulaze® (Cynosure Inc, MA, USA), is a commonly used laser-assisted subscision device on the market cleared by the FDA for cellulite treatment. This device is a 1440 -nm-wavelength Nd:YAG laser.[28,82] Laser therapies like Cellulaze® improve the appearance of cellulite by delivering energy in a targeted fashion to the dermis and subcutaneous tissue; this stimulates neocollagenesis and promotes local blood flow.[28] Numerous studies have shown established benefit of laser-assisted devices, with as many as 90% of patients experiencing persistent improvement through 6 months.[47,100,101] It has been proposed that laser-assisted devices result in less pain and bruising compared to manual and vacuum-assisted subscision.[47] However, remodeling of fibrous septae and lipolysis are limited with this technology.

Overall, the data for the subscision and subscision combination devices are promising, and as technology and precision evolve, this subset of cellulite treatments will likely continue to play a major role for patient treatment.

Conclusion

Cellulite can be extremely challenging to treat, due to the multifactorial and individualized nature in addition to complex pathophysiology of this condition. There are an increasingly wide variety of treatments appearing on the market, with a general shift toward targeted therapies. Each treatment has its drawbacks and even the most efficacious of treatments provide limited improvement and typically only for a short period of time, making patient counseling and expectation setting important.[62,102] Proper cellulite staging, grading, and appropriate patient selection are also crucial for the best outcomes; treating physicians should obtain a thorough history and physical examination to select the treatment that has the best chance for success.

With the advent of new evidence, numerous new technologies and devices are becoming available to treat cellulite. The future of cellulite is promising and treatment may lay in combination therapies; further investigation and development should be encouraged.

▶ MICRONEEDLING

Introduction

Microneedling, also termed percutaneous collagen induction (PCI) or collagen induction therapy, is an emerging dermatologic treatment modality in which an array of small needles creates microscopic punctures within the skin. An early version of the procedure gained traction in 1995 when Orentreich and Orentreich described subscision.[102] In this method, needles were utilized to disturb the connective tissue underlying wrinkles and scars.[103] In 1997, Camirand and Doucet treated scars with needle dermabrasion using a "tattoo pistol."[104] Fernandes later refined this technique in 2006 to create the basis for contemporary microneedling devices, employing a drum-shaped roller covered with embedded needles to produce numerous microchannels in the epidermis and dermis.[105] Current devices continue to utilize this process of focal microwounding to stimulate dermal remodeling, resulting in limited epidermal disturbance and tissue healing with low risks of consequent scarring.[106] Microneedling has since become recognized as a possible alternative to nonablative light-based treatments for scarring, striae, and facial rhytides. More recently, microneedling has also been proposed for alopecia and transdermal drug delivery. This section discusses the niche that microneedling occupies in current clinical practice and describes a practical guide for its use.

Devices

Numerous microneedling devices are now on the market and registered with the US FDA. According to the FDA, microneedling devices are instruments with needles, tips, or pins that are rolled or stamped over the skin.[107] They may have varying needle lengths and can be blunt or sharp. These devices may be termed microneedling instruments, needling instruments, dermal rollers, microneedle rollers, microneedle stamps, or dermal stamps.[107] Devices are primarily subdivided into two main categories: manual needle rollers and electric-powered pens.[108] Fixed needle rollers are cylindrical devices with embedded needles that pierce the skin in a rotating mechanism as the device passes over the desired treatment area. In contrast, electric-powered pens utilize spring-loaded needles to deliver repetitive, vertical "stamp-like motions" of modifiable speed and depth (Figure 10.7).[109] Generally, rollers and pens are moved over the skin in a perpendicular fashion with a pinpoint bleeding endpoint.[110] However, literature regarding exact depth, time, and number of passes is variable. Number of needles, needle length, diameter, and orientation may also vary across devices. In addition, operator pressure may influence treatment and end point.

Both device types create microscopic wounds within the epidermis and dermis (Figure 10.8), resulting in controlled injuries that stimulate new vessel formation and the release of dermal growth factors such as platelet-derived growth factor (PDGF), fibroblast growth factor (FGF), and transforming growth factors (TGF) alpha and beta.[111,112] Fibroblast activation with subsequent collagen and elastin deposition in the papillary dermis leads to improved cosmetic appearance as the tissue heals.[112-114]

Electric-powered pens offer certain theoretical advantages over traditional manual rollers, including more precise control in focal treatment areas, adjustable treatment depth, and decreased infection risk due to disposable needle tips (Table 10.5).[110] Electric pens may also allow treatment of smaller areas or lesions such as scars or upper cutaneous lip lesions.[110] Both home-use and medical-grade devices exist, with primary differentiation based on the depth of skin penetration.[114,115] Home devices are gaining increasing popularity among skincare consumers and typically feature shorter needle lengths; however, more penetrative devices are also available for purchase from various manufacturers. Individuals considering treatment with an at-home device should be cautioned regarding the risks of bleeding, infection, and scarring. As device use is pressure and operator dependent, the safety of home use devices is currently unclear.

In 2017, the US FDA issued a draft guidance for industry and FDA staff regarding microneedling and when it is determined to be classified as a medical device.[107] According to this draft, microneedles which claim to treat scars, wrinkles, deep facial lines, cellulite, stretch marks, dermatoses, acne, or alopecia meet device criteria. Those that stimulate collagen, stimulate angiogenesis, or promote wound healing also fall under that of a medical

FIGURE 10.7   Example of circular needle tip array.

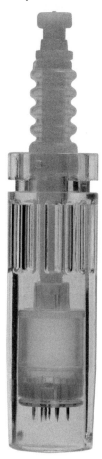

(Image courtesy of Eclipse.)

FIGURE 10.8   Schematic representation of microchannel created in the epidermis and dermis through microneedling.

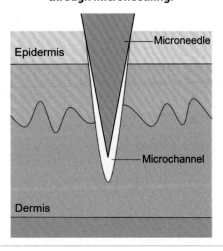

(Image adaptation courtesy of Sarika Uppaluri, University of Minnesota, Department of Dermatology.)

TABLE 10.5	Comparison of the Two Main Categories of Microneedling Devices	
	Manual Rollers	**Electric-Powered Pens**
Method of microinjury	• Fixed drum-shaped needle roller	• Electronic pen-shaped device with spring-loaded, disposable needles
Mechanism	• Tiny needles create epidermal and dermal microwounds	• Tiny needles create epidermal and dermal microwounds
Skin penetration	• Multidirectional	• Vertical
Advantages	• Minimal recovery time • Low risk of dyspigmentation	• Minimal recovery time • Low risk of depigmentation • Customizable treatment depth • Greater precision on focal small lesions/areas • Likely decreased infection risk due to disposable needles

device. Microneedling devices that do not penetrate the epidermis or dermis are not considered devices. This includes those that claim to exfoliate; improve skin appearance; or provide the skin with a smoother look, smoother feel, or luminous look. Marketing authorization may be obtained as class I or class II devices. Clinicians should be aware of their device's FDA status when seeking to purchase.[107]

Clinical Uses

Microneedling has been investigated as a noninvasive treatment alternative for numerous disease states, with evolving uses as clinicians gain additional experience with the procedure. The following subsections detail select uses for microneedling with associated literature on the topics. Notably, studies consist primarily of case reports and case series in addition to smaller randomized clinical trials; larger studies are needed to further establish the safety and efficacy of microneedling and compare its results to minimally invasive alternatives.[108]

Scarring

Microneedling is well known for its treatment of atrophic acne scars.[116] Multiple studies have highlighted the efficacy of fixed microneedle rollers in decreasing scar severity based on several established scarring scales, most commonly utilizing the Goodman and Baron global acne scarring classification. One of the more robust studies entailed a split-face, prospective trial by Alam et al., which demonstrated an average 41% perceived improvement in 15 patients with acne scarring at 6 months using manual needle rollers.[117] This efficacy appears to extend to patients of darker Fitzpatrick skin types (IV-VI) as well, with decreased risk of dyspigmentation and scarring as compared to traditional resurfacing devices such as ablative and nonablative laser treatments and chemical peels.[118] It has been proposed that improvement in ice-pick scars is less than that of box scars or rolling scars with microneedling.[110,115] Clinical results have been confirmed histologically. El-Domyati et al. performed punch biopsies on patients undergoing microneedling for postacne scarring at 1 and 3 months; significant increases in type I and III dermal collagen were seen at 3 months.[119] Additional scar types that may be responsive to microneedling include striae distensae, atrophic burn scars, and postsurgical scarring.[113,120,121] Microneedling appears to be a promising therapeutic alternative for these purposes with limited side effects.

Rejuvenation and Rhytides

Microneedling has become an attractive option for patients seeking skin rejuvenation given its minimal downtime and utility in reducing fine rhytides. Fabbrocini et al. performed two sessions of microneedling at 8-week intervals on 10 women with upper lip wrinkles; wrinkle severity decreased significantly after treatment using the Wrinkle Severity Rating Scale.[122] Another study by El Domyati et al. utilized fixed needle rollers on 10 patients with Glogau class II-III wrinkles at 2-week intervals. All patients showed objective clinical improvement in appearance of rhytides and skin texture, and subjectively reported high satisfaction with microneedling treatments. Histologic changes included significantly increased epidermal thickness with rete ridge development after 1 and 3 months.[123] Fabbrocini et al. demonstrated reduction in depth of neck rhytides with concurrent increase in skin thickness after two microneedling treatment sessions based on ultrasound images.[124] Results appear to be cumulative for the purposes of skin rejuvenation; Alster et al. have described three to six treatment sessions at 2 to 4 week intervals.[110]

Melasma

Melasma, a chronic dyspigmentation disorder, may be an additional condition amenable to microneedling (Figure 10.9A and B). In one study, Lima demonstrated that microneedling—followed by depigmentation formula 24 hours later—led to 100% patient satisfaction among 22 patients with refractory melasma.[125] Fabbrocini et al. performed two sessions of microneedling on 20 female patients with melasma in combination with depigmenting serum (containing rucinol and sephora-alpha) on one half of the face; solely depigmenting serum was applied on the other half. Combination therapy resulted in a greater reduction in Melasma Area Severity Index (MASI) versus topical serum alone.[126] A larger randomized controlled trial by Budamakuntla et al. utilized combination microneedling with tranexamic acid microinjections versus injections alone in sixty Chinese patients. Both groups saw decreased MASI scores with greater reduction demonstrated in the combination group.[127] It is unclear whether these combination studies would have noted similar achievements without the use of adjunct medications, yet these preliminary reports are encouraging for future melasma therapy.

FIGURE 10.9 **Patient photographs before (A) and after (B) one session of microneedling for melasma.**

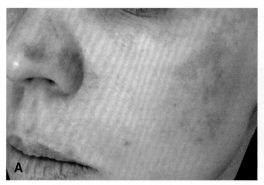 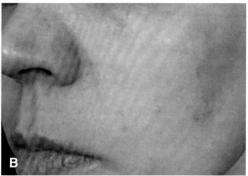

(Image courtesy of Ronda S. Farah, MD, University of Minnesota Department of Dermatology, MN, USA.)

Alopecia

Microneedling has recently been introduced in the literature as a possible tool to improve several types of alopecia, usually in combination with topical medications. Dhurat et al. found that use of minoxidil combined with weekly microneedling resulted in a mean change in hair counts that was greater at 12 weeks as compared to topical minoxidil only among 100 male participants with androgenetic alopecia.[128] However, comparison to a microneedling only group was lacking and subjects were instructed to use minoxidil between treatments, raising the possibility of a minoxidil only effect. In another study, four men with refractory androgenetic alopecia on finasteride and 5% minoxidil solution underwent microneedling over 6 months; improved satisfaction and hair density were reported.[129] In 2012, the effects of microneedling on female pattern hair loss were investigated along with the use of growth factors in 11 Korean women. In this study, microneedles were used to enhance penetration of growth factors across the stratum corneum on one half of the scalp and a significantly increased hair shaft density was found.[130] Additional articles have provided preliminary support for the use of microneedling among patients with alopecia. This literature is limited to case reports and series; further investigation for this purpose is warranted.[131,132]

Transdermal Drug Delivery

Microneedling has also newly been explored as a method for drug delivery as it results in physical disruption of the skin barrier without the use of light energy. Drug delivery may be accomplished through topical medication application following microneedling, drug administration through hollow needles, or the use of drug-coated microneedles themselves.[133] Of note, authors have suggested proceeding cautiously with nonsterilized medications due to an increased theoretical risk for entry of infectious microbes.[108] Further complicating drug delivery is the possibility for systemic absorption of topical medications, which may lead to potential toxicity. More research is needed demonstrating efficacy of transdermal drug delivery and investigating potential systemic effects before this technique becomes employed more widely.

Technique

As with all clinical procedures, patients interested in undergoing microneedling should receive appropriate counseling on treatment indications, alternatives, and associated risks and benefits. A thorough medical history and physical examination must be conducted to confirm that there are no major contraindications to proceeding with microneedling. A brief pretreatment visit or phone call should be initiated with patients 1 to 2 weeks prior to the procedure to ensure proper communication of necessary instructions. Specifically, clinicians should consider the patient's use of irritating products or medications including retinols, glycolic acid, salicylic acid, waxing, microdermabrasion, and abrasive scrubs. Of note, Alster et al. have recommended the use of retinoids, antioxidants, anticoagulants, and growth factors not be stopped prior to the procedure.[110] Certain clinicians suggest pretreatment prophylaxis with oral acyclovir/valacyclovir among patients with a history of herpes simplex or varicella infection.[110] Patients should be instructed to avoid excessive sun exposure and/or obtaining a tan prior to the procedure due to increased risk of hyperpigmentation.

A proposed outline for the electric-powered pen is described below (Table 10.6).[110] These procedural steps may not be applicable to all handheld electronic microneedling devices; furthermore, steps may vary based on practitioner preferences (Figure 10.10 and 10.11).

TABLE 10.6   Outline for Preparing and Performing a Typical Microneedling Procedure
Preparation
Consider antiviral medication prophylaxis prior to procedure.
Take baseline standardized photography.
Instruct patient to lie supine on treatment table, or alternative position, allowing for best visualization of treatment area.
Pull hair away from treatment area with towel or hairband.
Provide eye protection such as adhesive protective eyewear.
Remove product and makeup from skin with mild skin cleanser.
Review patient's allergies.
Consider use of topical anesthetic compound prior to procedure for pain control.
Clean skin with surgical antiseptic scrub.
Select device treatment settings. Recommended parameters depend on device being utilized, operator pressure, and number of passes; follow specific settings based on manufacturer guidelines and literature review.
Consider a test area prior to performing entire treatment.
Ensure personal protective equipment is worn by all personnel in treatment room such as eyewear, gloves, and masks.
Treatment
Reverify device treatment settings.
Apply gliding gel such as hyaluronic acid gel or other product as per manufacturer guidelines.
Place microneedling device perpendicular to treatment area.
Guide microneedling device in continuous passes over treatment area. Traditionally, three passes are performed over selected areas in alternative directions (e.g., horizontal, vertical, and oblique).[110]
Repeat treatment until desired end point (e.g., pinpoint bleeding; Figures 10.10 and 10.11) is observed.
Pursue treatment in new quadrant. Continue until all desired areas have been treated.
Document number and direction of passes in medical record.
Remove debris and/or excess bleeding with sterile gauze and solution. Any cooling solution should be sterile so as to minimize introduction of bacteria or other pathogens.
Apply pressure to any active bleeding.
Apply thin layer of postoperative topical (hyaluronic acid) as per manufacturer.

With regard to needle depth, thicker tissues can be treated with longer needles. On the face, cheeks, and perioral regions, Alster et al. have suggested needle depths of 1.5 to 3 mm.[110] Less aggressive depths of 0.5 to 1 mm are often preferred for thinner skin including the eyelids and nasal bridge. Clinicians should take caution when performing microneedling over periorbital regions due to risks of penetration to the eye. Also, there may be a theoretical increased risk when microneedling over bony prominences. Gliding gel, often composed of hyaluronic acid, is imperative for epidermal protection.

While there are no formal guidelines for postprocedure microneedling care, clinicians may consider having patients apply daily broad-spectrum, physical blocking sunscreen after the procedure site is healed. Makeup application should be avoided until 48 hours after the procedure.[110] The treatment area may be cleansed with a gentle daily facial

FIGURE 10.10   Patient photographs before microneedling treatment (A) and at clinical end point (B) with pinpoint bleeding. Mild serous discharge is present postprocedure on the right cheek with associated mild erythema.

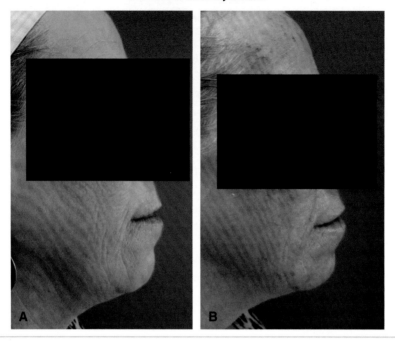

(Image courtesy of Ronda S. Farah, MD, University of Minnesota Department of Dermatology, MN, USA.)

FIGURE 10.11   Patient photograph demonstrating clinical endpoint of pinpoint bleeding on the lower face.

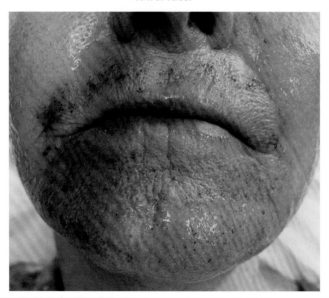

(Image courtesy of Ronda S. Farah, MD, University of Minnesota Department of Dermatology, MN, USA.)

cleanser, though clinicians may consider discontinuing harsh nonprescription skincare products—particularly abrasive scrubs or toners—which may overly irritate the skin in the following days. Transient erythema, swelling, and skin flaking within the first 72 hours are expected.[110] Patients should be advised that repeat treatments are likely necessary to achieve optimal results.[110]

Risks and Contraindications

As a minimally invasive procedure, microneedling is generally well tolerated with a low risk of adverse events. Swelling may be minimized with cold compresses and sleeping at an incline the first evening following the procedure. The risk of microneedling-induced hyperpigmentation is low, but can be further decreased through proper avoidance of sun exposure. As with all light-based procedures, patients with active tans should not be treated.

Burning, bruising, serous ooze, crusting, and scabbing have been reported.[116] Any signs or symptoms of blistering, bruising, pustules, pain, crusting, active bleeding, or increasing discomfort warrant immediate clinician notification and management. A case of undesired tram track scarring—or patterned scarring in alternating "crisscrossing" directions—following two sessions of microneedling therapy has also been described.[134] Other than daily sunscreen, patients should be advised to avoid application of topical products not recommended by their clinician due to an increased risk of hypersensitivity reactions.[110] Indeed, hypersensitivity reactions and development of foreign body granulomas have been reported with use of topical vitamin C.[135]

Clinicians should exercise caution or avoid performance of microneedling in patients with active acne lesions, history of keloid scarring, hypertrophic scarring, koebnerizing skin disease, facial verruca, active infection, untreated neoplasm, active chemotherapy, anticoagulant use, pregnancy, uncontrolled diabetes, or immunosuppression. Clinicians should also proceed carefully when performing microneedling near areas recently injected with botulinum toxin, as combination treatment may lead to toxin diffusion.[110] Anything considered nonsterile should not be applied onto the skin with open microchannels. Infection risk is low overall, as needle device tips are disposable or sterilizable and equipment is cleaned between patients. However, a case has been reported of a patient who contracted human immunodeficiency virus (HIV) in possible relation to a "vampire facial" (platelet-rich plasma [PRP] delivered via microneedling) from a spa in New Mexico.[136] Patients should ensure that they are visiting reputable centers with proper certifications prior to pursuing treatment with microneedling.

Conclusion

Microneedling is a relatively new treatment in the fields of dermatology and medical aesthetics. Given its overall promising efficacy, excellent side effect profile, and minimal recovery time, microneedling is becoming incorporated into many clinical practices. Common uses include atrophic acne scarring and skin rejuvenation, although newer applications such as androgenetic alopecia and transdermal drug delivery are also being investigated. Subsequent research defining more precise treatment parameters and focusing on the long-term effects of microneedling is needed moving forward.

▶ PLATELET-RICH PLASMA

Introduction

Platelet-rich plasma (PRP) has been described as autologous plasma with a platelet count higher than whole blood after centrifugation.[137] Initially defined by hematologists in the 1970s, this broad definition did not articulate the exact platelet concentration necessary to qualify product as PRP. Regardless, the use of PRP has since proliferated to various medical specialties with treatments involving wound healing, bone regeneration, musculoskeletal injuries, and anti-inflammation.[137] Long used in orthopedic medicine and made popular on social media, PRP also has science to support its use in dermatology.[138] This includes, but is not limited to, off-label uses for the management of alopecia, photoaging, facial revolumization, scar management, and ulcerations.[137] As these numerous applications are promising and rapidly growing within the United States, the associated literature has skyrocketed. Nevertheless, the precise mechanism of action of PRP and optimal parameters in many of these situations is unknown. Herein, we provide an overview of PRP therapy and discuss literature on its current cutaneous and aesthetic utilities.

Mechanism

While the exact mechanism of PRP remains unclear, it is hypothesized that PRP improves cell growth and tissue repair through platelet activation and release of a cocktail of growth factors that activate downstream signaling pathways. The conjecture is that the high concentration of platelets, often on the order of more than 1,000,000 platelets/μL, may play an important role in mediating tissue repair, wound healing, and stimulate angiogenesis.[139] Platelets are activated via a two-step process that involves platelet degranulation and subsequent release of growth factors from alpha granules, followed by cleavage of fibrinogen.[140] Once activation occurs, hundreds of growth factors may be secreted from alpha granules, including PDGF, TGF-β, vascular endothelial growth factor (VEGF), insulin-like growth factor 1 (IGF-1), and FGF.[139] Notably, variability of growth factor levels in PRP is one of the many factors that have been postulated to influence efficacy of PRP injections.

Preparation of Platelet-Rich Plasma

Through the 510(k) process, multiple devices have been FDA cleared to generate PRP from whole blood.[138] However, the injection of PRP is not currently regulated by the FDA. There are various protocols for producing autologous concentrations of PRP. No standardized protocol for PRP treatment presently exists, but all protocols follow a similar principle to obtain PRP (Figure 10.12). This process begins by drawing approximately 10 to 60 mL of a patient's whole blood into a test tube with a solution of anticoagulant such as sodium citrate or acid citrate dextrose, which also prevents platelet activation prior to injection.[141] Specific gravity drives the separation of cell types.[141,142] There are two general centrifugation methods used to separate cell types when obtaining PRP. These have been referenced as single-spin and double-spin methods (Figure 10.13). In the single-spin method, a single centrifugation step results in separation into three components: platelet-poor plasma (PPP), PRP, and red blood cells (RBCs) from top to bottom. The PPP is drawn off and PRP is collected. In the double-spin method, two centrifugation steps are required. In the first centrifugation step, the sample of whole blood is separated into two parts. The plasma-containing component is within the top portion and the red blood cell–containing component is within the bottom portion.[143] The plasma-containing

FIGURE 10.12 **Preparation of platelet-rich plasma (PRP) utilizing a single-spin system. PPP, platelet-poor plasma.**

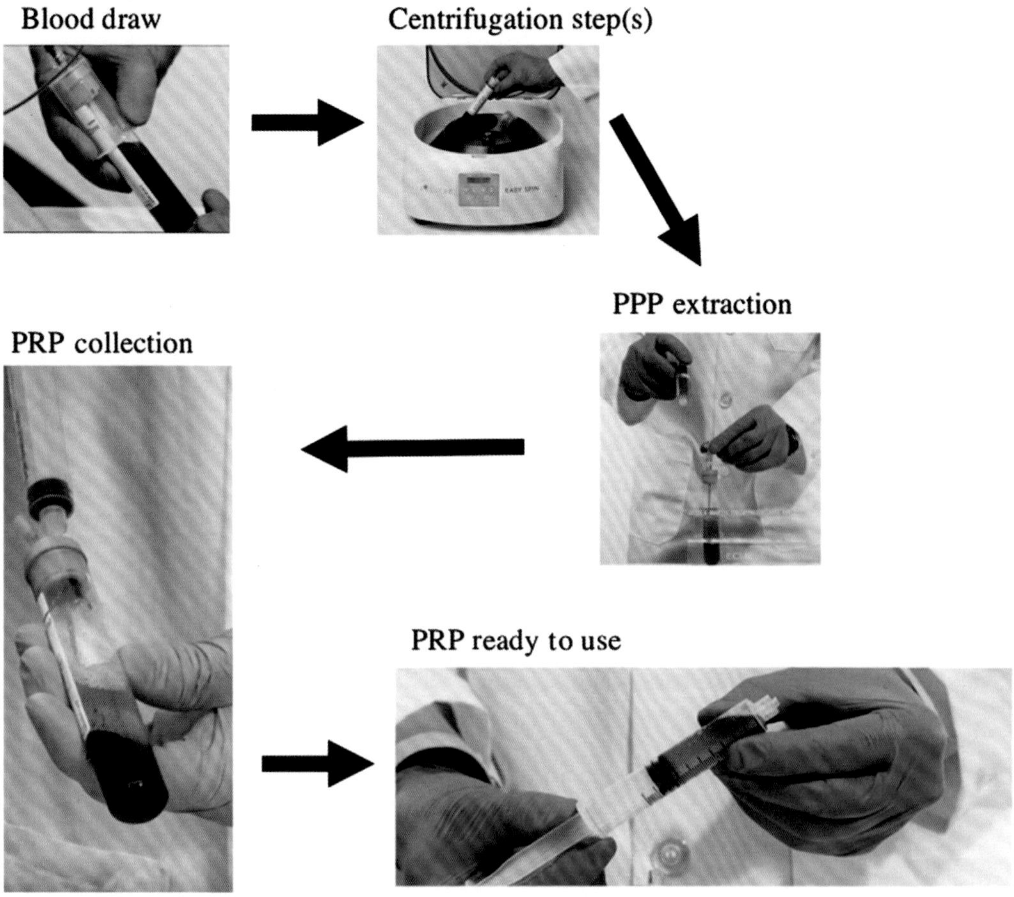

Blood draw

Centrifugation step(s)

PPP extraction

PRP collection

PRP ready to use

(Image courtesy of Eclipse.)

component is separated and transferred to a second tube and a second centrifugation step is completed. The PPP portion (top layer) is drawn off, leaving the clinician or investigator with the PRP (bottom layer). Some studies have suggested the double centrifugation method is superior to the single centrifugation method and possibly more efficacious in concentrating platelets.[143] While these two methods exist, there are several factors that remain variable in the PRP preparation process. The device type, anticoagulant used, amount of whole blood drawn, and temperature of blood product all may be additional variables that warrant further investigation. The optimal PRP concentration for various applications in dermatology, including alopecia and facial aesthetics, is unknown. Some report the optimal platelet concentration to induce angiogenesis in human endothelial cells is 1.5×10^6 platelets per microliter.[144] Others report that a platelet concentration of three times the platelet concentration in whole blood samples is optimal.[145]

Prior to injection, endogenous or exogenous platelet activation should be considered. Platelet activation results in alpha granules releasing growth factors, which are thought to be the basis of clinical improvement. Endogenous activators include components of extracellular matrix (ECM) which activate platelets once injected, such as host dermal collagen and thrombin.[141] Exogenous activators such as calcium chloride, calcium gluconate, bovine thrombin, an ECM product known as A-cell MatriStem^R, and microparticles such as Dalteparin protamine may also be added to PRP prior to injection.[146-150]

FIGURE 10.13   Schematic comparing single-spin (top) versus double-spin (bottom) methods. PRP, platelet-rich plasma; PPP, platelet-poor plasma.

Single-spin method

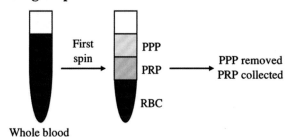

Double-spin method

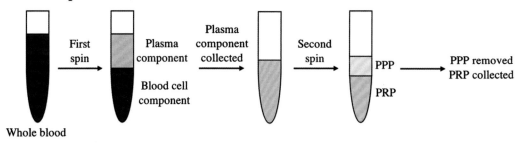

(Image courtesy of Ronda S. Farah, MD, University of Minnesota, Department of Dermatology, MN, USA.)

The addition of adipose-derived stem cells and follicular stem cells may mediate tissue regeneration following stimulation with various growth factors.[151-153] The conundrum of whether to activate with an exogenous product or allow for endogenous platelet activation has been discussed within the literature.[141,142,146,148] However, more research is needed to fully understand the mechanism of PRP and to determine whether or not exogenous activation is more efficacious, and if so, in which clinical situations and with which activators.

It should be noted that PRP is a blood product and, therefore, bears risk for exposure to blood-borne pathogens to employees and patients. This risk includes exposure to hepatitis B, hepatitis C, and HIV. There have been reports of consumers acquiring HIV from unsafe practices involving PRP in New Mexico in 2018.[154] Clinicians and consumers should be aware of the need for appropriate blood-borne pathogen training. As when using other blood products in a medical facility, strict protocols for blood-borne pathogen protection should be followed along with proper sterilization, disinfection, and proper use of materials during the process.

As with any novel minimally invasive procedure, the use of PRP within the clinical setting requires strict clinician assessment and application. Baseline clinical history and standardized photography should be collected. Risks should be reviewed, including, but not limited to, risk of bleeding, infection, pain, ecchymosis, edema, swelling, erythema, nerve injury, numbness, headache, vascular occlusion and blindness.[155] The possibility of no improvement, slight improvement, worsening, and need for multiple treatments should be discussed. Any off-label use should be revealed. Many physicians advocate for baseline complete blood count being obtained prior to injection. Patients with history of bleeding disorder, blood thinners, anemia, active malignancy, chemotherapy use, active radiation at the site, altered anatomy, or other hematological disease should avoid PRP or at minimum a thorough discussion with hematology or another treating physician should be considered. Also, great caution in those who are immunosuppressed, using nonsteroidal anti-inflammatory drugs (NSAIDs), with premalignant skin lesions, or being managed with corticosteroids should be taken. Garg et al.[139] suggest absolute contraindications include hemodynamic instability, active anticoagulant use, platelet dysfunction syndrome, hemodynamic instability, liver disease, active infection at the procedure site, sepsis, and low fibrinogen. Pain is expected with the procedure and clinicians have utilized topical and injectable local anesthetics, vibration, massage, sensory toys, music, and localized cooling devices to alleviate treatment discomfort.

Platelet-Rich Plasma and Alopecia

The off-label use of PRP for the management of alopecia has rapidly grown over the last decade. Overall, numerous studies in the literature have supported its efficacy, particularly for the treatment of androgenetic alopecia.[139,140,147,156-162] While the use of PRP in nonscarring alopecia is promising, there are limited publications examining applications in scarring alopecias.

The mechanism through which PRP results in clinical improvement in those with alopecia remains elusive. It is hypothesized that the release of growth factors and cytokines stimulates hair follicles and promotes new hair growth.[157] Growth factors, including PDGF, VEGF, TGF-β, epidermal growth factor (EGF), and FGF, interact with surface receptors on dermal papilla cells, increasing vascularization and promoting hair follicle formation.[163] Moreover, these growth factors promote cellular proliferation and differentiation of dermal papilla cells, thereby increasing downstream signaling effects, which allows the transition from the telogen phase to the anagen phase attributed to hair growth. However, in 2019, Rodrigues et al. called into question the growth factor hypothesis, with their study lacking a correlation with platelet counts or growth factor levels.[160] Furthermore, Li et al. reported increased survival of follicles through activation of extracellular signal-regulated kinase (ERK) and Akt signaling.[164] The precise mechanism of PRP and its effects on hair growth remain to be defined; therefore, additional investigation is warranted.

Nonscarring Alopecias

Nonscarring alopecias are a group of reversible hair loss diseases lacking scarring of the follicular ostia. Diagnoses include androgenetic alopecia (AGA), alopecia areata (AA), telogen effluvium (TE), and trichotillomania. The use of PRP for the management of nonscarring hair disease has grown in popularity over the last decade. AGA garners the most supportive literature and evidence for efficacy.[165] There are several randomized controlled trials evaluating PRP for AGA.[158-160,162,166] The majority of the literature reports improvement in pattern hair loss after PRP treatment. One study by Gentile et al.[167] compared nonactivated PRP and activated PRP in patients with AGA. They used a half-head approach in which one half of the patient's head was treated with either nonactivated or activated PRP and the other half received a placebo. Clinically improved hair counts and improved hair density were found on the treatment side for both nonactivated and activated PRP compared to placebo. This study also revealed disparities in platelet concentration between various collection systems.[167]

It should be noted that reports with lack of efficacy have also been published.[166] Disease severity, concomitant therapy, study size, study design, platelet concentration, and treatment regimen are just a few of possible reasons for efficacy variability. Most recently, Hausauer et al. suggested a uniform treatment regimen of monthly injections for 3 months followed by a booster injection 3 months later.[159] Continued investigations focused on these variables will likely lead to improved regimens and patient outcomes.

With regard to other nonscarring alopecias, several publications have investigated the use of PRP in AA. It is characterized as a T-cell–mediated autoimmune disease of the hair follicle.[168] A literature review and meta-analysis by Marchitto et al. suggested PRP as a promising and potential treatment option for AA.[169] Even with randomized clinical trials validating PRP treatment for AA, its use is still disputable. Studies have shown PRP to be ineffective in hair growth for some patients with AA.[170] The underlying reasons for variations in clinical outcomes have yet to be determined. As with AGA, contributing factors may include the clinical characteristics of the hair loss, disease duration, disease severity, past medical history, and PRP composition. Data on the use of PRP on other nonscarring alopecias, such as telogen effluvium or trichotillomania, are lacking (Figure 10.14).

Cicatricial Alopecias

Cicatricial alopecias result in destruction of follicular ostia and, traditionally, permanent loss of hair follicles. However, clinicians may note regrowth of hair with early intervention. In addition to physical symptoms, a patient can suffer from severe psychological and emotional distress.[171] Currently, cicatricial alopecias are difficult to manage as current treatments such as topical steroids, intralesional steroids, immunosuppressants, hydroxychloroquine, and oral antibiotics are a far cry from a cure. In the dermatology literature, cicatricial alopecias include lichen planopilaris (LPP), frontal fibrosing alopecia (FFA), discoid lupus, central centrifugal cicatricial alopecia (CCCA), dissecting cellulitis, and folliculitis decalvans. As with AGA, the use of PRP for management of scarring alopecias is not approved by the FDA. Few studies have investigated the management of scarring alopecias with PRP, with most of the literature focused on LPP. There are at least four case reports of PRP being used in the management of LPP. In 2016, there was an initial case report of a patient diagnosed with LPP treated with PRP and a microneedling device.[172] One patient was treated with three consecutive monthly treatments of PRP with complete regression of active LPP symptoms that were present prior to treatment. This case study was the first to report success of PRP for treating LPP,[172] although it is unclear whether

FIGURE 10.14   **Before (A) and after (B) photos of platelet-rich plasma (PRP) for male androgenetic alopecia.**

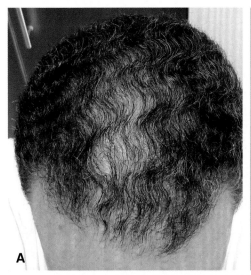
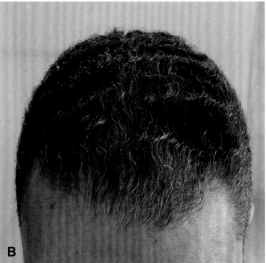

(Courtesy of Dr. Charles E Crutchfield III, Crutchfield Dermatology, Eagan, MN.)

this improvement was related to the PRP, the microneedling procedure, or a combination of the two. In the three remaining cases reported in 2018 and 2019, hair growth and hair thickening were demonstrated.[173-175] However, there is concern of lack of standardized photography in at least two of these case reports. Additional research with larger populations and longer term studies are needed. There are two additional case reports investigating scarring alopecia management with PRP. In the case of CCCA, which is described as hair loss in the crown of the head radiating in a circular pattern outward, there is one reported patient that demonstrated improvement.[175] With regard to FFA, a type of scarring alopecia resulting in the loss of frontal hair line and brows, there was one case report from 2019 where improvement was seen at 5 months follow-up after PRP treatment.[176]

Platelet-Rich Plasma and Aesthetics

Although not FDA approved, the use of PRP for the management of cosmetic concerns has gained popularity. Numerous studies and clinician anecdotal reports have recounted improvement in photoaging, texture, tone, revolumization, and scarring. On the review of the literature focused on photodamage, a study by Alam et al. investigated whether a single PRP injection could improve the visual appearance of photodamaged skin in 27 patients.[177] Each patient received PRP injections in one cheek and sterile injections of normal saline in the other cheek. After 6 months of PRP therapy, patients self-reported significantly improved appearance of wrinkles and skin texture in the PRP-treated side compared to the saline-treated cheek. However, physician evaluations showed no significant difference between PRP and normal saline.[177] Another study by Redaelli et al. evaluated the effects of PRP injections every 3 months on the face and neck.[178] Photographs from a dermoscope, digital camera, and photographic imaging system were used to evaluate the appearance of the face and neck after PRP treatment. They reported an average improvement of 24% for nasolabial folds, 33% for skin homogeneity and texture, 22.5% for skin tonicity, and 30% for periocular wrinkles.[178] While these studies are promising, additional investigations are needed to fully understand the impact of PRP on photoaging and skin texture.

PRP has also been proposed to be helpful for facial volume depletion. Revolumization is hypothesized to occur through the use growth factors within PRP that stimulate activity of fibroblasts and promote collagen production.[179] A study by Elnehrawy et al. examined the effects of a single PRP injection in 20 women with facial wrinkles.[180] Their results demonstrated statistically significant improvement in the appearance of the nasolabial folds.[180]

PRP used in combination with other well-established cosmetic therapies has also been reported. A study by Willemsen et al. showed that PRP, when added to a facial lipofilling procedure, decreases overall recovery time and improves aesthetic outcomes.[181] Yuksel et al. examined the effects of PRP on human facial skin.[182] PRP was applied with a derma roller three times, 2 weeks apart on the forehead, cheekbone, and jaw and also injected into crow's feet wrinkles. Dermatologists evaluated the outcomes and a statistically significant improvement was seen in skin firmness-sagging after three PRP treatment sessions.[182] Shin et al. compared combination PRP with fractional laser versus fractional laser alone in Korean women and found improvements in skin texture and skin elasticity.[183] A prospective study by Hersant et al. examined the effectiveness of combining PRP with hyaluronic acid through facial intradermal injections.[184] Significant improvement assessed on the FACE-Q scale was seen at 6 months, compared to baseline.[184] However, a comparison group to hyaluronic acid only was lacking. Overall, while these combination treatments within aesthetics are exciting, continued research is needed to fully understand effectiveness and parameters for clinical use.

Scarring due to acne is a concern for many patients, and PRP has also been used to attempt to treat it. PRP is an adjuvant therapeutic option for patients with acne scars and has been used as an adjunct therapy to current acne scar revision procedures. Deshmukh et al. compared the efficacy of PRP and subcision versus subcision alone as treatment for acne scars.[185] Subjects received PRP injections into the scar after subcision on the right side of their face and the left side received subcision only. PRP with subcision showed 32.08% in acne scarring versus 8.33% improvement with subcision alone.[185] Nofal et al. provided promising results for intradermal PRP injections when treating atrophic acne scars of varying grades.[186] Traumatic scars may also benefit from PRP.[187] PRP is also used as a therapeutic tool to aid in recovery because of its wound healing properties. Lee et al. examined the effects of PRP to enhance wound healing after carbon dioxide fractional resurfacing treatment for acne scars in 14 Korean patients.[188] They found that the half of the face treated with PRP after a laser resurfacing treatment recovered more quickly and with faster improvement in erythema. Decreased edema was also noted but did not reach statistical significance.[188]

Overall, the applications for PRP within the aesthetic arena are novel and rapidly expanding. However, numerous large randomized controlled trials are lacking. Furthermore, definitive understanding of the use of PRP for aesthetics—including optimal preparation, treatment intervals, and long-term safety and efficacy—are yet to be delineated.

Conclusion

As the use of PRP in the clinical setting expands, its testing in novel cutaneous medical scenarios also grows. To date, these uses include PRP in conjunction with hair transplantation, treatment of ulcerations, and management of vitiligo.[189-192] Overall, the potential for PRP within the medical arena is exponential and holds great promise for human disease. However, many variables remain to be elucidated prior to developing a standardized and effective PRP protocol for each application. Lack of standardization in PRP preparation and administration, along with limited understanding of the basic science, makes PRP an excellent target for future investigation. Additional studies are needed to fully understand the use of PRP injection therapy for our patients.

REFERENCES

1. El-Domyati M, Hosam W, Abdel-Azim E, Abdel-Wahab H, Mohamed E. Microdermabrasion: a clinical, histometric, and histopathologic study. *J Cosmet Dermatol*. 2016;15:503-513. doi:10.1111/jocd.12252.
2. Monteleone G. *Microdermabrasion with aluminum hydroxide powder in scar camouflaging*. In: *Proceedings of the 3rd Meeting of Southern Italy Plastic Surgery Association*. Benevento, Italy: 1988.
3. *The American Society for Aesthetic Plastic Surgery*. New York, NY: Cosmetic Surgery National Data Bank Statistics; 2017. Available at https://www.surgery.org/sites/default/files/ASAPS-Stats2017.pdf.
4. Karimipour DJ, Kang S, Johnson TM, et al. Microdermabrasion with and without aluminum oxide crystal abrasion: a comparative molecular analysis of dermal remodeling. *J Am Acad Dermatol*. 2006;54:405-410. doi:10.1016/j.jaad.2005.11.1084.
5. Bhalla M, Thami GP. Microdermabrasion: reappraisal and brief review of literature. *Dermatol Surg*. 2006;32:809-814. doi:10.1111/j.1524-4725.2006.32165.x.
6. Andrews SN, Zarnitsyn V, Bondy B, Prausnitz MR. Optimization of microdermabrasion for controlled removal of stratum corneum. *Int J Pharm*. 2011;407:95-104. doi:10.1016/j.ijpharm.2011.01.034.
7. Spencer JM. Microdermabrasion. *Am J Clin Dermatol*. 2005;6(2):89-92. doi:10.2165/00128071-200506020-00003.
8. Freedman BM, Rueda-Pedraza E, Waddell SP. The epidermal and dermal changes associated with microdermabrasion. *Dermatol Surg*. 2001;27:1031-1033. doi:10.1046/j.1524-4725.2001.01031.x.
9. Shim EK, Barnette D, Hughes K, Greenway HT. Microdermabrasion: a clinical and histopathologic study. *Dermatol Surg*. 2001;27:524-530. doi:10.1046/j.1524-4725.2001.01001.x.
10. Tan MH, Spencer JM, Pires LM, Ajmeri J, Skover G. The evaluation of aluminum oxide crystal microdermabrasion for photodamage. *Dermatol Surg*. 2001;27:943-949. doi:10.1046/j.1524-4725.2001.01120.x.

11. Fernandes M, Pinheiro NM, Crema VO, Mendonça AC. Effects of microdermabrasion on skin rejuvenation. *J Cosmet Laser Ther*. 2014;16:26-31. doi:10.3109/14764172.2013.854120.

12. Rajan P, Grimes PE. Skin barrier changes induced by aluminum oxide and sodium chloride microdermabrasion. *Dermatol Surg*. 2002;28:390-393. doi:10.1046/j.1524-4725.2002.01239.x.

13. Lew BL, Cho Y, Lee MH. Effect of serial microdermabrasion on the ceramide level in the stratum corneum. *Dermatol Surg*. 2006;32:376-379. doi:10.1111/j.1524-4725.2006.32076.x.

14. Small R, Hoang D, Linder J. *Chemical Peels, Microdermabrasion & Topical Products*. Philadelphia, PA: Lippincott Williams & Wilkins; 2013.

15. Lee WR, Shen SC, Wang KH, Hu CH, Fang JY. Lasers and microdermabrasion enhance and control topical delivery of vitamin C. *J Invest Dermatol*. 2003;121:1118-1125. doi:10.1046/j.1523-1747.2003.12537.x.

16. Loesch MM, Travers JB, Kingsley MM, Travers JB, Spandau DF. Skin resurfacing procedures: new and emerging options. *Clin Cosmet Investig Dermatol*. 2014;7:231-241. doi:10.2147/CCID.S50367.

17. Freedman BM. Hydradermabrasion: an innovative modality for nonablative facial rejuvenation. *J Cosmet Dermatol*. 2008;7:275-280 doi:10.1111/j.1473-2165.2008.00406.x.

18. Freedman BM. Topical antioxidant application enhances the effects of facial microdermabrasion. *J Dermatolog Treat*. 2009;20(2):82-87. doi:10.1080/09546630802301818.

19. Karimipour DJ, Karimipour G, Orringer JS. Microdermabrasion: an evidence-based review. *Plast Reconstr Surg*. 2010;125:372-377. doi:10.1097/PRS.0b013e3181c2a583.

20. Hernandez-Perez E, Ibiett EV. Gross and microscopic findings in patients undergoing microdermabrasion for facial rejuvenation. *Dermatol Surg*. 2001;27:637-640. doi:10.1046/j.1524-4725.2001.00291.x.

21. Tsai R-Y, Wang C-N, Chan H-L. Aluminum oxide crystal microdermabrasion: a new technique for treating facial scarring. *Dermatol Surg*. 1995;21:539-542. doi:10.1111/j.1524-4725.1995.tb00258.x.

22. Lloyd JR. The use of microdermabrasion for acne: a pilot study. *Dermatol Surg*. 2001;27:329-331. doi:10.1046/j.1524-4725.2001.00313.x.

23. Kolodziejczak A, Wieczorek AM, Rotsztejn HP. The assessment of the effects of the combination of microdermabrasion and cavitation peeling in the therapy of seborrhoeic skin with visible symptoms of acne punctata. *J Cosmet Laser Ther*. 2019;21:286-290. doi:10.1080/14764172.2018.1525751.

24. Waldman A, Bolotin D, Arndt KA, et al. ASDS Guidelines Task Force: consensus recommendations regarding the safety of lasers, dermabrasion, chemical peels, energy devices, and skin surgery during and after isotretinoin use. *Dermatol Surg*. 2017;43:1249-1262. doi:10.1097/DSS.0000000000001166.

25. Janda K, Tomikowska A. Cellulite – causes, prevention, treatment. *Ann Acad Med Stetin*. 2014;60(1):29-38.

26. Atamoros FMP, Pérez DA, Sigall DA, et al. Evidence-based treatment for gynoid lipodystrophy: a review of the recent literature. *J Cosmet Dermatol*. 2018;17(6):977-983. doi:10.1111/jocd.12555.

27. Khan MH, Victor F, Rao B, Sadick NS. Treatment of cellulite: part I. Pathophysiology. *J Am Acad Dermatol*. 2010;62(3):361-370. doi:10.1016/j.jaad.2009.10.042.

28. Sadick N. Treatment for cellulite. *Int J Womens Dermatol*. 2019;5(1):68-72. doi:10.1016/j.ijwd.2018.09.002.

29. Draelos ZD, Marenus KD. Cellulite: etiology and purported treatment. *Dermatol Surg*. 1997;23(12):1177-1781. doi:10.1111/j.1524-4725.1997.tb00468.x.

30. Avram MM. Cellulite: a review of its physiology and treatment. *J Cosmet Laser Ther*. 2004;6(4):181-185. doi:10.1080/14764170410003057.

31. Davis DS, Boen M, Fabi SG. Cellulite: patient selection and combination treatments for optimal results – a review and our experience. *Dermatol Surg*. 2019;45:1171-1184.

32. Scherwitz C, Braun-Falco O. So-called cellulite. *J Dermatol Surg Oncol*. 1978;4(3):221-229. doi:10.1111/j.1524-4725.1978.tb00416.x.

33. Nürnberger F, Müller G. So-called cellulite: an invented disease. *J Dermatol Surg Oncol*. 1978;4(3):221-229.

34. Hexsel D, Hexsel CL. Social impact of cellulite and its impact on quality of life. In: Goldman MP, Hexsel D, Leibaschoff G, Bacci PA, eds. *Cellulite Pathophysiology and Treatment*. Boca Raton, FL: CRC Press; 2006: 2-4.

35. Hexsel D, Fonte De Souza J, Weber M, Taborda ML. Preliminary results of the elaboration of a new instrument to evaluate quality of life in patients with cellulite: CELLUQOL. *J Am Acad Dermatol*. 2009;60(3):AB62. doi:10.1016/j.jaad.2008.11.285.

36. Rossi ABR, Vergnanini AL. Cellulite: a review. *J Eur Acad Dermatol Venereol*. 2000;14(4):251-262. doi:10.1046/j.1468-3083.2000.00016.x.

37. Barnhill W. *The Cellulite Myth*. *The Washington Post*. 1985. Available at https://www.washingtonpost.com/archive/lifestyle/wellness/1985/03/06/the-cellulite-myth/661b5726-da95-43ec-9459-dfabb505bbcf/?utm_term=.3fc5465a1ac4.

38. Ronsard N. *Cellulite: Those Lumps, Bumps and Bulges You Couldn't Lose Before*. New York, NY: Beauty and Health Publishing and Co; 1973.

39. *Cellulite Treatment*. *RealSelf.com*. 2019. Available at https://www.realself.com/cellulite-treatment/cost.

40. Goldman MP, Hexsel D. *Cellulite: Pathophysiology and Treatment (Basic and Clinical Dermatology)*. 2nd ed. Boco Raton, FL: CRC Press; 2010.

41. Emanuele E, Bertona M, Geroldi D. A multilocus candidate approach identifies ACE and HIF1A as susceptibility genes for cellulite. *J Eur Acad Dermatol Venereol*. 2010;24(8):930-935. doi:10.1111/j.1468-3083.2009.03556.x.

42. Emanuele E, Minoretti P, Altabas K, Gaeta E, Altabas V. Adiponectin expression in subcutaneous adipose tissue is reduced in women with cellulite. *Int J Dermatol*. 2011;50(4):412-416. doi:10.1111/j.1365-4632.2010.04713.x.

43. Rudolph C, Hladik C, Hamade H, et al. Structural gender dimorphism and the biomechanics of the gluteal subcutaneous tissue: implications for the pathophysiology of cellulite. *Plast Reconstr Surg.* 2019;143(4):1077-1086. doi:10.1097/PRS.0000000000005407.

44. Puddu P, Ventrice C, Pennasilico G, et al. An open randomized controlled study on the efficacy of low-sodium water intake evaluated by non-invasive methods in patients with cellulite. *Eur J Inflamm.* 2017;1(1):43-48. doi:10.1177/1721727x0300100109.

45. Piérard GE, Nizet JL, Piérard-Franchimont C. Cellulite: from standing fat herniation to hypodermal stretch marks. *Am J Dermatopathol.* 2000;22(1):34-37.

46. Mirrashed F, Sharp JC, Krause V, Morgan J, Tomanek B. Pilot study of dermal and subcutaneous fat structures by MRI in individuals who differ gender, BMI, and cellulite grading. *Skin Res Technol.* 2004;10(3):161-168. doi:10.1111/j.1600-0846.2004.00072.x.

47. Friedmann D, Vick G, Mishra V. Cellulite: a review with a focus on subcision. *Clin Cosmet Investig Dermatol.* 2017;10:17-23. doi:10.2147/CCID.S95830.

48. Curri S. *Las paniculopatías de estasis venosa: diagnostico clínico e instrumental.* Barcelona, Spain: Hausmann; 1991.

49. Draelos ZD. *Cellulite pathophysiology.* In: *Cellulite Pathophysiology and Treatment.* 2nd ed. New York, NY: Informa Healthcare; 2010.

50. Angelini F, Orlandi C, Di Fiore P, et al. *Medical therapy.* In: *Cellulite Pathophysiology and Treatment.* 2nd ed. New York, NY: Informa Healthcare; 2010.

51. Nikolis A, Enright KM. Methods of standardizing photography for cellulite in the buttocks and thighs. *Dermatol Surg.* 2019;45:1208-1210. doi:10.1097/DSS.0000000000001666.

52. Hexsel D, Hexsel CL, Dal'Forno T, Schilling de Souza J, Silva AF, Siega C. Standardized methods for photography in procedural dermatology using simple equipment. *Int J Dermatol.* 2017;56(4):444-451. doi:10.1111/ijd.13500.

53. Zerini I, Sisti A, Cuomo R, et al. Cellulite treatment: a comprehensive literature review. *J Cosmet Dermatol.* 2015;14(3):224-240. doi:10.1111/jocd.12154.

54. Hexsel DM, Dal'Forno T, Hexsel CL, Dal'forno T, Hexsel CL. A validated photonumeric cellulite severity scale. *J Eur Acad Dermatol Venereol.* 2009;23(5):523-528. doi:10.1111/j.1468-3083.2009.03101.x.

55. Hexsel D, Fabi SG, Sattler G, et al. Validated assessment scales for cellulite dimples on the buttocks and thighs in female patients. *Dermatol Surg.* 2019;45:S2-S11. doi:10.1097/dss.0000000000001993.

56. Hexsel D, Weber MB, Taborda ML, Forno TD, Dal'Forno T, Prado D. Celluqol® – a quality of life measurement for patients with cellulite. *Surg Cosmet Dermatol.* 2011;3(2):96-101.

57. Kutlubay Z, Songur A, Engin B, Khatib R, Calay Ö, Serdaroğlu S. An alternative treatment modality for cellulite: LPG endermologie. *J Cosmet Laser Ther.* 2013;15(5):266-270. doi:10.3109/14764172.2013.787801.

58. Tülin Güleç A. Treatment of cellulite with LPG endermologie. *Int J Dermatol.* 2009;48(3):265-270. doi:10.1111/j.1365-4632.2009.03898.x.

59. Collis N, Elliot LA, Sharpe C, Sharpe DT. Cellulite treatment: a myth or reality. A prospective randomized, controlled trial of two therapies, endermologie and aminophylline cream. *Plast Reconstr Surg.* 1999;104(4):1110-1114. doi:10.1097/00006534-199909020-00037.

60. Hexsel D, Soirefmann M. Cosmeceuticals for cellulite. *Semin Cutan Med Surg.* 2011;30(3):167-170. doi:10.1016/j.sder.2011.06.005.

61. Hexsel D, Zechmeister Ddo P, Goldman MP. *Topical management of cellulite.* In: *Cellulite Pathophysiology and Treatment.* 2nd ed. New York, NY: Informa Healthcare; 2010.

62. Khan MH, Victor F, Rao B, Sadick NS. Treatment of cellulite: part II. Advances and controversies. *J Am Acad Dermatol.* 2010;62(3):373-384. doi:10.1016/j.jaad.2009.10.041.

63. Lupi O, Semenovitch IJ, Treu C, Bottino D, Bouskela E. Evaluation of the effects of caffeine in the microcirculation and edema on thighs and buttocks using the orthogonal polarization spectral imaging and clinical parameters. *J Cosmet Dermatol.* 2007;6(2):102-107. doi:10.1111/j.1473-2165.2007.00304.x.

64. Kligman AM, Pagnoni A, Stoudemayer T. Topical retinol improves cellulite. *J Dermatol Treat.* 1999;10(2):119-125. doi:10.3109/09546639909056013.

65. Piérard-Franchimont C, Piérard GE, Henry F, Vroome V, Cauwenbergh G. A randomized, placebo-controlled trial of topical retinol in the treatment of cellulite. *Am J Clin Dermatol.* 2000;1(6):369-374. doi:10.2165/00128071-200001060-00005.

66. Sainio EL, Rantanen T, Kanerva L. Ingredients and safety of cellulite creams. *Eur J Dermatol.* 2000;10(8):596-603.

67. Belenky I, Margulis A, Elman M, Bar-Yosef U, Paun SD. Exploring channeling optimized radiofrequency energy: a review of radiofrequency history and applications in esthetic fields. *Adv Ther.* 2012;29(3):249-266. doi:10.1007/s12325-012-0004-1.

68. Beasley KL, Weiss RA. Radiofrequency in cosmetic dermatology. *Dermatol Clin.* 2014;32(1):79-90. doi:10.1016/j.det.2013.09.010.

69. Sadick NS, Malerich SA, Nassar AH, Dorizas AS. Radiofrequency: an update on latest innovations. *J Drugs Dermatol.* 2014;13(11):1331-1335.

70. Narsete T, Narsete DS. Evaluation of radiofrequency devices in aesthetic medicine: a preliminary report. *J Dermatol Ther Case Rep Eval.* 2017;1(1):5-8.

71. Kapoor R, Shome D, Ranjan A. Use of a novel combined radiofrequency and ultrasound device for lipolysis, skin tightening and cellulite treatment. *J Cosmet Laser Ther.* 2017;19(5):266-274. doi:10.1080/14764172.2017.1303169.

72. Fritz K, Salavastru C, Gyurova M. Clinical evaluation of simultaneously applied monopolar radiofrequency and targeted pressure energy as a new method for noninvasive treatment of cellulite in postpubertal women. *J Cosmet Dermatol.* 2018;17(3):361-364. doi:10.1111/jocd.12525.

73. Alexiades-Armenakas M, Dover JS, Arndt KA. Unipolar radiofrequency treatment to improve the appearance of cellulite. *J Cosmet Laser Ther.* 2008;10(3):148-153. doi:10.1080/14764170802279651.

74. Alexiades M, Munavalli G, Goldberg D, Berube D. Prospective multicenter clinical trial of a temperature-controlled subcutaneous microneedle fractional bipolar radiofrequency system for the treatment of cellulite. *Dermatol Surg.* 2018;44(10):1262-1271. doi:10.1097/DSS.0000000000001593.

75. Sadick N, Magro C. A study evaluating the safety and efficacy of the VelaSmooth system in the treatment of cellulite. *J Cosmet Laser Ther.* 2007;9(1):15-20.

76. Sadick NS, Mulholland RS. A prospective clinical study to evaluate the efficacy and safety of cellulite treatment using the combination of optical and RF energies for subcutaneous tissue heating. *J Cosmet Laser Ther.* 2004;6(4):187-190. doi:10.1080/14764170410003039.

77. Sadick NS. *VelaSmooth and VelaShape.* In: *Cellulite Pathophysiology and Treatment.* 2nd ed. New York, NY: Informa Healthcare; 2010.

78. Sadick N, Rothaus KO. Aesthetic applications of radiofrequency devices. *Clin Plast Surg.* 2016;43(3):557-565. doi:10.1016/j.cps.2016.03.014.

79. Sadick NS, Nassar AH, Dorizas AS, Alexiades-Armenakas M. Bipolar and multipolar radiofrequency. *Dermatol Surg.* 2014;40:S174-S179. doi:10.1097/DSS.0000000000000201.

80. Wanitphakdeedecha R, Sathaworawong A, Manuskiatti W, Sadick NS. Efficacy of multipolar radiofrequency with pulsed magnetic field therapy for the treatment of abdominal cellulite. *J Cosmet Laser Ther.* 2017;19(4):205-209. doi:10.1080/14764172.2017.1279332.

81. Goldberg DJ, Fazeli A, Berlin AL. Clinical, laboratory, and MRI analysis of cellulite treatment with a unipolar radiofrequency device. *Dermatol Surg.* 2008;34(2):204-209. doi:10.1111/j.1524-4725.2007.34038.x.

82. Luebberding S, Krueger N, Sadick NS. Cellulite: an evidence-based review. *Am J Clin Dermatol.* 2015;16(4):243-256. doi:10.1007/s40257-015-0129-5.

83. Modena DAO, da Silva CN, Grecco C, et al. Extracorporeal shockwave: mechanisms of action and physiological aspects for cellulite, body shaping, and localized fat—systematic review. *J Cosmet Laser Ther.* 2017;19(6):314-319. doi:10.1080/14764172.2017.1334928.

84. Hexsel D, Camozzato FO, Silva AF, Siega C. Acoustic wave therapy for cellulite, body shaping and fat reduction. *J Cosmet Laser Ther.* 2017;19(3):165-173. doi:10.1080/14764172.2016.1269928.

85. Knobloch K, Kraemer R. Extracorporeal shock wave therapy (ESWT) for the treatment of cellulite – a current metaanalysis. *Int J Surg.* 2015;24(2015):210-217. doi:10.1016/j.ijsu.2015.07.644.

86. Werschler WP. Evaluation of microfocused ultrasound with visualization (MFU-V) for lifting and tightening of facial and neck skin laxity using a customized, high-density and vectoring treatment approach. *J Am Acad Dermatol.* 2014;70(5):AB43. doi:10.1016/j.jaad.2014.01.177.

87. Goldberg D, Bard S, Kassim A, Payongayong L. *A Single-center, Prospective Study of the Efficacy and Safety of Micro-focused Ultrasound With Visualization for Lifting, Tightening, and Smoothing of the Buttocks and Thighs.* 2013. Available at https://onlinelibrary.wiley.com/doi/full/10.1002/lsm.22127.

88. Moreno-Moraga J, Valero-Altés T, Martínez Riquelme A, Isarria-Marcosy MI, Royo De La Torre J. Body contouring by non-invasive transdermal focused ultrasound. *Lasers Surg Med.* 2007;39(4):315-323. doi:10.1002/lsm.20478.

89. Casabona G, Pereira G. Microfocused ultrasound with visualization and calcium hydroxylapatite for improving skin laxity and cellulite appearance. *Plast Reconstr Surg Glob Open* 2017;5(7):1-8. doi:10.1097/GOX.0000000000001388.

90. Harris MO, Sundaram HA. Safety of microfocused ultrasound with visualization in patients with Fitzpatrick skin phototypes III to VI. *JAMA Facial Plast Surg.* 2015;17(5):355-357. doi:10.1001/jamafacial.2015.0990.

91. Ingargiola MJ, Motakef S, Chung MT, Vasconez HC, Sasaki GH. Cryolipolysis for fat reduction and body contouring. *Plast Reconstr Surg.* 2015;135(6):1581-1590. doi:10.1097/prs.0000000000001236.

92. Coleman KM, Pozner J. Combination therapy for rejuvenation of the outer thigh and buttock. *Dermatol Surg.* 2016;42:S124-S130. doi:10.1097/dss.0000000000000752.

93. Sadick NS, Goldman MP, Liu G, et al. Collagenase clostridium histolyticum for the treatment of edematous fibrosclerotic panniculopathy (cellulite): a randomized trial. *Dermatol Surg.* 2019;45:1047-1056. doi:10.1097/DSS.0000000000001803.

94. Jung TW, Kim ST, Lee JH, et al. Phosphatidylcholine causes lipolysis and apoptosis in adipocytes through the tumor necrosis factor alpha-dependent pathway. *Pharmacology.* 2018;101(3-4):111-119. doi:10.1159/000481571.

95. Mahmud K, Crutchfield CE. Lipodissolve for body sculpting: safety, effectiveness, and patient satisfaction. *J Clin Aesthet Dermatol.* 2012;5(10):16-19..

96. Eldsouky F, Ebrahim HM. Evaluation and efficacy of carbon dioxide therapy (carboxytherapy) versus mesolipolysis in the treatment of cellulite. *J Cosmet Laser Ther.* 2018;20(5):307-312. doi:10.1080/14764172.2017.1400175.

97. Hexsel DM, Mazzuco R. Subcision: a treatment for cellulite. *Int J Dermatol.* 2000;39(7):539-544. doi:10.1046/j.1365-4362.2000.00020.x.

98. Kaminer MS, Coleman WP, Weiss RA, Robinson DM, Coleman WP, Hornfeldt C. Multicenter pivotal study of vacuum-assisted precise tissue release for the treatment of cellulite. *Dermatol Surg.* 2015;41(3):336-347. doi:10.1097/DSS.0000000000000280.

99. Geronemus RG, Kilmer SL, Wall SH, et al. An observational study of the safety and efficacy of tissue stabilized–guided subcision. *Dermatol Surg*. 2019;45(8):1057-1062. doi:10.1097/dss.0000000000001911.

100. DiBernardo BE, Sasaki GH, Katz BE, et al. A multicenter study for cellulite treatment using a 1440-nm Nd:YAG wavelength laser with side-firing fiber. *Aesthet Surg J*. 2016;36(3):335-343. doi:10.1093/asj/sjv203.

101. Katz B. Quantitative & qualitative evaluation of the efficacy of a 1440 nm Nd:YAG laser with novel bi-directional optical fiber in the treatment of cellulite as measured by 3-dimensional surface imaging. *J Drugs Dermatol*. 2013;12(11):1224-1230.

102. Alster TS, Tehrani M. Treatment of cellulite with optical devices: an overview with practical considerations. *Lasers Surg Med*. 2006;38(8):727-730. doi:10.1002/lsm.20411.

103. Orentreich DS, Orentreich N. Subcutaneous incisionless (subcision) surgery for the correction of depressed scars and wrinkles. *Dermatol Surg*. 1995;21:543-549. doi:10.1111/j.1524-4725.1995.tb00259.x

104. Camirand A, Doucet J. Needle dermabrasion. *Aesthetic Plast Surg*. 1997;21:48-51. doi:10.1007/s002669900081

105. Fernandes D. Minimally invasive percutaneous collagen induction. *Oral Maxillofac Surg Clin North Am*. 2005;17:51-63. doi:10.1016/j.coms.2004.09.004

106. Ramaut L, Hoeksema H, Pirayesh A, Stillaert F, Monstrey S. Microneedling: Where do we stand now? A systematic review of the literature. *J Plast Reconstr Aesthetic Surg*. 2018;44:397-404. doi:10.1016/j.bjps.2017.06.006

107. U.S. Food & Drug Administration. *Regulatory Considerations for Microneedling Devices: Draft Guidance for Industry and Food and Drug Administration Staff*. Rockville, MD: Food & Drug Administration; 2017.

108. Iriarte C, Awosika O, Rengifo-Pardo M, Ehrlich A. Review of applications of microneedling in dermatology. *Clin Cosmet Investig Dermatol*. 2017;10:289-298. doi:10.2147/CCID.S142450

109. Mccrudden MTC, Mcalister E, Courtenay AJ, González-Vázquez P, Raj Singh TR, Donnelly RF. Microneedle applications in improving skin appearance. *Exp Dermatol*. 2015;24:561-566. doi:10.1111/exd.12723

110. Alster TS, Graham PM. Microneedling: A review and practical guide. *Dermatol Surg*. 2018;44:397-404. doi:10.1097/DSS.0000000000001248

111. Aust MC, Reimers K, Repenning C, et al. Percutaneous collagen induction: Minimally invasive skin rejuvenation without risk of hyperpigmentation – fact or fiction? *Plast Reconstr Surg*. 2008;122:1553-1563. doi:10.1097/PRS.0b013e318188245e

112. Fernandes D, Signorini M. Combating photoaging with percutaneous collagen induction. *Clin Dermatol*. 2008;26:192-199. doi:10.1016/j.clindermatol.2007.09.006

113. Aust MC, Knobloch K, Vogt PM. Percutaneous Collagen Induction Therapy as a Novel Therapeutic Option for Striae Distensae. *Plast Reconstr Surg*. 2010;126:219e-220e. doi:10.1097/prs.0b013e3181ea93da

114. Doddaballapur S. Microneedling with dermaroller. *J Cutan Aesthet Surg*. 2009;2:110-111. doi:10.4103/0974-2077.58529

115. Singh A, Yadav S. Microneedling: Advances and widening horizons. *Indian Dermatol Online J*. 2016;7:244-254. doi:10.4103/2229-5178.185468

116. Harris AG, Naidoo C, Murrell DF. Skin needling as a treatment for acne scarring: an up-to-date review of the literature. *Int J Womens Dermatology*. 2015;1:77-81. doi:10.1016/j.ijwd.2015.03.004

117. Alam M, Han S, Pongprutthipan M, et al. Efficacy of a needling device for the treatment of acne scars: a randomized clinical trial. *JAMA Dermatology*. 2014;150:844-849. doi:10.1001/jamadermatol.2013.8687

118. Cohen BE, Elbuluk N. Microneedling in skin of color: a review of uses and efficacy. *J Am Acad Dermatol*. 2016;74:348-355. doi:10.1016/j.jaad.2015.09.024

119. El-Domyati M, Barakat M, Awad S, Medhat W, El-Fakahany H, Farag H. Microneedling therapy for atrophic acne scars an objective evaluation. *J Clin Aesthet Dermatol*. 2015;8:36-42.

120. Aust MC, Knobloch K, Reimers K, et al. Percutaneous collagen induction therapy: An alternative treatment for burn scars. *Burns*. 2010;36:836-843. doi:10.1016/j.burns.2009.11.014.

121. Eilers RE, Ross EV, Cohen JL, Ortiz AE. A combination approach to surgical scars. *Dermatol Surg*. 2016;42:S150-S156. doi:10.1097/DSS.0000000000000750.

122. Fabbrocini G, De Vita V, Pastore F, et al. Collagen induction therapy for the treatment of upper lip wrinkles. *J Dermatolog Treat*. 2012;23:144-152. doi:10.3109/09546634.2010.544709.

123. El-Domyati M, Barakat M, Awad S, Medhat W, El-Fakahany H, Farag H. Multiple microneedling sessions for minimally invasive facial rejuvenation: an objective assessment. *Int J Dermatol*. 2015;54:1361-1369. doi:10.1111/ijd.12761.

124. Fabbrocini G, De Vita V, Di Costanzo L, et al. Skin needling in the treatment of the aging neck. *Skinmed*. 2011;9(6):347-351.

125. Lima Ede A. Microneedling in facial recalcitrant melasma: report of a series of 22 cases. *An Bras Dermatol*. 2015;90(6):919-921. doi:10.1590/abd1806-4841.20154748.

126. Fabbrocini G, De Vita V, Fardella N, et al. Skin needling to enhance depigmenting serum penetration in the treatment of melasma. *Plast Surg Int*. 2011;2011(6):158241. doi:10.1155/2011/158241.

127. Budamakuntla L, Loganathan E, Suresh D, et al. A randomised, open-label, comparative study of tranexamic acid microinjections and tranexamic acid with microneedling in patients with melasma. *J Cutan Aesthet Surg*. 2013;6(3):139-143. doi:10.4103/0974-2077.118403.

128. Dhurat R, Sukesh M, Avhad G, Dandale A, Pal A, Pund P. A randomized evaluator blinded study of effect of microneedling in androgenetic alopecia: a pilot study. *Int J Trichology*. 2013;5(1):6-11. doi:10.4103/0974-7753.114700.

129. Dhurat R, Mathapati S. Response to microneedling treatment in men with androgenetic alopecia who failed to respond to conventional therapy. *Indian J Dermatol*. 2015;60(3):260-263. doi:10.4103/0019-5154.156361.

130. Lee YB, Eun YS, Lee JH, et al. Effects of topical application of growth factors followed by microneedle therapy in women with female pattern hair loss: a pilot study. *J Dermatol.* 2013;40(1):81-83. doi:10.1111/j.1346-8138.2012.01680.x.

131. Mysore V, Chandrashekar B, Yepuri V. Alopecia areata – successful outcome with microneedling and triamcinolone acetonide. *J Cutan Aesthet Surg.* 2014;7(1):63-64. doi:10.4103/0974-2077.129989.

132. Harris AG, Murrell DF. Combining microneedling and triamcinolone-a novel way to increase the tolerability of intralesional corticosteroid delivery in children with alopecia areata. *Australas J Dermatol.* 2015;56:40-41. doi:10.1111/ajd.12337.

133. Hou A, Cohen B, Haimovic A, Elbuluk N. Microneedling: a comprehensive review. *Dermatol Surg.* 2017;43:321-339. doi:10.1097/DSS.0000000000000924.

134. Pahwa M, Pahwa P, Zaheer A. "Tram track effect" after treatment of acne scars using a microneedling device. *Dermatol Surg.* 2012;38:1107-1108. doi:10.1111/j.1524-4725.2012.02441.x.

135. Soltani-Arabshahi R, Wong JW, Duffy KL, Powell DL. Facial allergic granulomatous reaction and systemic hypersensitivity associated with microneedle therapy for skin rejuvenation. *JAMA Dermatol.* 2014;150:68-72. doi:10.1001/jamadermatol.2013.6955.

136. Howard J. *"Vampire facial" may have exposed spa clients to HIV, New Mexico health officials say.* 2018. Cable News Network (CNN). https://www.cnn.com/2019/04/30/health/vampire-facial-hiv-cases-new-mexico-bn/index.html. Accessed July 16, 2019.

137. Alves R, Grimalt R. A review of platelet-rich plasma: history, biology, mechanism of action, and classification. *Skin Appendage Disord.* 2018;4(1):18-24. doi:10.1159/000477353.

138. Crutchfield CE III, Shah N. *PRP: What Dermatologists Should Know.* 2018. https://practicaldermatology.com/articles/2018-oct/prp-what-dermatologists-should-know. Accessed November 25, 2019.

139. Garg S, Manchanda S. Platelet-rich plasma – an 'Elixir' for treatment of alopecia: personal experience on 117 patients with review of literature. *Stem Cell Investig.* 2017;4:64. doi:10.21037/sci.2017.06.07.

140. Cavallo C, Roffi A, Grigolo B, et al. Platelet-rich plasma: the choice of activation method affects the release of bioactive molecules. *Biomed Res Int.* 2016;2016:6591717. doi:10.1155/2016/6591717.

141. Hesseler MJ, Shyam N. Platelet-rich plasma and its utility in medical dermatology: a systematic review. *J Am Acad Dermatol.* 2019;81(3):834-846. doi:10.1016/j.jaad.2019.04.037.

142. Dhurat R, Sukesh M. Principles and methods of preparation of platelet-rich plasma: a review and author's perspective. *J Cutan Aesthet Surg.* 2014;7:189-197. doi:10.4103/0974-2077.150734.

143. Nagata MJH, Messora MR, Furlaneto FAC, et al. Effectiveness of two methods for preparation of autologous plateletrich plasma: an experimental study in rabbits. *Eur J Dent.* 2010;4(4):395-402. doi:10.1055/s-0039-1697859.

144. Giusti I, Rughetti A, D'Ascenzo S, et al. Identification of an optimal concentration of platelet gel for promoting angiogenesis in human endothelial cells. *Transfusion.* 2009;49(4):771-778. doi:10.1111/j.1537-2995.2008.02033.x.

145. Graziani F, Ivanovski S, Cei S, Ducci F, Tonetti M, Gabriele M. The in vitro effect of different PRP concentrations on osteoblasts and fibroblasts. *Clin Oral Implants Res.* 2006;17(2):212-219. doi:10.1111/j.1600-0501.2005.01203.x.

146. Everts PAM, Knape JTA, Weibrich G, et al. Platelet-rich plasma and platelet gel: a review. *J Extra Corpor Technol.* 2006;38(2):174-187. Available at http://www.ncbi.nlm.nih.gov/pubmed/16921694.

147. Takikawa M, Nakamura S, Nakamura S, et al. Enhanced effect of platelet-rich plasma containing a new carrier on hair growth. *Dermatol Surg.* 2011;37(12):1721-1729. doi:10.1111/j.1524-4725.2011.02123.x.

148. Gupta AK, Versteeg SG, Rapaport J, Hausauer AK, Shear NH, Piguet V. The efficacy of platelet-rich plasma in the field of hair restoration and facial aesthetics – a systematic review and meta-analysis. *J Cutan Med Surg.* 2019;23(2):185-203. doi:10.1177/1203475418818073.

149. Delong JM, Russell RP, Mazzocca AD. Platelet-rich plasma: the PAW classification system. *Arthroscopy.* 2012;28:998-1009. doi:10.1016/j.arthro.2012.04.148.

150. Rose P. Hair restoration surgery: challenges and solutions. *Clin Cosmet Investig Dermatol.* 2015;8:361-370. doi:10.2147/CCID.S53980.

151. Zhang L, Zhang B, Liao B, et al. Platelet-rich plasma in combination with adipose-derived stem cells promotes skin wound healing through activating Rho GTpase-mediated signaling pathway. *Am J Transl Res.* 2019;11:4100-4112.

152. Tobita M, Tajima S, Mizuno H. Adipose tissue-derived mesenchymal stem cells and platelet-rich plasma: stem cell transplantation methods that enhance stemness. *Stem Cel Res Ther.* 2015;6(1):215. doi:10.1186/s13287-015-0217-8.

153. Gentile P, Scioli MG, Bielli A, et al. Platelet-rich plasma and micrografts enriched with autologous human follicle mesenchymal stem cells improve hair re-growth in androgenetic alopecia. Biomolecular pathway analysis and clinical evaluation. *Biomedicines.* 2019;7(2):27. doi:10.3390/biomedicines7020027.

154. New Mexico Department of Health. *Free Testing for Persons Who Received Any Injections.* Available at https://nmhealth.org/news/alert/2019/4/?view=762. Accessed November 25, 2019.

155. Kalyam K, Kavoussi SC, Ehrlich M, et al. Irreversible blindness following periocular autologous platelet-rich plasma skin rejuvenation treatment. *Ophthal Plast Reconstr Surg.* 2017;33:S12-S16. doi:10.1097/IOP.0000000000000680.

156. Alves R, Grimalt R. Randomized placebo-controlled, double-blind, half-head study to assess the efficacy of platelet-rich plasma on the treatment of androgenetic alopecia. *Dermatol Surg.* 2016;42:491-497. doi:10.1097/DSS.0000000000000665.

157. Gentile P, Garcovich S, Bielli A, Scioli MG, Orlandi A, Cervelli V. The effect of platelet-rich plasma in hair regrowth: a randomized placebo-controlled trial. *Stem Cell Transl Med.* 2015;4(11):1317-1323. doi:10.5966/sctm.2015-0107.

158. Gkini M-A, Kouskoukis A-E, Tripsianis G, Rigopoulos D, Kouskoukis K. Study of platelet-rich plasma injections in the treatment of androgenetic alopecia through an one-year period. *J Cutan Aesthet Surg.* 2014;7(4):213-219. doi:10.4103/0974-2077.150743.

159. Hausauer AK, Jones DH. Evaluating the efficacy of different platelet-rich plasma regimens for management of androgenetic alopecia. *Dermatol Surg.* 2018;44(9):1191-1200. doi:10.1097/DSS.0000000000001567.

160. Rodrigues BL, Montalvão SAL, Cancela RBB, et al. Treatment of male pattern alopecia with platelet-rich plasma: a double-blind controlled study with analysis of platelet number and growth factor levels. *J Am Acad Dermatol.* 2019;80(3):694-700. doi:10.1016/j.jaad.2018.09.033.

161. Schiavone G, Raskovic D, Greco J, Abeni D. Platelet-rich plasma for androgenetic alopecia. *Dermatol Surg.* 2014;40(9):1010-1019. doi:10.1097/01.DSS.0000452629.76339.2b.

162. Starace M, Alessandrini A, D'Acunto C, et al. Platelet-rich plasma on female androgenetic alopecia: tested on 10 patients. *J Cosmet Dermatol.* 2019;18(1):59-64. doi:10.1111/jocd.12550.

163. Gupta AK, Carviel J. A mechanistic model of platelet-rich plasma treatment for androgenetic alopecia. *Dermatol Surg.* 2016;42(12):1335-1339. doi:10.1097/DSS.0000000000000901.

164. Li ZJ, Choi H-I, Choi D-K, et al. Autologous platelet-rich plasma: a potential therapeutic tool for promoting hair growth. *Dermatol Surg.* 2012;38(7 pt 1):1040-1046. doi:10.1111/j.1524-4725.2012.02394.x.

165. Lotti T, Goren A, Verner I, D'Alessio PA, Franca K. Platelet rich plasma in androgenetic alopecia: a systematic review. *Dermatol Ther.* 2019;32(3):e12837. doi:10.1111/dth.12837.

166. Mapar MA, Shahriari S, Haghighizadeh MH. Efficacy of platelet-rich plasma in the treatment of androgenetic (male-patterned) alopecia: a pilot randomized controlled trial. *J Cosmet Laser Ther.* 2016;18(8):452-455. doi:10.1080/1476417 2.2016.1225963.

167. Gentile P, Cole J, Cole M, et al. Evaluation of not-activated and activated PRP in hair loss treatment: role of growth factor and cytokine concentrations obtained by different collection systems. *Int J Mol Sci.* 2017;18(2):408. doi:10.3390/ijms18020408.

168. Xing L, Dai Z, Jabbari A, et al. Alopecia areata is driven by cytotoxic T lymphocytes and is reversed by JAK inhibition. *Nat Med.* 2014;20(9):1043-1049. doi:10.1038/nm.3645.

169. Marchitto MC, Qureshi A, Marks D, Awosika O, Rengifo-Pardo M, Ehrlich A. Emerging nonsteroid-based procedural therapies for alopecia areata. *Dermatol Surg.* 2019;45(12):1484-1506. doi:10.1097/DSS.0000000000002053.

170. Khademi F, Tehranchinia Z, Abdollahimajd F, Younespour S, Kazemi-Bajestani SMR, Taheri K. The effect of platelet rich plasma on hair re-growth in patients with alopecia areata totalis: a clinical pilot study. *Dermatol Ther.* 2019;32:e12989. doi:10.1111/dth.12989.

171. Hunt N, McHale S. The psychological impact of alopecia. *BMJ.* 2005;331(7522):951-953. doi:10.1136/bmj.331.7522.951.

172. Bolanča Ž, Goren A, Getaldić-Švarc B, Vučić M, Šitum M. Platelet-rich plasma as a novel treatment for lichen planopilaris. *Dermatol Ther.* 2016;29(4):233-235. doi:10.1111/dth.12343.

173. Jha AK. Platelet-rich plasma for the treatment of lichen planopilaris. *J Am Acad Dermatol.* 2018;79(5):e95-e96. doi:10.1016/j.jaad.2018.05.029.

174. Jha AK. Platelet-rich plasma as an adjunctive treatment in lichen planopilaris. *J Am Acad Dermatol.* 2019;80(5):e109-e110. doi:10.1016/j.jaad.2018.09.013.

175. Dina Y, Aguh C. Use of platelet-rich plasma in cicatricial alopecia. *Dermatol Surg.* 2019;45(7):979-981. doi:10.1097/DSS.0000000000001635.

176. Özcan D, Tunçer Vural A, Özen Ö. Platelet-rich plasma for treatment resistant frontal fibrosing alopecia: a case report. *Dermatol Ther.* 2019;32(5). doi:10.1111/dth.13072.

177. Alam M, Hughart R, Champlain A, et al. Effect of platelet-rich plasma injection for rejuvenation of photoaged facial skin. *JAMA Dermatol.* 2018;154(12):1447. doi:10.1001/jamadermatol.2018.3977.

178. Redaelli A, Romano D, Marcianó A. Face and neck revitalization with platelet-rich plasma (PRP): clinical outcome in a series of 23 consecutively treated patients. *J Drugs Dermatol.* 2010;9(5):466-472.

179. Elghblawi E. Platelet-rich plasma, the ultimate secret for youthful skin elixir and hair growth triggering. *J Cosmet Dermatol.* 2018;17:423-430. doi:10.1111/jocd.12404.

180. Elnehrawy NY, Ibrahim ZA, Eltoukhy AM, Nagy HM. Assessment of the efficacy and safety of single platelet-rich plasma injection on different types and grades of facial wrinkles. *J Cosmet Dermatol.* 2017;16(1):103-111. doi:10.1111/jocd.12258.

181. Willemsen JCN, van der Lei B, Vermeulen KM, Stevens HPJD. The effects of platelet-rich plasma on recovery time and aesthetic outcome in facial rejuvenation: preliminary retrospective observations. *Aesthet Plast Surg.* 2014;38(5):1057-1063. doi:10.1007/s00266-014-0361-z.

182. Yuksel EP, Sahin G, Aydin F, Senturk N, Turanli AY. Evaluation of effects of platelet-rich plasma on human facial skin. *J Cosmet Laser Ther.* 2014;16(5):206-208. doi:10.3109/14764172.2014.949274.

183. Shin M-K, Lee J-H, Lee S-J, Kim N-I. Platelet-rich plasma combined with fractional laser therapy for skin rejuvenation. *Dermatol Surg.* 2012;38(4):623-630. doi:10.1111/j.1524-4725.2011.02280.x.

184. Hersant B, SidAhmed-Mezi M, Niddam J, et al. Efficacy of autologous platelet-rich plasma combined with hyaluronic acid on skin facial rejuvenation: a prospective study. *J Am Acad Dermatol.* 2017;77(3):584-586. doi:10.1016/j.jaad.2017.05.022.

185. Deshmukh NS, Belgaumkar VA. Platelet-rich plasma augments subcision in atrophic acne scars. *Dermatol Surg.* 2019;45(1):90-98. doi:10.1097/DSS.0000000000001614.

186. Nofal E, Helmy A, Nofal A, Alakad R, Nasr M. Platelet-rich plasma versus CROSS technique with 100% trichloroacetic acid versus combined skin needling and platelet rich plasma in the treatment of atrophic acne scars: a comparative study. *Dermatol Surg.* 2014;40(8):864-873. doi:10.1111/dsu.0000000000000091.

187. Cervelli V, Nicoli F, Spallone D, et al. Treatment of traumatic scars using fat grafts mixed with platelet-rich plasma, and resurfacing of skin with the 1540 nm nonablative laser. *Clin Exp Dermatol.* 2012;37(1):55-61. doi:10.1111/j.1365-2230.2011.04199.x.

188. Lee JW, Kim BJ, Kim MN, Mun SK. The efficacy of autologous platelet rich plasma combined with ablative carbon dioxide fractional resurfacing for acne scars: a simultaneous split-face trial. *Dermatol Surg.* 2011;37(7):931-938. doi:10.1111/j.1524-4725.2011.01999.x.

189. del Pino-Sedeño T, Trujillo-Martín MM, Andia I, et al. Platelet-rich plasma for the treatment of diabetic foot ulcers: a meta-analysis. *Wound Repair Regen.* 2018;27:170-182. doi:10.1111/wrr.12690.

190. Garg S, Dosapaty N, Arora AK. Laser ablation of the recipient area with platelet-rich plasma – enriched epidermal suspension transplant in vitiligo surgery. *Dermatol Surg.* 2019;45(1):83-89. doi:10.1097/DSS.0000000000001641.

191. Ibrahim ZA, El-Ashmawy AA, El-Tatawy RA, Sallam FA. The effect of platelet-rich plasma on the outcome of short-term narrowband-ultraviolet B phototherapy in the treatment of vitiligo: a pilot study. *J Cosmet Dermatol.* 2016;15(2):108-116. doi:10.1111/jocd.12194.

192. Westerhof W. Treatment of vitiligo with UV-B radiation vs topical psoralen plus UV-A. *Arch Dermatol.* 1997;133(12):1525-1528. doi:10.1001/archderm.1997.03890480045006.

11

Minimally Invasive Aesthetic Surgical Procedures

Christopher J. Rizzi, MD, and John J. Chi, MD, MPHS

Chapter Highlights

- Although the popularity of minimally invasive aesthetics continues to rise, dramatic improvement in appearance at times requires a more invasive, surgical approach.
- Blepharoplasty, facelift, and neck lift are surgical procedures that can offer more noticeable rejuvenation than noninvasive techniques.
- Thread lifts are gaining in popularity and are an alternative to open surgical procedures to address the aging face and neck.

Facial rejuvenation can be achieved with nonsurgical, noninvasive modalities with astounding results; however, patients with more advanced signs of aging will see limited results from those interventions. For better or for worse, these patients require surgical intervention. It is important for the aesthetic facial surgeon to be competent in multiple surgical techniques to treat the aging face. Surgical treatment of the aging face can result in dramatic postoperative results, but also require more investment from the patient and the provider—time, effort, costs, and risks. Adoption of these surgical techniques into practice requires a thorough knowledge of the underlying anatomy and technical maneuvers specific to each modality of treatment. This chapter will succinctly discuss several important procedures for the aesthetic facial surgeon—blepharoplasty, facelift, neck rejuvenation, and thread lift.

▶ BLEPHAROPLASTY

The importance of addressing the periorbital region in the aging face cannot be understated. The eyelid and brow complex often show the earliest signs of aging, and the appearance of this region can distract from the benefits of other aesthetic interventions of the face.[1] To this end, it is imperative for the aesthetic physician to be competent in the evaluation and treatment of the periorbital region. Blepharoplasty is an excellent method to address excess skin laxity and eyelid fullness and to redefine the eyelid crease. Both upper and lower lid blepharoplasty have the ability to create dramatic improvements in the appearance of the periorbital area and midface.[1] The technique and anatomy of upper eyelid blepharoplasty are relatively straightforward with minimal variability. In contrast, lower eyelid blepharoplasty anatomy, technique, and possible complications require a much more thorough understanding and experience. Only upper eyelid blepharoplasty will be discussed in this chapter. With the appropriate preoperative evaluation, attention to detail, and operative technique, dramatic results can be achieved with minimal risk.

Preoperative Evaluation

In order to maximize aesthetic results and minimize postprocedural complications, a thorough preoperative evaluation of blepharoplasty candidates is imperative. Not only do these patients need to be assessed for candidacy for the surgical procedure, attention must be paid to the risk of potential complications related to the health of the eye. Patients at risk for postoperative dry eye, lagophthalmos, and ptosis can be identified preoperatively and counseled accordingly.[2] It is also important to understand the eyes in the greater context of the brow-eyelid complex.[3] Addressing redundant upper eyelid skin without addressing eyebrow ptosis can lead to unhappy patients and need for revision procedures. A ptotic eyebrow should always be corrected prior to the upper eyelid as correcting the brow ptosis will have an impact on the upper eyelid. Some providers elect to perform these procedures in the same setting, while others will perform a brow lift followed by a staged upper eyelid blepharoplasty.[4]

Candidates for upper eyelid surgery will commonly present with excess upper eyelid skin and upper lid fullness and complain about the appearance of fatigue. Thinning and redundancy of the upper eyelid skin commonly occur with age. Laxity of the orbital septum with fat herniation and hypertrophy of the orbicularis oculi muscle often leads to fullness of the upper lid. As with any other cosmetic procedure, it is important to understand the patient's motivation for surgery in order to adequately address their specific concerns. An ophthalmologic history should also be taken, specifically regarding symptoms of dry eye, other ocular complaints, and prior procedures. If concerns arise, formal ophthalmologic evaluation will be necessary.

Physical Examination

The examination must not only concentrate on the underlying pathology, but also assess the patient's risk for postoperative complication or poor aesthetic outcome. The periorbital region must also be evaluated in the greater context of facial rejuvenation. Upper eyelid dermatochalasis (excess upper eyelid skin) is present to a varying degree in the majority of older patients. This must be distinguished clinically from blepharochalasis. This is a recurrent inflammatory pathology of the eyelid resulting in recurrent edema and fullness of the upper lid. Blepharochalasis leads to stretching, thinning, and redundancy of the upper eyelid tissue through a different mechanism. Although patients with both of these pathologies can benefit from upper blepharoplasty, a thorough history and examination is necessary to distinguish between the two etiologies. During evaluation of the upper eyelid, the presence of excess upper eyelid skin, orbicularis hypertrophy, and pseudoherniated orbital fat should be assessed. With thinning of the orbital septum, pseudoherniation of the medial and central fat compartments commonly leads to upper lid fullness and must be addressed for the optimal outcome. The locations of upper eyelid fullness should be documented at the preoperative visit and any asymmetry noted.

To avoid postoperative complications, attention must be paid to the function of the eye. A general ophthalmologic examination is indicated, specifically if the patient has any complaints related to the eye.[5] Unrecognized upper eyelid ptosis can lead to poor functional outcomes, need for revision surgery, and worsening of ptosis. Secondary signs of ptosis may include a hyperfunctioning frontalis muscle on the affected side. The patient should be asked to close the eyes and gently open without aggressively raising the eyebrow to reveal compensated ptosis. If ptosis is present, the patient should be referred to an oculoplastic surgeon prior to performing upper lid blepharoplasty. Although this may result in loss of the patient referral, postblepharoplasty ptosis is a feared complication of upper blepharoplasty and can be difficult to correct.[4] If there is clinical concern, dry eye and visual field testing may be indicated. The Schirmer test is commonly used to assess for dry eyes. The patient may also be referred for formal visual field testing prior to upper blepharoplasty if required. This is usually required prior to insurance approval for functional blepharoplasty.

Appropriate photographic documentation is essential in the evaluation of all cosmetic surgery patients and blepharoplasty is no different. Preoperative and postoperative photographs should include the five standard views depicted in Figure 11.1. In addition, close-up frontal and lateral views of the eyes should be taken with the eyes in primary gaze, squinting, looking up, and closed.[6]

Anatomy

Thorough understanding of the anatomy of the upper eyelid is crucial to performing effective blepharoplasty. Adequate knowledge of the underlying anatomy is necessary both to

FIGURE 11.1   **Standard photo array for a patient undergoing facial rejuvenation. (A) Right lateral, (B) right oblique, (C) frontal, (D) left oblique, and (E) left lateral views.**

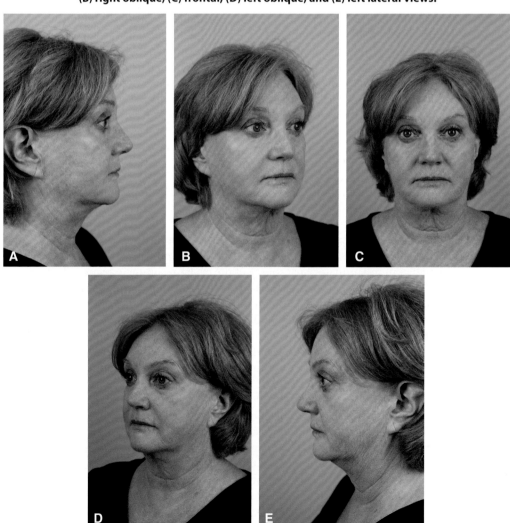

FIGURE 11.2   Eyelid anatomy. Sagittal section through the eyelid depicting the lamellar anatomy. Note that dissection through the supratarsal upper lid will proceed through the skin, orbicularis, orbital septum, and into the orbital fat. The orbital fat overlies the levator aponeurosis and Muller muscle, which should not be disturbed during upper blepharoplasty.

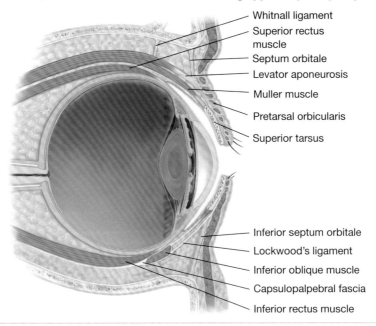

Whitnall ligament
Superior rectus muscle
Septum orbitale
Levator aponeurosis
Muller muscle
Pretarsal orbicularis
Superior tarsus

Inferior septum orbitale
Lockwood's ligament
Inferior oblique muscle
Capsulopalpebral fascia
Inferior rectus muscle

(Reprinted with permission from Chung KC, van Aalst J, Mehrara B, et al. *Flaps in Plastic and Reconstructive Surgery.* 1st ed. Philadelphia, PA: Wolters Kluwer; 2019.)

determine which patients would benefit from operative intervention and to formulate a comprehensive surgical plan. The anatomic layers of the eyelids are depicted in Figure 11.2. The layers of the upper eyelid vary dependent on the location relative to the tarsal plate. Generally, all blepharoplasty incision and dissection are performed superior to this important landmark. The layers of the upper lid in this region include the skin, orbicularis oculi muscle, levator aponeurosis, and Muller muscle. Above the levator aponeurosis, the orbital septum and orbital fat compartments lie deep to the orbicularis oculi. The supratarsal crease, usually 8 to 10 mm above the lid margin, is an important surface landmark in blepharoplasty. This crease is created by the insertion of fibers from the levator aponeurosis into the skin. This is minimally present in the Asian eyelid and is generally recreated for westernization of the upper eyelid. Deep to the orbital septum in the upper eyelid lie the medial (nasal) and central fat pads and laterally lies the lacrimal gland (Figure 11.3). Fat within the central compartment often drapes over the medial fat compartment and therefore superior retraction of the central fat will permit visualization of the medial fat pad. In addition, the medial fat is typically paler in color than the yellow central fat.

Surgical Technique

Instrumentation

A general soft tissue instrumentation set with a #15 blade scalpel, curved tissue scissor, skin hook retractors, needle driver, and forceps will suffice for upper blepharoplasty. Many surgeons prefer to use the Westcott surgical scissors as these can provide more cutting accuracy and tactile feedback. A monopolar or bipolar electrocautery should also be available.

FIGURE 11.3   Orbital fat compartments. Orbital septum and preaponeurotic fat pads in a right-sided orbit.

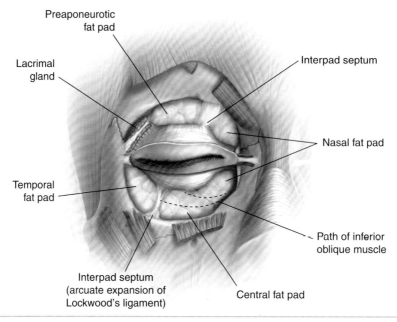

Preaponeurotic fat pad

Lacrimal gland

Interpad septum

Nasal fat pad

Temporal fat pad

Path of inferior oblique muscle

Interpad septum (arcuate expansion of Lockwood's ligament)

Central fat pad

(Reprinted with permission from Chung KC, Disa JJ, Gosain A, et al. *Operative Techniques in Plastic Surgery*. 1st ed. Philadelphia, PA: Wolters Kluwer; 2019.)

Anesthesia

Local anesthesia is typically sufficient for upper eyelid blepharoplasty although general anesthesia may be used depending on patient comfort or the need to perform concurrent procedures. Approximately 1 to 2 mL of lidocaine with epinephrine should be injected in the subcutaneous plane over both eyelids. If a corneal shield is utilized, topical tetracaine drops may be applied for patient comfort.

Incision Marking

Appropriate marking of the skin to be excised is a crucial part of the blepharoplasty procedure. Inadequate resection of upper lid skin can lead to suboptimal cosmetic result or need for revision procedures. Overaggressive skin excision can lead to significant morbidity including lagophthalmos, scleral show, and keratitis.[7] Marking should always be performed with the patient in the upright position and prior to the injection of a local anesthetic. The inferior incision should be placed at the level of the supratarsal crease, usually 8 to 10 mm above the lid margin at the mid-pupil. In Asian blepharoplasty, this incision is placed at the desired supratarsal crease. A pinch technique can then be performed to determine the amount of excess skin present. To do this, the excess skin is grasped with a smooth forceps and pulled to the point just prior to lid eversion. The superior incision and skin to be excised are then marked. This should be done at multiple points along the eyelid to determine the appropriate amount of skin excision. A general rule of thumb is that there should be 20 mm of skin present between the lid margin and the thicker eyebrow skin to avoid lagophthalmos. An elliptical skin excision is then marked utilizing the superior and inferior markings previously made. The incision should taper medially and not extend beyond the medial canthus to prevent

FIGURE 11.4   Upper blepharoplasty incision marking. Elliptical incision marking for standard upper blepharoplasty. The inferior incision is made along the supratarsal crease. The ellipse is tapered medially and does not extend beyond the medial canthus. The ellipse extends longer laterally and tapers at or just beyond the lateral orbital rim.

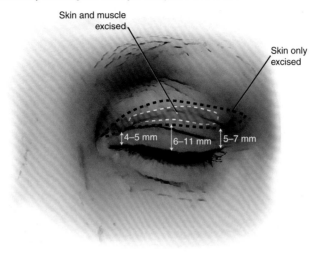

(Reprinted with permission from Larrabee WF Jr, Ridgway J, Patel S. *Master Techniques in Otolaryngology – Head and Neck Surgery: Facial Plastic Surgery.* 1st ed. Philadelphia, PA: Wolters Kluwer; 2017.)

webbing in this region. Laterally, the incision may extend to the lateral orbital rim and may curve slightly upward into a skin crease if required for excision of standing cone deformity. The markings should be evaluated for symmetry. An example of appropriate skin marking is depicted in Figure 11.4.

Procedure

After appropriate skin marking has been confirmed, a local anesthetic is injected and the skin incisions are made. Incision is made through the skin only, preserving the underlying orbicularis. Resection of the orbicularis oculi may lead to orbital hollowing in some patients and consideration should always be given to preserving it. Starting laterally, the skin is dissected from the underlying orbicularis muscle and removed. At this point, a strip of orbicularis muscle may be removed within the middle of the skin excision if indicated to reduce upper eyelid fullness. Hemostasis is achieved with a cautery. If only skin excision is to be performed, closure is performed at this time (Figure 11.5).

If it has been determined that the patient requires fat excision, the orbital septum is identified and incised medially. This incision can be extended laterally over the central portion of the eyelid. The central fat is then readily identified and can be debulked, if indicated. Conservative removal of central fat will reduce the risk of postoperative A-frame deformity and hollowed upper eyelids.[8] Gentle pressure may be applied to the globe to visualize redundant fat. Prior to removal of fat, a local anesthetic should be injected directly into the fat and an electrocautery is used for hemostasis. Retracting the central fat pad superiorly and laterally will reveal the pale colored medial fat. Again, gentle pressure is placed on the globe and the medial fat is cauterized and excised. Single layer closure is then typically performed with a 6-0 prolene suture in a running fashion. Care must be taken to perform a meticulous closure both medially and laterally to prevent medial webbing and standing cone deformity, respectively. To avoid lateral standing cone deformity,

FIGURE 11.5   Intraoperative blepharoplasty. (A) Preoperative excision marking, (B) after skin excision with excised skin pictured above, and (C) after skin closure.

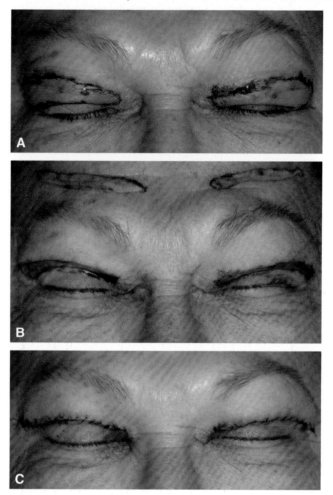

many surgeons close the lateral angle of the incision first—as the aesthetics of the central portion of the incision can accommodate mild to moderate skin redundancy. An ophthalmic antibiotic ointment is then applied to the incision. Pre- and postoperative photos are depicted in Figure 11.6.

Postoperative Care

The patient may be discharged after the procedure. Cold compress application during the first 24 hours is essential to reduce swelling and ecchymosis. An ophthalmic antibiotic ointment should be applied to the incisions three to four times daily to reduce the risk of infection. Pain should be controlled with acetaminophen and a low dose narcotic may be required. NSAIDs should be avoided for 7 days postoperatively. Physical exercise should be avoided for at least 10 days. Prolene sutures should be removed in approximately 5 days. At the time of suture removal, close attention should be paid to the incision as partial dehiscence is not uncommon. A steri-strip may be placed over the lateral portion of the incision after suture removal to provide additional support for 24 to 48 hours after suture removal.

FIGURE 11.6 **Preoperative and postoperative blepharoplasty. Both patients underwent upper blepharoplasty. (A and C) Preoperative photographs. (B and D) Postoperative results. Note the improvement in lateral hooding and tarsal platform show.**

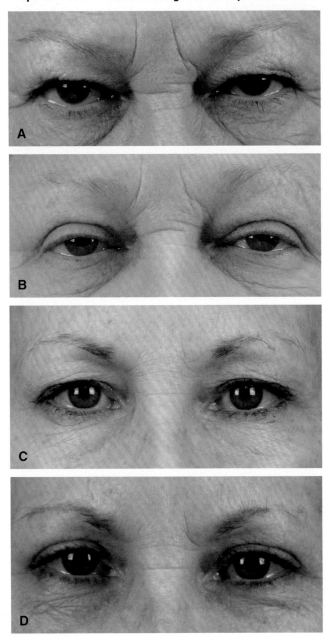

Complications

Most complications can be prevented by appropriate preoperative evaluation, surgical marking, and intraoperative hemostasis. Incisional erythema, sensation of tightness of the upper lid, tearing, and mild lagophthalmos are usually self-resolving. Hematoma is rare following upper lid blepharoplasty but may be heralded by increasing pain and swelling immediately postprocedure (Figure 11.7). Temporary lagophthalmos is not

FIGURE 11.7   **Postblepharoplasty hematoma. Preseptal hematoma following both upper and lower blepharoplasty.**

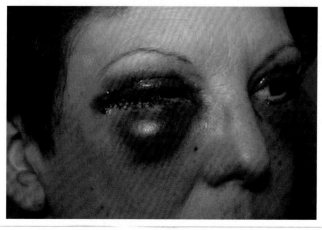

(Reprinted with permission from Rosen CA, Johnson JT. *Bailey's Head and Neck Surgery – Otolaryngology Review.* 1st ed. Philadelphia, PA: Wolters Kluwer; 2014.)

uncommon after blepharoplasty and should be treated with lubricating eye drops and eye taping. Referral to an ophthalmologist may be required if the patient becomes increasingly symptomatic and persistent lagophthalmos may require secondary skin grafting.[9] Blindness after upper lid blepharoplasty is rare and is generally secondary to unrecognized hematoma.[10] Overaggressive fat resection, specifically in the central compartment, may lead to an A-frame hollowing within the central eyelid. This is a difficult problem to correct and may require revision surgery, fat or filler injection.

▶ FACELIFT

Rejuvenation of the midface and lower face may be accomplished with both noninvasive techniques and surgical approaches. Since the first facelifts were performed in the early 1900s, our understanding of anatomy and surgical technique has evolved. Early techniques involved dissection and resuspension of the facial skin only. This limited approach led to an unnatural operated appearance and a rapid recurrence of facial ptosis. Lambros simply stated, "A young face is not an old face with tight cheek skin."[11] The major breakthrough in facelift understanding occurred in the 1970s when the superficial musculoaponeurotic system (SMAS) was described by Mitz and Peyronie in 1976.[12] Since this anatomic tissue structure was described, facelift techniques have concentrated on its dissection and suspension. With this evolution, contemporary facelift surgery is able to produce a natural appearing, long-lasting, dramatic result in appropriately selected patients. Many different techniques have been developed and further added to the mystique and confusion surrounding facelift surgery.[13] It is important to realize that effective results can be achieved with multiple different facelift techniques and philosophies. For the developing aesthetic surgeon, the specific facelift technique performed is not as important as possessing a thorough understanding of anatomy, a strict attention to detail, and appropriate patient selection.

Patient Evaluation

As with all cosmetic surgery patients, it is important to understand and appropriately address the patient's specific cosmetic concerns. Many patients requesting a facelift may be better suited for nonsurgical treatment with injectable fillers or neuromodulators. In contrast, other patients may have significant signs of facial aging that requires a more aggressive open surgical approach to achieve a reasonable aesthetic result. It is important to understand the patient's specific goals and risk tolerance. In contrast to many minimally invasive techniques, facelift patients can expect significant downtime and the risk of serious complications should be discussed.

A thorough medical history should be taken for each patient including previous interventions, medical comorbidities that may put them at higher risk of complication, and any medications that could result in higher risk of bleeding. Patients with medical conditions, which may affect wound healing should be counseled as such, although surgery may still be performed. Smoking puts patients at high risk of healing issues and skin flap necrosis. Most surgeons will not perform facelift in currently smoking patients and will require that the patient abstain from all nicotine products in the perioperative period.[14]

Physical examination should involve evaluation of the patient's general facial appearance and skin quality. Specific attention should be paid to the jowl and prejowl area, as this area can be dramatically improved with most facelift techniques. The neck should also be examined to determine whether the patient would benefit from concurrent submentoplasty or direct neck lift. The midfacial soft tissues are difficult to address with the facelift techniques described in this chapter and the patient should be counseled as such. Ideal facelift candidates have well-projected bony anatomy and adequate skin elasticity. Specifically, patients with prominent cheekbones and an appropriately projected chin are likely to see the best results. Those patients without adequate bony anatomy may be candidates for augmentation with silicone malar or chin implants. It is important to recognize these patients preoperatively, as outcomes from soft tissue repositioning alone can be suboptimal.

Anatomy

Understanding the tissue planes of the face is imperative to perform a safe and effective facelift. The layers of the face in the region of the parotid gland include the skin, subcutaneous fat, SMAS, parotid fascia, and parotid gland. Anterior to the parotid gland, the masseter muscle underlies the SMAS. Deep to the masseter lies the periosteum and bone. Traversing through these layers and attaching the periosteum directly to the skin are the facial retaining ligaments. These include the orbicularis, zygomatic, and mandibular retaining ligaments.[15] Release of these ligaments in the sub-SMAS plane leads to an increase in the amount of lift achieved. These layers are depicted in Figure 11.8.

The motor nerves of the face are all deep to the SMAS plane. These travel within the parotid gland posteriorly, and on top of the masseter muscle anterior to the parotid gland. The temporal and marginal mandibular branches are at greatest risk for injury as these nerves exit the parotid gland more posteriorly and do not have as many redundant branches. Both nerves are found deep to the SMAS throughout their course. The temporal branch traverses over the zygomatic arch approximately 1.5 to 2.0 cm preauricular and is just deep to the SMAS. The location of the nerve can also be approximated by Pitanguy line. This is a line drawn starting 5 mm inferior to the tragus and extending superiorly to a point 1.5 cm superior to the lateral extent of the eyebrow.[16] With the conservative sub-SMAS dissection techniques described in this chapter, these nerves should not be encountered. With more aggressive sub-SMAS dissection techniques, specifically the deep plane techniques, these nerves are at higher risk of injury and care must be taken to either identify or avoid these structures. The great auricular nerve is the most commonly injured nerve in facelift procedures.[17] This nerve provides sensation to the postauricular skin, auricle, and lobule. It lies in the immediate sub-SMAS plane, superficial to the sternocleidomastoid muscle in the postauricular region. Care must be taken when raising the posterior skin flap to avoid traumatizing this nerve.

FIGURE 11.8   Facial tissue planes. Soft tissue planes in the face. The facial nerve branches run immediately deep to the SMAS plane.

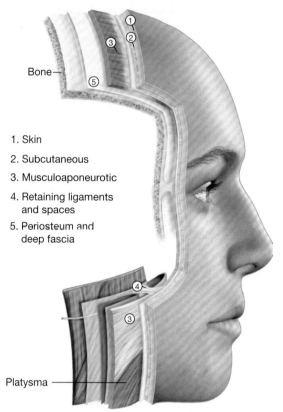

Bone

1. Skin
2. Subcutaneous
3. Musculoaponeurotic
4. Retaining ligaments and spaces
5. Periosteum and deep fascia

Platysma

(Reprinted with permission from Brown DL, Borschel GH, Levi B. *Michigan Manual of Plastic Surgery*. 2nd ed. Philadelphia, PA: Wolters Kluwer; 2014.)

Surgical Technique

Instrumentation

A standard soft tissue set can be utilized for performing facelift. The importance of a quality facelift scissor cannot be understated as this increases both efficiency and accuracy in dissecting the tissue planes. Lighted retractors or a headlight should be utilized to illuminate the surgical field as the facelift flaps are being elevated. Electrocautery and judicious hemostasis are essential to reduce the risk of postoperative hematoma and ecchymosis.

Anesthesia

Facelift can be performed with a combination of local anesthesia and IV sedation. The patient's cardiorespiratory status should be monitored throughout the procedure whenever sedation is used. Smaller less invasive "tuck-up" procedures can potentially be performed with oral sedation and local anesthesia in the awake patient. Given the large surgical area and length of the procedure, local anesthetic amounts must be recorded to avoid lidocaine toxicity. It is helpful to utilize anesthetic tumescent solution to hydrodissect, anesthetize, and vasoconstrict. Many surgeons prefer general anesthesia for patient comfort. This must be done without the use of muscle relaxant as the facial nerve activity must be visible intraoperatively.

Incision Marking

Many of the stigmata of facelift can be avoided by diligent incision marking. Specific attention should be paid to the temporal hair tuft, preauricular skin, and postauricular sulcus.[18,19] The anterior marking is made around the temporal hair tuft and extended posteriorly to the root of the helix. The anterior incision should then extend inferiorly within a preauricular skin crease. In female patients, a posttragal incision may be used to disguise the preauricular incision. In male patients with sideburns, a pretragal incision should be made to avoid transposing hair-bearing skin into the ear canal. The incision should then loop around the auricular lobule. It is helpful to leave 1 to 2 mm of skin between the lobular insertion and the incision to preserve the lobular attachment. The postauricular incision is then marked along the posterior portion of the auricle, above the postauricular sulcus. Therefore, with healing and scar contracture, the incision will lie within the sulcus. The incision is then extended posteriorly along the hairline (Figure 11.9).

Procedure

After surgical marking, a local anesthetic tumescent solution should be injected into the subcutaneous plane of the face throughout the region of planned dissection. Liberal injection in this area can serve to partially hydrodissect the subcutaneous plane and to distribute the vasoconstrictive agent throughout the operative field. The skin incision is then made in its entirety. The incision may be beveled at the posterior hairline to avoid injury to the hair follicles.

The skin flap is then raised in the subcutaneous plane. Starting posteriorly, a scalpel is used to enter the subcutaneous plane and begin raising the skin flap. With the aid of retraction, a facelift scissor can then be used to raise the skin flap off the underlying sternocleidomastoid muscle. The skin in the postauricular region is more densely adherent

FIGURE 11.9 **Common facelift incision variations. Variation may occur with relation to the temporal hair tuft, preauricular incision, and posterior hairline incision.**

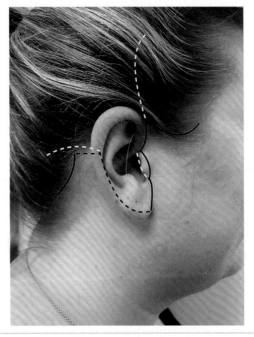

to the mastoid fascia and sharp dissection is generally required. The great auricular nerve may be visualized at this time and all dissection should be superficial to this structure. Dissection should proceed inferiorly and anteriorly within this plane to the attachment of the lobule. The anterior skin flap is then raised in a similar fashion. Adequate retraction and assistant countertraction are essential to performing this efficiently. The preauricular skin flap should be elevated anteriorly beyond a line joining the lateral canthus and mandibular angle. Inferiorly, this subcutaneous pocket is connected with the postauricular pocket previously dissected (Figure 11.10B). If a submental dissection has already been performed, dissection proceeds anteriorly to connect the submental and postauricular dissection pockets. Meticulous hemostasis should then be achieved with bipolar electrocautery. After the skin flap is fully raised, the underlying SMAS is visualized and can be manipulated. Multiple techniques exist for manipulation of the SMAS.[13]

Superficial Musculoaponeurotic System Imbrication/Plication

A simple but effective technique to elevate and lift the SMAS is plication or imbrication. SMAS plication is performed by grasping the anterior SMAS and lifting in a posterior-superior vector. The redundant SMAS is then folded upon itself and secured with multiple 3-0 permanent sutures, approximately 1 cm anterior to the tragus. A running suture can then be placed across the plication to avoid external contour deformities. This technique is beneficial as it does not involve incising the SMAS or risking branches of the facial nerve. SMAS imbrication involves excising the redundant portion of SMAS and suturing the opposing edges together in a similar fashion (Figure 11.10). This has also been termed a SMAS-ectomy with excision of the redundant SMAS and reapproximation of the cut edges. For an increased SMAS lift, a sub-SMAS dissection can be performed anterior to the SMAS incision. This provides greater mobility of the SMAS flap. Extensive anterior dissection of the SMAS can produce the most dramatic lift and is necessary to affect the nasolabial fold and medial face (Figure 11.11). This extended deep-plane lift puts the facial nerve branches at higher risk for injury and should only be performed by surgeons comfortable with this anatomy.

Purse-String Lift

The purse-string technique can also be utilized to lift the SMAS. The first purse-string technique was described by Saylan in 1999 with the advantages of a small preauricular incision and with the use of local anesthesia without sedation.[20] This involves the placement of two concentric purse-string sutures within the SMAS to provide lift. The sutures are first anchored to the periosteum of the posterior zygomatic arch. The first purse-string suture is then placed in a U-shaped pattern from the zygomatic arch inferiorly to grasp the upper platysma. The second purse-string suture is then placed through the zygomatic arch periosteum and multiple small bites of the SMAS and parotid fascia taken in an O-shape. This is then secured to provide the SMAS lift. Excess bunching of SMAS can be excised directly thereafter. Modifications to this technique were described by Brandy in 2004 to include a postauricular dissection and a more vertically oriented lift.[21] These modifications permitted a greater ability to address the jowl line and upper neck.

Minimal Access Cranial Suspension Lift

The short scar minimal access cranial suspension (MACS) lift was first described by Tonnard in 2007.[22] This lift involves a preauricular incision extending around the temporal hair tuft. A subcutaneous flap is then raised in a fashion similar to the other facelift techniques described. Three separate purse-string sutures are then placed. In contrast to the purse-string lift, these sutures are anchored to the deep temporal fascia instead of the zygomatic

FIGURE 11.10 **SMAS facelift. (A) Incision marking, (B) raising of the skin flap with marking of SMAS incision, (C) raising of the SMAS flap, (D) imbrication of redundant SMAS anteriorly, (E) posterior advancement of the redundant SMAS to the mastoid periosteum, (F) skin trimming, and (G) final incision closure with drain placement.**

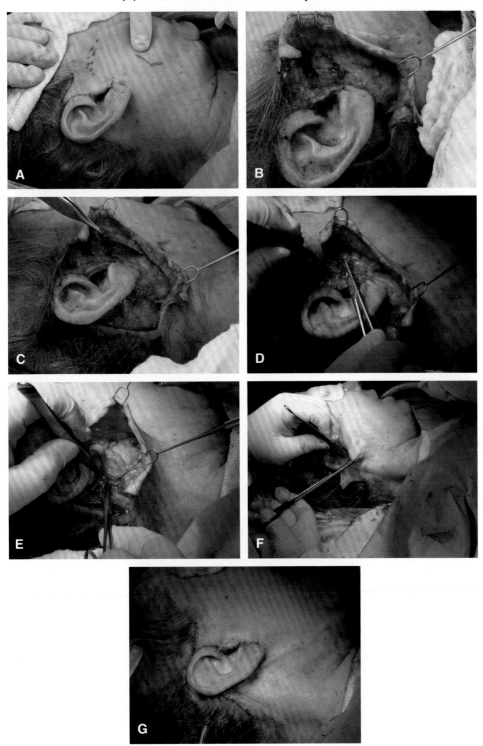

FIGURE 11.11   Preoperative and postoperative facelift. (A) Preoperative and (B) postoperative photos of a patient undergoing deep plane facelift with autologous fat injection to the malar fat pad. Note the improvement in volumization of the midface in addition to smoothing of the neck contour.

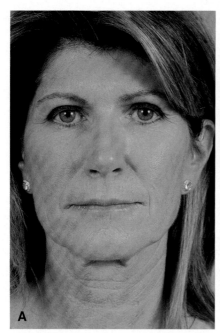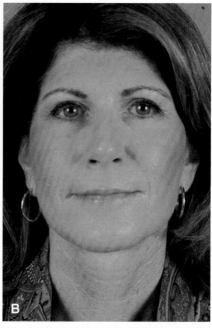

(Reprinted with permission from Chung KC, Thorne CH, Sinno S. *Operative Techniques in Facial Aesthetic Surgery.* 1st ed. Philadelphia, PA: Wolters Kluwer; 2020.)

arch. A U-shaped vertical suture is placed, followed by an O-shaped oblique suture. In addition to these two purse-string sutures, the MACS lift employs a third malar loop. This loop is anchored within the deep temporal fascia just lateral to the lateral orbital rim and serves to lift the malar fat pad. Skin redraping is then performed in a vertical vector to avoid the necessity of a postauricular incision. The MACS lift employs a more vertical vector than the standard purse string or SMAS techniques. Proponents of this lift argue that the vertical lift vector reduces the risk of stigmata of lateral sweep associated with other facelift techniques. This procedure can also be performed under local anesthesia with reduced recovery time and morbidity compared to other more aggressive facelift procedures.

Skin Closure

Irrespective of the SMAS technique utilized, meticulous skin trimming and closure is paramount to a good aesthetic outcome. After the SMAS has been secured, the skin should be laid down flat without tension for trimming. A scissor is used to make a cut in the redundant skin perpendicular to the original incision (Figure 11.10G). This can be done at multiple points and the skin is temporarily stapled. After the amount of redundant skin to be removed has been determined, the skin is trimmed and a multilayer closure is performed. A small suction drain may be placed in the wound bed but is not always required. It is imperative that the skin not be closed under tension. Rather, the skin should be laid down and not pulled tightly when excised. Undue skin tension can lead to widened scars and an operated appearance. A standing cone deformity may need to be excised at the temporal tuft. The incision can be extended anteriorly along the hairline for this purpose if required. Conservative skin excision with minimal tension is most important in the region of the lobule to avoid distortion of the earlobe. Care should be taken to match the preoperative appearance of the lobular attachment. Posteriorly, the hairline should realign to avoid obvious step-offs.

Dressing

A circumferential compressive head wrap may be placed after facelift. This reduces postoperative edema, ecchymosis, and the risk of hematoma. This should be replaced on the first postoperative day to examine for hematoma or other complications.

Complications

Hematoma is the most common complication, occurring in 1% to 15% of patients, and must be identified promptly (Figure 11.12A).[23,24] This may be heralded by increased pain in the postoperative period with concomitant fullness. Any asymmetric pain or swelling should be closely evaluated for hematoma. Meticulous intraoperative hemostasis is necessary but not always sufficient to prevent hematoma formation. The vast majority of acute hematomas can be treated with needle aspiration and pressure dressing but reoperation may be required.[25]

Unrecognized and untreated hematoma can lead to necrosis of the skin flap, resulting in delayed healing and poor scar appearance. Male gender, hypertension, smoking, and perioperative use of antiplatelet therapy have been associated with increased hematoma risk.[26] Perioperative blood pressure control is also vital to prevent this complication.[27]

FIGURE 11.12   Facelift complications. (A) Immediate postoperative facelift hematoma. (B) Postoperative pixie ear deformity with inferior displacement of the lobule and visible preauricular incision.

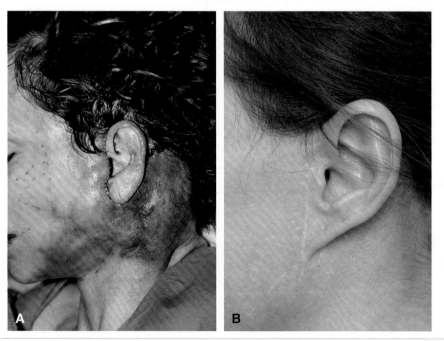

(Reprinted with permission from Larrabee WF Jr, Ridgway J, Patel S. *Master Techniques in Otolaryngology – Head and Neck Surgery: Facial Plastic Surgery.* 1st ed. Philadelphia, PA: Wolters Kluwer; 2017.)

Skin flap necrosis can result from hematoma, excessive tension on wound closure, raising the flap too thin, or other patient-related factors. Deep-plane techniques reduce the risk of skin flap necrosis as the SMAS is left attached to the skin flap distal to the SMAS incision. Smoking increases the risk of skin necrosis 12-fold and therefore patients should abstain from nicotine intake in the perioperative period. Some surgeons perform a urine cotinine test on the day of surgery preoperatively to ensure patient compliance. Skin necrosis is usually managed conservatively with wound care and healing is allowed to occur by secondary intention. Scar revision or resurfacing can be performed at a later time if required.

Avoiding the stigmata of facelift is an important consideration. Although these patients may achieve an improved overall appearance, an unnatural look is undesirable. Most of these stigmata can be avoided by appropriate incision marking and meticulous closure. Specific attention should be paid to elevation of the temporal hair tuft above the helical root as this appears unnatural and is indicative of facelift. Satyr ear (pixie ear deformity) can occur if the earlobe is closed under tension (Figure 11.12B). As healing and contraction occur, the earlobe is pulled inferiorly. This is a difficult complication to fix and will require reoperation. The posterior hairline must also be closed meticulously to avoid a step-off in this region. Patients who have an unnatural posterior hairline will be required to modify their hair styling to make this less obvious. The lateral sweep facelift deformity was much more common in the days of skin-only lift and is largely prevented by the use of SMAS techniques.[28] However, excess skin tension in the lateral direction can lead to lateral sweep appearance if not identified intraoperatively.

Nerve injury is rare after facelift but is one of the most feared complications. The most commonly injured nerve during facelift surgery is the great auricular nerve. This provides cutaneous sensation to the auricle, earlobe, and postauricular skin. The paresthesia improves over time; however, permanent paresthesia of the lobule may occur if the nerve is severed. Motor nerve injury is much less common, with the temporal and marginal mandibular branches the most commonly affected. If this is identified intraoperatively, microscopic repair should be performed; however, this is rarely the case. If identified postoperatively, approximately 85% will resolve spontaneously.[29] Therefore, reassurance is essential for these patients.

Adjunctive Procedures

Facial aging not only involves descent of facial soft tissues, but also loss of facial volume.[1] This occurs both in the soft tissue and at the bony level. Fat injection is commonly performed at the time of facelift to provide volumization to the malar, temporal, and periorbital regions. Malar or chin implants may be placed at the time of facelift to improve bony projection. Laser skin resurfacing can also be performed concomitantly with facelift. Laser resurfacing should only be performed in cases where a minimal ($\sim$3.0 cm) cutaneous flap is raised to minimize the risk of skin necrosis.[30] It is appropriate to stage resurfacing until after the facelift has healed to preserve the vascular integrity of the skin flap.

▶ NECK LIFT

In order to achieve a balanced outcome in rejuvenation of the aging face, evaluation and management of the neck are imperative. In fact, many patients present primarily requesting improvement in neck appearance and contour. It is important for any aesthetic facial surgeon to be comfortable in addressing excess submental tissue and laxity. A broad range of surgical techniques have been described and the intervention selected should be a product of the patient's pathology and the surgeon's comfort level. Many noninvasive skin-tightening modalities are available; however, these are out of the scope of this chapter.

Patient Evaluation

The neck and submental region should be assessed on every patient presenting with concerns of facial aging. Some patients will volunteer specific concerns regarding the neck appearance. Others, with more significant pathology, may be distracted by other aspects of their facial aging. Failure to address the neck while addressing the remainder of the face can lead to unnatural appearances and suboptimal outcomes. A thorough history should be taken regarding previous rejuvenation intervention for the neck, as well as radiation therapy or prior parotid surgery. The patient should be examined for any scars that might indicate prior intervention. Platysmal banding, excess skin laxity, and excess subcutaneous fat should be noted. Patients with a large amount of excess skin may be better candidates for a direct neck lift. The quality and thickness of the skin should also be evaluated to determine the ability to camouflage incisions. The cervicomental angle must be evaluated on lateral view as this is the region where evidence of aging is most apparent. The location of the hyoid bone should be noted as patients with a relatively low and anterior lying hyoid bone may be suboptimal candidates for submentoplasty. Examination should also include palpation of the neck soft tissues to determine the elasticity and pliability of the neck skin. Standard aesthetic photographs should be taken. In addition to the standard sequence, a lateral view with the head in flexion and extension can be useful if intervention on the neck is planned.

Anatomy

The anatomic layers of the neck are analogous to the layers encountered in facelift. The platysma muscle is an extension of the facial SMAS and is present deep to the subcutaneous fat. This muscle is often deficient or dehiscent in the midline. With most submentoplasty techniques, a subcutaneous plane will first be developed, followed by a subplatysmal plane. This is analogous to the planes developed in a sub-SMAS facelift. As in the face, all vital neurovascular structures lie deep to this muscular layer. These include the marginal mandibular branch of the facial nerve, the external jugular, and the anterior jugular veins. Within the submental region, the digastric muscles are present deep to the platysmal layer. In the midline between the digastric muscles lies the deep submental fat.[31] This deep fat compartment is separate from the subcutaneous fat and often needs to be addressed. The submandibular glands also lie deep to the platysma muscle, between the anterior and posterior bellies of the digastric. Submandibular gland management may be necessary for achieving an appropriately contoured lower face and neck. Partial submandibular gland excision is practiced in varying degrees.[14]

Procedures

Submental Liposuction

Younger patients with a mild amount of subcutaneous submental fat are excellent candidates for submental liposuction. The procedure involves a small submental incision, can be done comfortably under local anesthesia, results in minimal downtime, and can provide excellent results in the correct patient. Patient selection is very important as the ability for the skin to retract and redrape after submental liposuction will lead to the best results. Older patients with an excessive amount of skin laxity are not good candidates for this procedure. The ideal candidates for submental liposuction have elastic, healthy skin and a high posterior hyoid bone position.

Technique

Areas of excess fat to be removed should first be marked prior to injection of a local anesthetic. The local anesthetic tumescent solution is infiltrated throughout the anterior neck between the sternocleidomastoid muscles. The submental crease is marked and a small (4-8 mm) incision centered around the midline is made in this crease. A subcutaneous plane is then elevated with a 4- or 6-mm liposuction cannula between the sternocleidomastoid muscles and inferiorly to the cricoid. The extent of this dissection is predicated on the excess fat distribution of the patient. After tunnels have been created, negative pressure is applied to the liposuction cannula and the subcutaneous fat is removed. The sharp side of the cannula should be facing away from the dermis, toward the subcutaneous fat to prevent thinning of the overlying dermis, puckering, and scar formation. Once the excess areas of fat have been addressed, the cannula is removed and the incision is closed in layers. A compressive neck dressing may be placed postoperatively to reduce ecchymosis and edema.

Submentoplasty/Platysmaplasty

For patients with more excessive subcutaneous fat and platysmal laxity, submental liposuction alone will not yield an ideal result. To achieve optimal results in these patients, the platysma and submental fat must be directly addressed. The addition of platysmaplasty to submental liposuction serves to recreate and tighten the muscular sling that supports the deep neck contents. This is often performed in conjunction with facelift, which allows excess neck skin to be excised laterally. In patients with more elastic skin, submentoplasty with platysmaplasty may be performed and the excess skin is allowed to contract with healing. In some patients, direct excision of the anterior neck redundancy may be required. Failure to address this excess skin can lead to a turkey gobbler deformity.

Technique

Prior to performing local anesthesia, the submental crease and anterior platysmal bands should be marked. An anesthetic tumescent solution should be injected throughout the anterior neck as in submental liposuction. In addition, a concentrated local anesthetic should be injected into the submental crease. A 3- to 4-cm horizontal incision is marked in the submental crease and the incision is made through the epidermis and dermis. A subcutaneous plane, superficial to the platysma muscle, is then elevated sharply in a similar fashion to facelift. Submental open liposuction is performed at this time. The platysma is then grasped with forceps, incised, and a subplatysmal plane is developed sharply. This should be done under direct visualization when possible, facilitated by placement of a retractor in the submental incision. Prominent blood vessels can be present in the immediate subplatysmal plane and hemostasis is achieved with bipolar cautery. The limits of this dissection are the anterior borders of the SCM muscles laterally and the cricoid inferiorly.

After the platysmal flap has been raised, redundant platysma muscle may be excised or plicated in the midline (Figure 11.13). If deep submental fat is to be excised, the anterior digastric bellies are identified at this time. Deep cervical fat may be excised between these muscles down to the mylohyoid. A vertical corset platysmaplasty is then performed. The medial edges of the platysma are sutured together in a running fashion. The running suture starts superiorly at the submentum, proceeds inferiorly to the limit of dissection, and back superiorly to be tied. Any redundant platysma is then excised in the midline to prevent anterior contour deformity (Figure 11.14). The submental incision is then closed in layers and a compressive neck dressing is placed.

FIGURE 11.13   Platysmaplasty. Vertical corset platysmaplasty. The platysma is reapproximated in the midline and excess platysma removed. Small lateral relaxing incisions in the platysma may be made to divide platysmal bands.

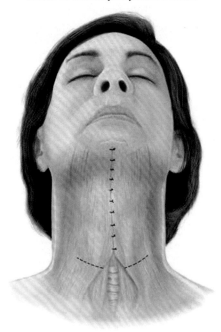

(Reprinted with permission from Chung KC, Thorne CH, Sinno S. *Operative Techniques in Facial Aesthetic Surgery*. 1st ed. Philadelphia, PA: Wolters Kluwer; 2020.)

Direct Neck Lift

The most aggressive technique to address neck skin laxity is the direct neck lift. This involves direct excision of excess skin and subcutaneous tissue by an anterior midline neck incision. Patient selection is of vital importance when considering direct neck lift as the incision will be visible and poor wound healing can lead to a poor aesthetic outcome. Direct neck lift specifically addresses the excess midline neck skin that is not addressed by the submental approach. Older male patients are generally the best candidates for this procedure, although some female patients may benefit as well. This may also be done as a second-stage procedure if suboptimal skin elasticity results in redundant anterior neck skin after platysmaplasty.

Technique

Prior to injection of a local anesthetic, the redundant anterior neck skin is marked with two vertical incisions in an elliptical fashion. Horizontal incisions are then marked at the submental crease and an inferior neck crease just above the sternal notch (Figure 11.15A). The local anesthetic is then infiltrated into the marked incisions and subcutaneous plane. Full thickness incisions are made through the skin and the excess skin excised (Figure 11.15B and C). This approach provides unparalleled exposure to the subcutaneous fat and platysma for modification as described for platysmaplasty. After the platysma has been closed, the neck incision is closed (Figure 11.15D). Multiple techniques exist to excise the standing cone deformities that develop adjacent to the horizontal incisions.[32] To prevent postoperative webbing of the vertical incision, it is beneficial to create a z-plasty at the cervicomental angle for skin closure. This reorients the scar into the horizontal position, prevents postoperative webbing, and helps to define the cervicomental angle. Meticulous, tension-free closure is necessary to minimize the appearance of the scar (Figure 11.16).

FIGURE 11.14   Submentoplasty with platysmal plication. (A) Excess platysma and fat are identified after subcutaneous plane has been raised. (B) Redundant platysma is cross-clamped and a running suture is placed to approximate remnant platysma in the midline. (C) Excess platysma excised after reapproximation.

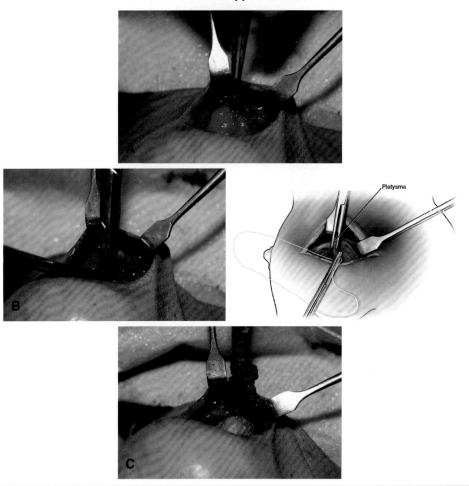

(Reprinted with permission from Larrabee WF Jr, Ridgway J, Patel S. *Master Techniques in Otolaryngology – Head and Neck Surgery: Facial Plastic Surgery.* 1st ed. Philadelphia, PA: Wolters Kluwer; 2017.)

Complications

Hematoma is a relatively rare complication of submentoplasty, occurring in 1% to 3% of cases.[33,34] As in facelift, meticulous hemostasis, avoidance of antiplatelet medications, and perioperative blood pressure management are important for hematoma prevention. In contrast to facelift, skin necrosis secondary to hematoma is rare in submentoplasty. When hematoma does occur, it can lead to delayed healing and increased infection risk. Hematomas should be drained when recognized either by needle aspiration or by surgical evacuation with placement of a pressure dressing.

Contour irregularities are more common after neck rejuvenation than many other facial cosmetic procedures. Persistent platysmal bands will be present if not addressed at the initial procedure with platysmaplasty. Excess removal of subcutaneous fat can lead to the cobra neck deformity. This deformity presents with persistent bilateral anterior

FIGURE 11.15   Direct neck lift. (A) Incisional marking. The area to be excised is marked with two vertical incisions. An incision is marked in the submental crease and z-plasty incisions are marked laterally. (B) Skin incisions are made and a subcutaneous plane is raised. (C) Platysma is left intact deep to the excision and is reapproximated in the midline. (D) Skin closure performed with z-plasty at the cervicomental angle.

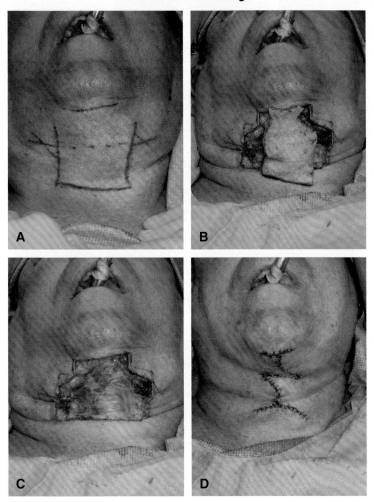

platysmal bands in the setting of excessive fat removal in the submentum. This usually requires revision surgery with platysmaplasty for correction. Uneven removal of subcutaneous fat can also lead to contour irregularities and lumping of fatty deposits, resulting in an unnatural appearance. This can be prevented by use of a small caliber (4-6 mm) liposuction cannula with attention paid to the homogeneity of fat removal.

▶ THREAD LIFTING

Thread lifting is a relatively fast, inexpensive technique for midfacial lifting developed in the early 1990s. This technique involves placement of multiple suspension sutures in the subcutaneous plane in order to rejuvenate the face, primarily by elevating the midface. In contrast to many other facial rejuvenation procedures, thread lifting does not entail

FIGURE 11.16   Neck lift preoperative and postoperative photos. This patient underwent submentoplasty in combination with facelift. Note the improvement in neck skin laxity and jawline definition. (A) Preoperative, (B) digital imaging, and (C) postoperative photo.

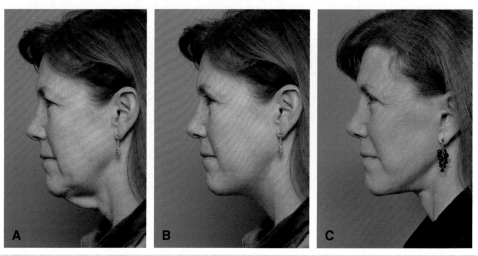

(Reprinted with permission from Larrabee WF Jr, Ridgway J, Patel S. *Master Techniques in Otolaryngology – Head and Neck Surgery: Facial Plastic Surgery.* 1st ed. Philadelphia, PA: Wolters Kluwer; 2017.)

removal of redundant tissue. Lifting is performed only in the subcutaneous plane without any lift of the underlying SMAS or facial musculature. Multiple techniques have been described to perform the thread lift procedure, with most of the variation and development regarding the different suture materials utilized for the procedure.[14] Many different suture materials are currently available. The most commonly used at this time are permanent barbed sutures; however, temporary sutures have also been utilized. These barbed sutures catch the subcutaneous tissues along multiple unidirectional or bidirectional barbs in order to distribute the lifting tension along the entire length of the suture. A minimal surrounding fibrosis then occurs around the suture, which is postulated to lead to long-lasting results even if the sutures are no longer present.[35]

Patient Evaluation

As with any other facial rejuvenation evaluation, a complete facial analysis should be performed and the patient's expectations are understood. Any previous history of facial procedures should be elucidated as subdermal scar tissue can cause difficulty passing the threads. Because thread lifting does not provide as dramatic of a result as a facelift, good candidates will have early-stage mild to moderate soft tissue ptosis. Patients younger than the age of 50 will have the best results.[36] An excessive amount of soft tissue redundancy will not be well corrected with thread lifting because excess subcutaneous tissue is not removed. Thread lifting is mainly able to address the melolabial and labiomandibular folds and patients with primary complaints regarding this area will be the best candidates. Any reactivity to suture material or history of excessive fibrosis should be discussed.

Technique

The major benefit of thread lifting is minimal patient discomfort, downtime, and efficiency with which the procedure is performed. Generally, the procedure can be completed in 1 hour and the patient may return to work the same day. The suture placement and angle of suspension will be patient specific and should be decided prior to the procedure. Patients with predominantly lower facial mandibular ptosis will require a more superior direction of suspension. A small depot of local anesthetic is injected into the facial skin 1 to 2 cm anterior to the tragus. A puncture is then made in this region with a large (18-21 gauge) needle. A long cannula holding the thread is then inserted through the puncture and tunneled in the subdermal plane to an area approximately 1 cm beyond the fold to be corrected. The cannula is then slowly removed, leaving the thread in place. The excess thread can then be gently pulled to visualize the vector of lift achieved. Pressure is placed along the course of the thread to engage the suture barbs. The thread is then cut flush with the skin to remove the excess length.

Complications

Complications of thread lifting can be related to both surgical technique and the foreign body reaction to implanted threads. Immediate postprocedural complications include ecchymosis and edema along the thread tracts. This is usually self-limited and resolving. Puckering of the skin may also occur as a result of superficially placed threads.[37] Given the dynamic nature of facial musculature, relaxation or breaking of threads may occur over time. This can result in asymmetry and the potential need for revision procedures. One major issue with thread lifting is that removal of barb threads is very difficult and may require a much more extensive or disfiguring procedure.

Outcomes

Thread lifting is limited by both the degree of effect that can be achieved and the length of time for which this effect is observed. Although the minimal fibrosis and collagen remodeling that occur around the threads are postulated to increase the longevity of results beyond the lift of the thread, the longevity of effect is debated. The few studies evaluating the longevity of the thread lift have had mixed results. One such study, published by Sulamanidze et al.[38] which evaluated 186 undergoing thread lifting with permanent sutures concluded that improvement was persistent in most patients with a follow-up of 2 to 30 months. However, no objective criteria for evaluation or definitive data were presented. In contrast, a study by Bertossi et al.[39] on 160 patients treated with thread lifting demonstrated that although an instantaneous effect of thread lifting was evident, improvement in facial ptosis is no longer apparent after 1 year. Currently, this is an area of some debate and little data are available. The general consensus at this time is that a short-term benefit is achieved with thread lifting; however, the longevity of the results is not comparable to facelift.

▶ CONCLUSION

For patients with a significant amount of redundant skin and soft tissue ptosis, open surgical approaches may be necessary to provide the desired correction. Blepharoplasty, facelift, and neck lift each addresses different regions of the face and can lead to dramatic improvement. Thread lifting is another modality that may be utilized; however, the longevity of the lift and potential complications have not led to widespread adoption as an alternative to facelift. Appropriate patient evaluation, anatomic knowledge, and technical ability are all necessary to provide patients with the ideal outcome.

REFERENCES

1. Chi JJ. Periorbital surgery – forehead, brow and midface. *Facial Plast Surg Clin North Am*. 2016;24:107-117.
2. Hartstein ME, Don K. How to avoid blepharoplasty complications. *Oral Maxillofacial Surg Clin North Am*. 2009;21(1):31-41.
3. Shadfar S, Perkins SW. Surgical treatment of the brow and upper eyelid. *Facial Plast Surg Clin North Am*. 2015;23(2):167-183.
4. Hahn S, Holds JB, Couch SM. Upper lid blepharoplasty. *Facial Plast Surg Clin N Am*. 2016;24:119-127.
5. Burke AJC, Wang T. Should formal ophthalmologic evaluation be a preoperative requirement prior to blepharoplasty? *Arch Otolaryngology Head Neck Surg*. 2001;127(6):719-722.
6. Henderson JL, Larrabee WF, Krieger BD. Photographic standards for facial plastic surgery. *Arch Facial Plast Surg*. 2005;7(5):331-333.
7. Whipple KM, Korn BS, Don OK. Recognizing and managing complications in blepharoplasty. *Facial Plast Surg Clin North Am*. 2013;21(4):625-637.
8. Zoumalan CI, Roostaeian J. Simplifying blepharoplasty. *Plast Reconstr Surg*. 2016;137(1):196e-213e.
9. Shorr N, Goldberg RA, McCann JD, Hoenig JA, Li TG. Upper eyelid skin grafting: an effective treatment for lagophthalmos following blepharoplasty. *Plast Reconstr Surg*. 2003;112(5):1444-1448.
10. Callahan MA. Prevention of blindness after blepharoplasty. *Ophthalmology*. 1983;90(9):1047-1051.
11. Lambros V. Models of facial aging and implications for treatment. *Clin Plast Surg*. 2008;35:319-327;discussion 317.
12. Mitz V, Peyronie M. The superficial musculo-aponeurotic system (SMAS) in the parotid and cheek area. *Plast Reconstr Surg* 1976;58(1):80-88.
13. Derby BM, Codner MA. Evidence-based medicine: face lift. *Plast Reconstr Surg*. 2017;139(1).151c-167e.
14. Stacey D, Warner JP, Duggal A, et al. International interdisciplinary rhytidectomy survey. *Ann Plast Surg*. 2010;64(4):370-375.
15. Alghoul M, Codner MA. Retaining ligaments of the face:review of anatomy and clinical applications. *Aesthet Surg J*. 2013;33(6):769-782.
16. Pitanguy I, Ramos AS. The frontal branch of the facial nerve: the importance of its variations in face lifting. *Plast Reconstr Surg*. 1966;38:352-356.
17. Lefkowitz T, Hazani R, Chowdhry S, Elston J, Yaremchuk MJ, Wilhelmi BJ. Anatomical landmarks to avoid injury to the great auricular nerve during rhytidectomy. *Aesthet Surg J*. 2013;33(1):19-23.
18. Webster RC, Nabil F, Smith RC. Male and female face-lift incisions. *Arch Otolaryngol*. 1982;108:299-302.
19. Johnson CM, Adamson PA, Anderson JR. The face-lift incision. *Arch Otolaryngol*. 1984;110:371-373.
20. Saylan Z. The S-lift: less is more. *Aesthet Surg J*. 1999;19(5):406-409.
21. Brandy DA. The QuickLift: a modification of the S-lift. *Cosmet Dermatol*. 2004;17:351-360.
22. Tonnard P, Verpaele A. The MACS-lift short scar rhytidectomy. *Aesthet Surg J*. 2007;27(2):188-198.
23. Zoumalan R, Rizk S. Hematoma rates in drainless deep-plane face-lift surgery with and without the use of fibrin glue. *Arch Otolaryngol*. 2008;10(2):103-107.
24. Perkins SW, Williams JD, Macdonald K, et al. Prevention of seromas and hematomas after face-lift surgery with the use of postoperative vacuum drains. *Arch Otolaryngol*. 1997;123:743-745.
25. Chaffoo RAK. Complications in facelift surgery: avoidance and management. *Facial Plast Surg Clin North Am*. 2013;21(4):551-558.
26. Gupta V, Winocour J, Shi H, Shack RB, Grotting JC, Higdon KK. Preoperative risk factors and complication rates in facelift: analysis of 11,300 patients. *Aesthet Surg J*. 2015;36(1):1-13.
27. Ramanadham SR, Mapula S, Costa C, et al. Evolution of hypertension management in face lifting in 1089 patients: optimizing safety and outcomes. *Plast Reconstr Surg*. 2015;135:1037-1043.
28. Miller TR, Eisbach KJ. SMAS facelift techniques to minimize stigmata of surgery. *Otolaryngologic Clin North Am*. 2007;40(2):391-408.
29. Kamer FM. One hundred consecutive deep plane face-lifts. *Arch Otolaryngol Head Neck Surg*. 1996;122(1):17-22.
30. Achauer BM, Adair SR, VanderKam VM. Combined rhytidectomy and full-face laser resurfacing. *Plast Reconstr Surg*. 2000;106(7):1608-1611.
31. Hatef DA, Koshy JC, Sandoval SE, Echo AP, Izaddoost SA, Hollier LH. The submental fat compartment of the neck. *Semin Plast Surg*. 2009;23(4):288-291. © Thieme Medical Publishers.
32. Bitner JB, Friedman O, Farrior RT, Cook TA. Direct submentoplasty for neck rejuvenation. *Arch Facial Plast Surg*. 2007;9(3):194-200.
33. Koehler J. Complications of neck liposuction and submentoplasty. *Oral Maxillofacial Surg Clin North Am*. 2009;21(1):43-52.
34. Jasin ME. Submentoplasty as an isolated rejuvenative procedure for the neck. *Arch Facial Plast Surg*. 2003;5(2):180-183.
35. de Pinho Tavares J, Oliveira CACP, Torres RP, Bahmad F Jr. Facial thread lifting with suture suspension. *Braz J Otorhinolaryngol*. 2017;83(6):712-719.
36. Kalra R. Use of barbed threads in facial rejuvenation. *Indian J Plast Surg*. 2008;41(suppl):S93-S100.
37. Sardesai MG, Zakhary K, Ellis DAF. Thread-lifts: the good, the bad, and the ugly. *Arch Facial Plast Surg*. 2008;10(4):284-285.
38. Sulamanidze MA, Fournier PF, Paikidze TG, Sulamanidze GM. Removal of facial soft tissue ptosis with special threads. *Dermatol Surg*. 2002;28(5):367-371.
39. Bertossi D, Botti G, Gualdi A, et al. Effectiveness, longevity, and complications of facelift by barbed suture insertion. *Aesthet Surg J*. 2018;39(3):241-247.

Index

Note: Page numbers followed by "f" indicate figures and "t" indicate tables.